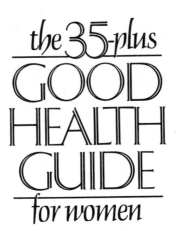

the 35-plus GOOD HEALTH GUIDE for women

ALSO BY JEAN PERRY SPODNIK

The 35-Plus Diet for Women (with Barbara Gibbons)

the 35-plus GOOD HEALTH GUIDE for women

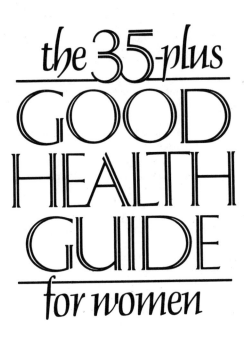

The Prime of Life Program for Women Over 35

JEAN PERRY SPODNIK, M.S., R.D., L.D.
and DAVID P. COGAN, M.D.

with JULIE HOUSTON

1817

An Edward Burlingame Book

HARPER & ROW, PUBLISHERS, New York
Grand Rapids, Philadelphia, St. Louis, San Francisco
London, Singapore, Sydney, Tokyo

Grateful acknowledgment is made for the following:

Chapter 5: Information on sunscreens from "Sunscreens," copyright 1988 by Consumers Union of the United States, Inc., Mount Vernon, N.Y. 10553. Excerpted by permission from Consumer Reports, June 1988.

Chapter 7: Information on mousses from "Mousses," copyright 1988 by Consumers Union of the United States, Inc., Mount Vernon, N.Y. 10553. Excerpted by permission from Consumer Reports, October 1988.

Chapter 12: Information on calcium from "The Truth About Calcium," copyright 1988 by Consumers Union of the United States, Inc., Mount Vernon, N.Y. 10553. Excerpted by permission from Consumer Reports, May 1988.

Chapter 13: Information on radial keratotomy from "Goodbye Glasses?" copyright 1988 by Consumers Union of the United States, Inc., Mount Vernon, N.Y. 10553. Excerpted by permission from Consumer Reports, January 1988.

Chapter 16: "Benefits of Exercise During Pregnancy" from "Exercise During Pregnancy," reprinted from the November 1988 issue of American Family Physician, copyright 1988 by the American Academy of Family Physicians.

"Exercise Guidelines for Pregnancy and Postpartum and Pregnancy Only" from the American College of Obstetricians and Gynecologists: "Exercise During Pregnancy and the Postnatal Period" (ACOG Home Exercise Program). Washington, D.C., ACOG, 1985, p. 4. Reprinted by permission.

Chapter 24: Charts on calories spent per hour, target zones, sample walking program and sample jogging program [Level 1], from Exercise and Your Heart, copyright 1984 by the American Heart Association. Reproduced by permission.

FIRST EDITION

Designed by Joan Greenfield

Library of Congress Cataloging-in-Publication Data

Spodnik, Jean Perry.
    The 35-plus good health guide for women: a prime of life program for women over 35/by Jean Perry Spodnik and David P. Cogan, with Julie Houston.—1st ed.
        p.   cm.
    Includes index.
    ISBN 0-06-016111-6
    1. Middle age women—Health and hygiene.   I. Cogan, David P. II. Houston, Julie.   III. Title.
RA778.S74   1989   88-45907
613'.04244—dc20

89 90 91 92 93 DT/RRD 10 9 8 7 6 5 4 3 2 1

CONTENTS

CONTENTS

FOREWORD

SOME MONTHS AFTER JEAN SPODNIK'S BOOK, *The 35-Plus Diet for Women* came out, one of my patients came in for a regular visit. This patient had a long and complicated medical history; her forty-seven years were marked by serious hormonal problems and a battle with cancer. She had also long been troubled by chronic overweight and had tried a variety of plans—including modified fasting—with no lasting success. As I entered the exam room, she greeted me with a smile, and I saw a woman not only more slender, but more relaxed and composed than I had ever seen her. With little prompting, she told me how she had carefully followed Jean's diet, had lost twenty pounds, and had sustained that dramatic loss on Jean's maintenance program. She paused and added—very seriously—words to this effect: "You know, Doctor, this plan is different. Within three days I knew it was working, and would work—and that was almost scary. I knew this would succeed, and now I had to decide if *I* wanted to succeed."

Her point was clear. Many people make dieting their chronic occupation, a never-ending, no-win job. Study after study shows a high percentage of women and men who regain weight one year after they lose it. For some, dieting becomes the whole ball game, with time, effort, money, and conversation constantly revolving around weight and appearance. My patient had found a plan that was really effective, and she understood that to succeed was to give up the old job—for her and for many others, an unsettling prospect.

Over the years I have sent Jean a continuous stream of new patients for consultations. We've worked on a collaborative approach to problems of nutrition, overall health and weight management, both uncomplicated and complicated by the problems that can develop in maturity—hypertension, high cholesterol, diabetes. When Jean walked over to my office one gray winter afternoon to talk about another book, one that would cover the broader health concerns of 35-plus women, I was naturally interested. We constantly work together on problems of health management in the reality of daily medical practice where not all is as we would like it, where whatever problems we solve one day will be replaced by a new set the next. We don't know everything and couldn't cover every area in this book, but we can provide the reflection and scope that comes only with years of clinical experience.

What follows reflects our belief in the principle my patient so vividly demonstrated: that for most people, the way to good health lies within their own hands, in appropriate partnership with broadly trained health professionals. Good health is not a matter of extreme beliefs and practices, but of good sense and what I think of as a standard of reasonableness. Jean Spodnik and I are "mainstream" in the best sense of the word, in that our skill has grown out of traditional medical and nutritional training and has broadened and matured as we have grown, matured, and learned from our work with our patients.

David P. Cogan

INTRODUCTION

IN MORE WAYS THAN ONE MY INTEREST in midlife health issues
is personal. When I was growing up, nobody knew anything about cholesterol or many of the other issues we now know are central to good health
and long life. I began my career in nutrition determined that my family
would avoid the kinds of health problems that beset my mother and my
aunts just a generation before me.

I started out in the 1950s as a research dietitian at the Cleveland Clinic,
studying the relationship between diet and cardiovascular disease. I set up
a research kitchen and had two cooks, Martha and Mary, to help test
recipes I developed for our studies. Even then *cholesterol* was a word only
a few people had heard. Butter was king and was used not only as a table
spread but in cooking as well. There was no such thing as polyunsaturated
margarine, so we made our own—from a special soybean oil Proctor and
Gamble supplied for the project. Once we got the recipe down, we taught
our patients how to make it at home.

What a long way we've come! Since then, I've kept my whole family on
a low cholesterol, low saturated fat diet. The spring before I was married, I
convinced my husband to have a fasting cholesterol test done. His count
was 240 milligrams per dilliliter—and he was a young man. In his most
recent test, more than thirty years later, the count was down at 150 milligrams, as it has been for many years.

Being prudent about what you eat does pay off.

This was brought home again in a big way with the development of the
35-plus diet. I created it out of a personal sense of urgency—my own rapid,
seemingly relentless weight gain after a full hysterectomy. My post-opera-

tive condition accelerated what other women experience over the course of the perimenopausal years—changes that begin, for most women, at age thirty-five. Like so many who had tried diet after diet without results, I felt a sense of helplessness as I watched my figure rounding out. But after years of working out diets for women with a wide variety of nutritional needs, I had too much practical experience not to be confident that, with a little luck, I could find an approach that really would tackle the problem of midlife weight gain. By working out a regimen that specifically dealt with the metabolic changes that occur during these years, I found a diet that succeeded. And I was lucky in having David Cogan as a colleague; he helped track the results of the diet in my first controlled study, and his continuing interest in women's health issues led him to collaborate with me on this new book.

Because it had worked for me, for the women who participated in the controlled study, and for many other patients since then, the enthusiastic response The 35-Plus Diet for Women received didn't surprise me. Women across the country wrote to relate their success with the diet. What I didn't really anticipate was how many would come to me with questions about other aspects of their health and well-being during midlife.

That interest helped spur the creation of the book you're holding in your hands. In many ways anticipation is a key idea here. All of us remember the enormous changes we went through during puberty. Those changes may have been more dramatic, but the changes you're going through now are nearly as numerous, and they can have a big impact on your present quality of life and on your future. We have two aims in this book: one is to help you anticipate and steer clear of problems down the road; the other is to provide what you need to know to be as healthy and attractive as you can be right now. Prime of life is no euphemism: midlife really can be the most productive and satisfying years of a woman's life. We hope that possibility becomes a reality for you.

Jean Perry Spodnik

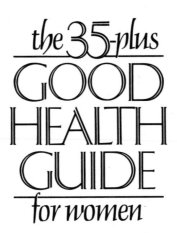

the 35-plus
GOOD
HEALTH
GUIDE
for women

PART ONE

Starting with a Clean Bill of Health

THIS BOOK WAS WRITTEN for one person only: you, the 35-plus woman. It was written with one goal in mind—to help you make your middle years the healthiest and happiest time of your life, starting right now.

You certainly deserve it. If you are between the ages of 35 and 55, you are among today's most accomplished members of society. You and your peers have achieved concurrent goals never dreamed of by women your age in the past: furthering your education, establishing professional careers, ensuring financial independence, and starting new families. At the same time, you've met these expanded objectives with the spirit of giving that has activated generations of women before you—generously nurturing children, encouraging spouses, pitching in to work overtime, lending a hand in your community, helping aging parents, and supporting friends and family in their times of need. You've reached out to help others in countless ways; now it is time to focus some attention on taking care of yourself and your own good health.

Like most women your age, you probably know it's time. Your body is telling you in subtle ways that you're ready for a midlife program for good health. The odds may seem stacked against all of us with new threats of cancer; newly discovered risks of sexually transmitted disease; compelling proof for the need to quit smoking, drinking, leading a sedentary life-style. If one part of you asks what's left to enjoy, another part of you counters with the answer you know is right: a lot. It all depends on how you arrange your midlife priorities. At this pivotal juncture, making intelligent choices that put your health first will bring real rewards in the way you look and

1

feel *right now*. It will also be the sound basis for decades of vigor still to come.

In her book *Passages*, Gail Sheehy explores the evolving phases of adulthood and maps out the enormous potential the future now holds for you. She describes the process of pulling away from "the trying twenties"—the time when we do what's supposed to be done in order to give shape to our grown-up lives—and moving toward what we want to do. This process brings with it a new sense of empowerment, a willingness perhaps to take risks. Now is the time to gear up for these changes, improving and extending your good health to fully savor what may be the most productive, enjoyable years of your life.

CHAPTER 1

David Cogan on Rating Your Health Professionals

IN THE PAST, IT WAS RARE FOR a woman to choose her own doctor, much less question his competence. Chances are she wasn't paying the medical bills, but even if she was, too often the message that filtered down from the male-dominated field of medicine was that she needn't worry herself with complicated details; she was to leave that to the doctor, and not take up his time with questions.

It would be good if we could say that this has altogether changed, but at least it's the exception rather than the rule. Most women now make their own informed choices about the quality of their medical care and who supplies it. Not only are there more doctors to choose from, but the curtains are wide open on once-shrouded areas of medicine that are a measure of a doctor's competence. Today's good doctors willingly share this information with their patients and prospective patients, including when and where they went to medical school and did their residency; and they will candidly assess their own limitations and, when needed, give their recommendations on where competent specialists may be found.

In addition to competence, you have every right to expect good rapport and adult-to-adult interaction with your health professionals. You may even have intervened on behalf of aging parents who still have passive attitudes toward medical care, to be sure all their needs are being met. More to the point, you should feel free to intervene on your own behalf, openly asking questions about treatments and procedures your doctor recommends.

As you come to this book, we hope you are completely satisfied with your own doctor and that you can count on continuing good care in the

3

years to come. Studies have shown a generally diminished public confidence in American medical care and also indicate greater satisfaction among people who have a regular doctor, one who knows them well. But in our transient society, changes often occur. Your doctor may retire or relocate, your own medical needs may change, or you may simply become dissatisfied with the care you are getting. If you're faced with any of these situations, how do you judge whether a doctor is a good one?

Competence

Many people base their assessment of a physician's competence not on medical school, residency training, or board certification but on some other estimate of the physician's professional experience. For some, this is an assessment based on reputation within the community, or among friends and family members. For others, it is a personal assessment based on their own experience of office visits. Although this process has the ring of authenticity and real-world assessment, the danger is that a physician can project an aura of competence without substance, since many highly competent and compassionate physicians are quiet and self-effacing.

There is no magic formula in making an evaluation of one's own doctor, but prospective patients seeking good personal physicians must try to use all data at hand and combine it with personal or shared experiences.

Specialty

Most doctors today are specialists. This means that in addition to their broad experience and education as medical doctors, they have chosen a certain area of medicine such as internal medicine, gastroenterology, or obstetrics-gynecology, and this specialty becomes the focal point of expertise in their practice. Should a patient's individual needs fall outside that specialty, a good physician will candidly state that this is the case, and will make a referral—most likely to a colleague with whom he has worked and whose reputation he trusts.

The first step in choosing a doctor, then, should be to evaluate his or her special area of competence in light of your own physical condition and basic concerns. All things being equal, we recommend an internist or a residency-trained family practitioner as the 35-plus woman's personal physician. Good programs in internal medicine or family practice prepare a physician for serving patients with a broad range of primary medical care, as well as with guidance in areas that are served by specialists. When an internist does not have the expertise needed, she or he will have a clear sense of when and to whom to make a referral.

If you have used your gynecologist as your primary physician up until now, it is definitely time for a more broadly trained physician to be involved in your health-care decisions. This does not mean leaving your gynecologist but rather adding an internist or family practitioner.

Medical School

While elite medical schools such as Harvard and Stanford do get the students with the most impressive college credentials, think twice before concluding that a doctor with such credentials is the only one for you.

As it turns out, many students from these schools today do not seek out general internal medicine or family practice as their specialty but instead gravitate to subspecialty practice. For routine care and prevention, much of your choice depends on the pool of available physicians in your area, including doctors who have studied at lesser-known schools but who are just as competent as their elite counterparts. Most medical schools in this country offer four-year programs, and they receive students who have completed a four-year undergraduate degree program. Moreover, all U.S. medical schools are subject to frequent formal and informal review; in fact, they have similar courses of study based on similar admission requirements and the expectation (sometimes built into the advancement structure) that their graduates will pass the sequence of exams given by the National Board of Medical Examiners.

Graduates from foreign medical schools deserve consideration too, since 20 percent of current practicing physicians in this country are U.S.- or foreign-born physicians who have graduated from schools in other countries. While the curricula and quality of foreign schools are difficult to evaluate against our standards, for their graduates to enter and ultimately practice in the United States, they must pass special exams that establish a certain level of technical knowledge before they begin their residency training. All graduates of foreign medical schools must do residency training (usually a minimum of three years) in this country, not simply to acquire the needed skills but also to ensure acculturation. After residency training, foreign graduates must pass the same certification exams taken by their American counterparts.

Information on schooling is readily available, and you should certainly look into it—but then look further before making your choice.

Residency and Board Certification

While you're at it, review your doctor's residency training and subsequent board certification. In general, hospitals affiliated with medical schools have the highest quality programs, with the residency programs of the various medical-school hospitals themselves accorded the highest status.

Board certification is increasingly common and a real plus in providing one more tangible indication of a physician's competence. This is a fairly new standard of medicine that does not apply to many older doctors, who have long been in practice. But lack of board certification in a specialty area, especially when the physician is fairly young, must raise questions. As long as you have a choice, we advise seeking a board-certified internist or family practitioner as your personal physician.

A competent physician won't squirm when asked about professional background or board certification, nor will he or she become defensive (or offensive!) when therapies are questioned or specific data need to be reviewed, perhaps involving a second opinion. If a second opinion is requested by you or your family, a good doctor won't make you feel guilty nor resent it. Instead, he or she will be receptive to this avenue for gaining extra professional expertise, at the same time giving you greater confidence in the plan of treatment. In fact, many health insurance policies actually require a second, and in some cases even a third, opinion before the company will reimburse a patient for certain procedures. In this regard, it's wise to check the details of your own policy in advance.

As defined, competence begins with a solid base of knowledge and the ability to use that knowledge well in a difficult situation. Ultimately, competence must also include good communications skills and be linked to the soul of a medical practice: compassion.

Compassion

In the description of what a typical physical examination entails, you may catch a glimpse here and there of that intangible, all-important quality of a good doctor: her or his compassion. Compassion has different meanings to different people. For me, it connotes kindness; reasonable patience on days that are wearisome both to patient and physician; general friendliness—and sometimes friendship—as the relationship unfolds; and true, consistent courtesy that extends over the years.

On some occasions, it may include an embrace; on others, a firm handshake as the visit begins or ends; and on still others, it may mean holding a hand and sharing a prayer, as happened with an 80-year-old patient of mine who was dying of cancer. Toward the very end, when she was hospitalized and our visits became daily "rounds," I recall one morning sitting next to her bed, holding her hand, and having her thank *me* for my help—so uncalled for when I had no wisdom or strength that would ever measure up to what she shared with me each day. On that morning she asked if we could pray together, and afterward, I realized that it was I who had received her compassion, that she had comforted me as she was dying.

On all occasions, compassion will be marked by words of support and encouragement, whatever the task and however the problem unfolds. While there are other attributes of compassion in addition to those I have described, there are also many technically competent physicians who don't display many of them. Thus it is up to each woman to observe and evaluate medical competence *vis à vis* her own idea of compassion, and use it to decide, ultimately, if this is the doctor for her.

Life-and-death situations in which a doctor's true self becomes apparent are few and far between, but in the course of building a working doctor-patient relationship there are a few modest but telling indications of how your doctor defines compassion. The most obvious of these fall into the category of what we might call "medical courtesy."

TIMELINESS.   The physician who is chronically, significantly late is discourteous in a very concrete way and lacks one of the components of compassion—mutual respect.

TONE OF VOICE.   The physician who communicates by "talking down" to you, insisting on your using his or her title while referring to you on a first-name basis, and who speaks from the farthest corner of the room or with a hand on the doorknob is telling you more than she or he may realize.

MANNER.   This is another area that can reveal much about your doctor's compassion. Issues that may be thought of as "procedural," such as the manner of responding to special requests, coping with unanticipated needs, and acting under pressure, properly fit into this area, as does candor, which is a real part of compassion and a true kindness in a medical professional.

While it may be nice to consider your doctor a friend, once you are in the examining room, don't expect to get into heated discussions about issues in the news or compare notes on the trips you took last summer. This situation usually calls for putting your personal conversation aside and mutually concentrating on your needs as a patient. In this type of equal partnership, rapport is best defined as professional rapport—a comfortable, candid give-and-take of information relating to your health.

Choosing a Nutritionist

If ever there were a fine tool of preventive health it is nutrition. Genes notwithstanding, good or bad nutrition can make the difference in your health and well-being. We believe that a personal doctor should be receptive to a patient's inquiry about finding a nutritionist, and be willing to make a referral to a good one. You can find a good nutritionist on your own, however, by evaluating competence as follows:

1. A baccalaureate graduate from a reputable university with a degree in nutrition.
2. Indication of an M.S. (masters in nutrition) or Ph.D. (doctorate of nutrition) following the name.
3. The letters R.D. (registered dietitian) following the B.S., M.S. or Ph.D., which indicate the person has passed a comprehensive test to certify him or her for registration nationally.
4. An L.D. (licensed dietitian) after the other credentials is further assurance that the person has met your state's standards to practice as a nutritionist, although some states do not require this procedure.

Don't assume that your doctor knows everything there is to know about nutrition. In fact, if your doctor advises treatment of a certain condition that involves only nutrition, query the source of his or her information. You may be given trustworthy information from the American Heart Association or American Diabetes Association, for example, but you have every right to ask questions about it. If large amounts of vitamins or minerals are suggested without adequate justification, get another opinion.

Women (and men) today rightfully expect their health professionals to combine technical competence with candor, good rapport, and compassion. Certainly you deserve nothing less in a trusted personal doctor. When you make the right choice—an informed choice—all else will fall securely into place, including competent referrals to specialists and other health professionals that may be required as need arises.

CHAPTER 2

The Midlife Medical Checkup

OUR MIDLIFE HEALTH program begins with a complete physical examination—we explain what it should include for every woman over thirty-five, why certain procedures are included, and how they are done. Your doctor may conduct the examination in a different sequence or manner, but what you will find here is certainly typical of the thorough going-over you should expect from this important "well visit" to your doctor's office.

If you feel you are in good health, the time and expense for a full medical examination may seem like a big investment. But it's a sound one. If you haven't had a checkup in the last five years, take the time to do so now. Coming through a complete exam with a clean bill of health—or with specific and reassuring help in dealing with your health problems—can be a surprisingly positive experience, a welcome release from nagging health questions and concerns you may have avoided confronting, postponing them, like Scarlett, to another day. If a physical did nothing more than relieve low-grade health anxieties, it would be therapeutic. But the real value comes from the education both you and your doctor get about your health: what shape you are in now, and what conditions might pose future health risks. While your education is paramount—it's the base from which you'll build a sound health program—educating your doctor about *you* is also important.

In the pages that follow, David Cogan will walk you through a complete physical. Having a basic understanding of procedures and tests will help demystify the experience and also help balance the scales; knowing something about what's going on goes a long way toward making your relationship with your doctor a true partnership. Don't be shy about asking questions during and after the procedure, and don't be afraid to ask for repetitions in lay terms. If past experience tells you that you'll forget half the things you wanted to ask once they've got you into that drafty exam-room gown, make a list before you leave home and take it with you into the examining room.

Making Your Appointment

We believe all adults should have a complete (baseline) physical and a follow-up physical at least every five years unless their doctor directs otherwise. Women should also have an annual blood-pressure check, pap test, pelvic exam, and breast exam.

If you haven't had a complete physical exam by your primary physician within the last five years (or if you're starting with a new doctor), don't depend on a friendly reminder from your doctor or the chidings of loved ones. Make this appointment now, not when you are sick.

When you call for your appointment, specify that you are requesting a complete physical so that the doctor blocks off ample time. If your gynecologist is someone other than your regular doctor, make that appointment now, too, if you haven't been examined in the last twelve months.

DAVID COGAN'S COMPLETE PHYSICAL EXAMINATION

Your "complete physical" is the best way to establish a medical record—a baseline for present and future health. The exam includes a history of past or present medical problems, a physical examination, and appropriate tests.

CHECKING IN.   Your doctor will probably ask you to arrive at his or her office in a fasting state, which means no food for twelve hours prior to the exam, although water is permitted. Your complete physical will begin with your filling out a basic information sheet. In our office, the front sheet of the chart is completed for each complete physical, whether you are a new patient or not. This is not busy paperwork but, rather, a helpful way of getting updated information relating to marital status and employment—items of real importance to the doctor in looking at you as a total patient.

PREPARING FOR YOUR EXAM.   After checking in, you may be asked to put on an examination gown so that there will be no break between your doctor's taking your history and the physical exam, or the interview may take place first and then you'll change and go into the exam room. In any case, before the examination a medical assistant will weigh you, take your temperature, and take your blood pressure. This simple screen—especially the blood-pressure check—is very important and is done in many offices even for brief medical appointments.

WORKING WITH YOUR DOCTOR. Rapport is established when your doctor joins you in the exam room. Your initial contact with each other can give you a good indication of your doctor's style and attitude in working with his or her patients—and how comfortable you are with that style. Is there a discreet warning, a gentle tap on the door to let you know the doctor's making an appearance, or does your doctor burst into the room as if he or she has just made a landing? A direct introduction, a handshake, and an initial greeting using your surname with a Miss or Mrs. preceding it clearly establishes an equal working relationship, whereas being called by your first name can sound condescending, particularly if this is an initial visit. It's different if the physician expects to be addressed by his or her first name, but interestingly, this rarely is the case.

TAKING YOUR HISTORY. Your doctor will usually begin the "history" by asking what prompted you to schedule the physical. This is a crucial first question, and your physician should be highly attuned to your response. Be candid. Explain whether you view this as just a routine or introductory exam, or if there is something bothering you that you especially want your doctor to address during the examination. If you describe a specific illness or concern, your doctor will note it as "the chief complaint," which leads to what then is described as "the history of the present illness," often abbreviated HPI. For many patients, the initial explanation for the visit is a general concern for wellness, while later on, in "the review of systems," specific concerns will surface. That's fine.

Because your medication history is particularly important, very early on in the interview your doctor will probably ask whether you take any prescription or over-the-counter medications, vitamins, or mineral supplements, and whether you have any specific allergies to medications.

Questions about your past medical history will include significant illnesses, both as a child and an adult, including overnight hospitalizations and surgical procedures, if any. Questions about your family history will include not only the health and death information of your parents and siblings but also the current health status of your spouse, if you are married, and that of your children, if you have any. Your doctor should also ask you about genetic history, particularly any incidence in parents or siblings of colon or breast cancer, both of which have strong family connections, as well as diabetes or hypertension, which also appear to run in families. Be prepared with as much specific information as you can give.

"Social and nutritional histories" are more important than they may sound. Your doctor can learn a lot about you from what you do for a living and how many hours you work. (With some people in our society, it can be an astonishing fifty to sixty or seventy hours a week.) The physician can also determine a great deal from your diet and the type of food you eat (how it is cooked, how regularly you eat certain foods, whether you eat between meals, whether you drink coffee or tea, as well as specific details on alcohol use or smoking). Even questions about your type of housing (whether you live on one floor or three, do your own housecleaning or lawn work, or even whether you consider your neighborhood safe or not) can be important. These are aspects of your daily life and capacities and all clearly are areas that have an impact on your overall health.

For similar reasons, your doctor may ask what you choose to do with your "free time": whether you lead an active social life or prefer social isolation; participate in club, synagogue, or church activities. You may smile or laugh if you are asked what you do for fun. Read books? Bake bread? Keep bees or roller skate? Travel with your husband? Get your child's swing going high, and then get on one yourself?

In addition to satisfying a normal curiosity about who you are as a person, the answers all contribute to a picture of good health and social interaction, or possibly a pattern of isolation and depression—key health determinants, especially in establishing a healthy, vigorous attitude about aging.

All the while your doctor is taking your history, he or she is observing your general appearance: your manner, mental alertness, memory, skin color—even whether you are slumped over or sitting comfortably erect. A good clinician—doctor or nurse—can gain an overall perception of wellness or malaise in a patient merely by observation.

THE REVIEW OF SYSTEMS. This phase of the exam usually follows the history, and it consists of a series of questions about specific head-to-toe physical functions and possibly ailments, starting literally with the eyes, ears, and nose and going all the way down to the feet. This is where topics of importance you may have forgotten to mention earlier or perhaps were reluctant to discuss will come to light. One typical area is sexual performance and dysfunction, which many men and women won't discuss until specific related issues are brought up. To some extent, the information you give in your medical history can help shed light on specific health problems now. For example, if you have intestinal problems, they could relate to something you described about your diet. The review of systems concludes taking your history, and the physical exam comes next.

The Physical Exam

Your doctor will use the information he or she has accumulated to this point throughout the rest of the examination. The physical usually begins with a review of your head, eyes, ears, nose, and throat, although many doctors routinely start with a blood-pressure check, even if the blood pressure has been recorded as normal by the medical assistant.

HEAD. While looking at your head, your doctor will specifically look at and feel (palpate) your scalp, looking for general shape, areas of tenderness, rashes, and, with the condition of the hair, whether there are any signs of hair loss.

EYES. The eye exam includes an assessment of your pupils, comparing one with the other to see if they are approximately equal in size; assessing their reactivity to light, and then the general ability of your eyes to move through a range of motion, called extraocular movement.

Examining the whites of your eyes, or sclerae, your doctor will check their color and, if you have not had a recent ophthalmological exam, will examine the fundus—the part of the eye seen through the pupil—using an ophthalmoscope to magnify the area. This is a useful assessment because the small arteries and veins of the retina are the only part of the body where such vessels can be seen, and thus they provide valuable information about your body's general vascular status.

Your doctor may advise you to have an ophthalmologic eye exam (the kind in which the pupils are dilated and a more thorough exam is done), and may suggest you have a glaucoma check (or may do these him- or herself, although this is not often the case).

EARS. The ear examination starts with a review of the outer ear: the pinna and the lobe. Using an otoscope, your doctor will then examine the outer ear and the ear canal, as well as the eardrum, or tympanic membrane. This checks for wax and, more important, for any abnormalities of the eardrum, such as perforation, as well as any indirect evidence of middle ear problems, such as fluid in the ear.

NOSE. Examining your nose, your doctor may look up both sides, or nares, to examine for polyps and see if the nasal septum—the divider between the right and left nostrils—is either perforated (has a hole in it) or deviated (bent in an unnatural or unusual way).

MOUTH AND TONGUE. Using a tongue blade and light source, your doctor will check your teeth and gums, a screen which may lead to dental referral. The doctor will look at the tongue carefully, paying close attention to its underside and side margins—particularly if you are a smoker, since smoking creates real potential for cancer in these areas—then he or she will observe the general condition and appearance of your throat.

NECK. Examination of your neck is done by palpation, feeling for any enlarged lymph nodes (often incorrectly referred to as glands), as well as checking for increased thyroid size or a lump in the thyroid, called a thyroid nodule.

In patients over 40, the carotid arteries, which carry blood to the brain and are located on the right and the left sides of the neck, are routinely checked for pulse strength. They are rated from 0 to 4, with 0 indicating absence, 1 weakness, 2 and 3 average or high normal, and 4 a bounding pulse (so strong it is virtually abnormal). Obviously this is an important checkpoint in the exam, because if the pulse is diminished or even absent, it is an implication of partial or even complete blockage of circulation to part of the brain. Your doctor may want to listen to the carotid arteries with a stethoscope for signs of noise (bruit), which in some cases is benign but in others can indicate a narrowing or obstruction.

CHEST AND BACK. The examination of your chest and back begins with a general look, or inspection, of the back and whether there's a proper spine curvature. Using a stethoscope, your doctor will then examine your lungs by auscultation—in lay terms, listening to the sounds you make when you breathe. The intent is to listen for sounds that don't belong: *wheezes* (whistling noises) common in asthma and emphysema; *rhonchi* or sounds of mucus that can occur in the lungs with an acute infection; and sometimes *rales*, the audible signs of fluid or infection in the lungs. The complete absence of sound, or what might be termed dullness, indicates the presence of a very large amount of fluid or some dense consolidation in the lungs.

HEART. Examination of the heart traditionally was taught as beginning with a combination of palpation and percussion (the latter actually tapping out the heart's border). However, in recent years, with the advent of routine X-rays and sophisticated techniques such as echocardiograms used to examine heart size, the value of percussion and even palpation has decreased, and thus is not done as often. As with the lungs, once again your doctor will use a stethoscope (and auscultation) to routinely examine your heart, listening for heart sounds in a certain pattern down the left and right sides of the breastbone, called the sternum, and then usually over to the left, under the left nipple. The usual normal sounds are termed the S-1 and S-2, corresponding to the opening and shutting of the valves, but any extra noises (murmurs) that might be made as blood goes through the heart valves will be picked up as well. In many cases, such sound signals a valve problem. In some people, however, it may be an "innocent murmur"—no cause for particular concern, but like all murmurs, a cause for further investigation.

Your doctor likewise will listen for what are termed "extra sounds": clicks or rubs that have special significance in certain illness states. Your heartbeat can be checked with the stethoscope to see if it is regular or if there are extra beats, and your heart rate can also be checked; in most patients, the normal range is between 60 and 100 beats per minute.

While all of this general information about your heart can be gleaned from simply listening to it, evidence of coronary artery disease or recent heart attack cannot be picked up and requires more sophisticated methods of detection. They can, however, be indirectly hinted at with lab tests that will follow your physical exam—for example, if cholesterol levels are shown to be high or the electrocardiogram (EKG) is abnormal.

BREASTS. For all 35-plus women, the breast examination is an important part of the physical. It begins with "inspection from the sitting or standing position," whereby your doctor observes the appearance of your breasts when you are in a normal sitting or standing position: seeing whether they are symmetrical and whether they appear to be approximately the same in size and configuration.

Thorough palpation is next, and that is done when you lie down. Many doctors, myself included, use the methods taught by the American Cancer Society for the most thorough exam. In this case, your doctor will ask you to raise the arm on the side of the breast being examined, thus pulling the breast upward a little to help make the examination more accurate. The best examining technique starts at the outside of the breast and uses a moderate amount of pressure and a circular, rotating motion of the fingers to transcribe a series of concentric circles on the breast tissue. The first, or outer, circle transcribes the outer part of the breast, and then the fingers move inward to make a second, third, and in some cases even a fourth circle, depending on the size of the breast. There is no rushing a breast exam. All breasts have what is called "a tail," which extends up to the underarm; that, too, is part of a thorough examination, as are the underarms themselves, because this is frequently where there is lymph-node swelling in breast disease.

It's a good idea to review the breast examination with your doctor each step of the way. If she or he hands you a written review sheet of breast-exam techniques at the end of the exam, this is not simply so that you will have a souvenir of your office visit or a nice diagram of your breasts; rather, it provides further encouragement and guidelines for you to do your own breast exams at home.

Use these techniques often—at least once a month or more—because they are your first and best step toward detecting breast cancer at the earliest possible stage, when its cure rate is highest. Even if you doubt your ability to detect a lump, a self-exam of the breasts done on a regular basis will give you such close knowledge of your normal breast tissue that you will become highly attuned to even the slightest signs of change. Self-exam guidelines are available from the American Cancer Society.

During the breast exam, your doctor may advise you to make an appointment for a mammogram, if you have not already had one. However, do not wait for the subject to come up; ask about it specifically. Studies continue in Europe and in this country to determine the optimal frequency of mammography, but the diagnostic value of a baseline mammogram has been documented, even for women in their thirties.

ABDOMEN.   As with the breasts, examining your abdomen begins with observation and then palpation. The purpose of such an exam is to check the size of the liver and spleen, to see that they are normal, and also to feel for unusual tenderness or lumps. Once again using a stethoscope, your doctor will listen for the normal, gurgling sounds of the bowels, and then move the stethoscope over the kidney areas, listening for an audible sign (a bruit) of artery narrowing.

THE EXTREMITIES.   With the abdominal examination completed, attention moves from your torso out to the "extremities": the lower legs and feet, but also the arms, hands, and wrists. Your doctor will look at your legs for any swelling or fluid retention (edema); and he or she will check for signs of varicose veins on your legs. She or he may check the blood-vessel pulsations of the feet, first the dorsalis pedis pulse on top of the feet and then the posterior tibialis artery pulsation near the Achilles tendon. As with the carotid artery, pulsations are graded 0 to 4, with 4 being a bounding, or extremely strong, pulse and 0 being an absent pulse. A pulse of 2 or 3 usually indicates good vascular health. The arch of the foot and skeletal structure, color, and general temperature of the feet are also checked, since they are good indications of how efficiently blood is circulating. Your doctor will be assessing whether your toenails look healthy and whether there are signs of fungal growth in the nails. Normal hair growth on the feet is a sign of good vascular health. A check between the toes can reveal tinea pedis, or athlete's foot, a condition that often goes undetected. Analogous to the ankle and foot exam, the pulse is checked at the wrist (radial pulse), and hands and fingers are palpated for signs of poor circulation or arthritis.

JOINTS.   To check joints, your doctor will probably guide you through simple range-of-motion exercises to see that your joints are functioning properly, particularly your weight-bearing knees and hip joints. He or she will also feel the joints for signs of arthritis, acute or chronic.

CENTRAL NERVOUS SYSTEM.   The neurological examination for most patients consists of a brief screen of "general motor and sensory function," assessing first the normal strength and activity of your muscles (motor function), and then whether the sensations of a light touch, vibration, or even a pinprick elicit a response (sensory function) in the arms and legs. Gait—the way one walks—is often checked, as is sense of balance.

Assessment of your general "mental status" actually progresses all through the general procedures, at least when the intent, as described here, is a screening exam. As with any other area that might present specific problems, the mental status "checkup" can be more detailed as need arises.

PELVIC EXAM. The pelvic and rectal exams usually conclude your physical. The pelvic is always done with a medical assistant in the room so that you will feel comfortable and your physician will have some assistance with slides and speculum. A commentary during the examination not only helps it go quickly but also provides straightforward information about your uterus and vagina. Ask your doctor to tell you what's going on as you are being examined, and don't feel embarrassed about asking questions.

The pelvic exam begins with an examination of the vulva, the external genitals, and then with a speculum, proceeds to an exam of the vagina and the cervix, with the doctor routinely checking for any sign of discharge and taking a pap smear both of the endocervix and of the vagina. The exam concludes with the bimanual exam. As with the breast exam, the bimanual exam of the pelvis should be thorough and deliberate, since it acts as a screen for certain gynecological cancers (pages 254–256). With the gloved fingers of one hand, usually two fingers only, your doctor will reach inside your vagina to palpate the cervix and, feeling with the other hand on your lower abdomen, gauge the condition of the uterus: its size, whether there is any tenderness when palpated, and if there are any fibroid tumors. This bimanual portion of the exam is also used to check the ovaries, again looking for any possibility of a mass on the ovary or an enlarged ovary. As with breast cancer, the chance of successfully treating ovarian cancer greatly increases the earlier it is detected. Such a check is of greatest value with slender women. If a woman is markedly obese, it is very unlikely the ovaries could be felt in a standard bimanual exam.

RECTAL EXAM. Changing gloves, your doctor then proceeds to do a rectal examination, checking for both masses or polyps, and also taking a stool sample that will later be checked chemically for any sign of blood.

Testing Procedures

What are considered the "standard tests" associated with a complete physical examination will vary, depending on your physician's preferences. In some offices, a huge number of tests may be done and in others, only a few. What follows is a rundown of the tests that in my opinion provide an ideal baseline in all 35-plus women seen on a "well visit."

COMPLETE BLOOD COUNT (CBC). This test has three main components. The *white blood cell count* in most people is between 5,000 and 10,000. The *hemoglobin* is a check of the red cell count to help determine whether or not you're anemic. The count is usually between 12 and 14 grams in women but can be a bit lower if a woman is actively menstruating. In an *estimate of the platelets*, sometimes the number of platelets is given —usually between 150,000 and 400,000—but other times on a CBC slip they are simply estimated to be adequate or not.

CHEMISTRY TESTS. In some offices, physicians will simply order what's called an SMA-20, which is an assortment of approximately twenty chemistry tests, including everything from blood sugar to thyroid function. Usually the physician targets several chemistry tests that experience has shown to be most valuable. These include a *blood-sugar level*, which in a fasting state usually is between 80 and 110; an *alkaline phosphatase*, which is a test of liver function; a *creatinine*, which shows kidney function; a *uric acid*, which is often associated with gout, if significantly elevated; and a *calcium test*, which can be elevated in certain problems that affect the bone.

In addition, your doctor might make it a practice to do a complete *lipid panel*: a profile gleaned from a collection of tests that measure levels of cholesterol, triglyceride, HDL cholesterol, and LDL cholesterol (discussed in Chapter 8).

VDRL. If there is no test for syphilis, called the VDRL, on your medical record, your doctor may want to do that. It should be negative, of course, but it is important to know that a patient who has been correctly treated for syphilis and cured may continue to show a positive VDRL—in the majority of cases, for a lifetime, but the test need not be repeated every time a patient has a physical.

URINALYSIS. This should always be done with a physical examination. It gives a valuable return for the money not only as a good, general screen of kidney function but also in checking whether there is glucose or protein in the urine. Either of the latter can indicate certain problems, with glucose relating to diabetes and protein as a nonspecific screen for certain types of kidney disease. Often a microscopic evaluation of the urine is called for, whereby a technician looks under a microscope to see if there are any white blood cells. In the context of a urine test, this can often indicate infection, while red blood cells (again, in the context of the urine) can signal inflammation, infection, and even, in some cases, cancer. Neither the urinalysis nor the pap smear can be done if the patient is menstruating the day of the exam.

CHEST X-RAY. If you are a new patient, your doctor most likely will want you to have at least one chest X-ray, both front and side views, which can serve as a valuable baseline for heart size and lung status. If you have had a recent chest X-ray and if you are a nonsmoker, this certainly need not be an annual requirement.

ELECTROCARDIOGRAM (EKG). The EKG is another test your doctor should suggest. Even if you don't have another one for another ten years, this baseline record is useful to have on file should there be any future testing and is especially important to refer to if there are any future questions of heart problems.

STRESS TEST. This test (see page 88) may also be warranted, especially if there are particular concerns about the health of your heart or if you are starting a new exercise program. If needed, the stress test usually is scheduled separately from your "well-visit" physical.

TB SKIN TEST. As part of the basic physical examination, some doctors will want to establish whether you have a positive or negative skin test for tuberculosis. Of course this is unnecessary if there is a history of clinical TB, or if there had been a BCG vaccination for TB, which is especially common overseas. Otherwise, learning whether the patient is either positive or negative is an important part of baseline information.

ADDITIONAL TESTS. Other issues of a baseline exam include *immunization update, mammography,* and *sigmoidoscopy* decisions, but usually these surface during the physical itself or in connection with specific complaints. (In a sigmoidoscopy, a flexible tube is passed into the rectum and lower colon to check for polyps or cancerous growths.)

Concluding the Complete Physical Exam

Once completed, your general examination has given your doctor the chance to evaluate aspects of your health and concerns about illness that you have shared with him or her. The general exam also gives you and your doctor adequate time to just sit and think for a few minutes about your general health. This thorough review is not something you need to do annually, but if you only visited the office when you were sick, there would never be the luxury of time to address the big picture: updating immunizations, deciding on mammography, health counseling, and so forth. A whole variety of positive accomplishments can be gained through a periodic physical exam, which is why we urge you to arrange for a complete physical with the person who is going to be your personal physician. It will provide both of you with a good initiation into a working relationship toward your good health—at 35-plus and well beyond.

THE OPTIMUM SCHEDULE FOR 35-PLUS MEDICAL APPOINTMENTS

Whom to See and When

Internist or Family Practitioner (Primary Physician)—After initial 35-plus baseline exam, a complete physical at least every five years, or more frequently if indicated.

Gynecologist—Annual visit for breast exam, pelvic exam, and pap smear, if not done by internist or family practitioner.

Nutritionist—As needed, unless under a nutritionist's care.

Dentist—At regular four- to six-month intervals.

Eye Doctor—Every two years if there are no intervening problems.

Special Tests and Immunizations

Mammogram—Baseline mammogram between ages 35 and 40. Between ages 40 and 50, you may want to have one every other year. Discuss this with your physician, particularly if you're at increased risk. When over age 50, mammogram every year, as recommended by the American Cancer Society.

Cholesterol/Lipid Study—Baseline and thereafter (if it's in a good range) every two years. If elevated, follow more frequently.

Blood Pressure Check—With every complete physical and also at yearly intervals.

Tetanus Immunization—Every ten years.

Flu Shots—Optional, but yearly if desired. Women with specific health problems should discuss the pros and cons with their doctors, particularly if allergic reactions are a possibility. Pneumonia vaccine is advised for everyone over age 65, and for anyone with lung problems.

PART TWO

What You See in the Mirror

IN THE CHAPTERS THAT follow, beginning with the principles of Jean Spodnik's revolutionary metabolism diet for 35-plus women, we'll show you how to take control over what you see in the mirror—improving the shape of your body by maintaining your optimum weight; adjusting to the changing needs of your skin so you give it the best care possible; maintaining healthy teeth and gums—in short, making all the head-to-toe improvements (right down to grooming your hair and nails) that will enhance your overall appearance. While a few of these concerns are primarily cosmetic, they are all inextricably linked with your total body health—and are of course a part of your overall sense of well-being.

CHAPTER 3

Maintaining Optimum Weight

WE WANT EVERY 35-PLUS woman to look and feel her best—within her optimum weight range. Although there are occasional extremes of high obesity or anorexia, the overwhelming majority of 35-plus women we see in clinical practice know exactly what optimum weight means for them. Assessment of their "target zone" is not based on model perfection, as in the teens and twenties when hairstyle, body contour, and even length and shape of fingernails are often judged by how closely they match the current ideal. Acknowledging that genes play a role in determining bone structure and overall weight distribution, most 35-plus women today resist media images and pat formulas—including the standard charts and graphs that attempt to pigeonhole people by age and height—and rely on their own intuition in judging their optimum weight.

While genetic predisposition to obesity may sound like a no-win situation, even here scientists are making some headway—discovering new connections among fat cells, appetite, behavior, and the brain, and possible ways to alter them. In one recent study, mice who were obese for genetic or metabolic reasons exhibited lower than normal levels of adipsin, a protein substance made by fat cells that is released into the bloodstream and consequently travels to the brain, where it may influence eating patterns and food metabolism. Comparisons of adipsin levels in humans are currently underway to determine whether there is a corollary between low adipsin levels and the predisposition to become fat. The outcome of all this is being watched very closely, since gains in treating certain types of obesity may prove enormous.

Most women, however, don't inherit the tendency to become obese.

Rather, they head into middle age facing a predictable, double-pronged challenge to maintaining their weight: the normal slowdown of basal metabolism which occurs in *both* sexes, coupled with the effects of specific female hormonal activity.

BMR

Basal metabolism is defined as the lowest rate at which a person turns food into the fuel, or energy, needed to maintain life. Basal metabolic rate (BMR) is determined when a person is at "digestive rest"—that is, having eaten no food for fourteen hours; at physical rest—lying still; and at emotional rest—free of stress.

One's basal metabolic rate varies throughout his or her life span. It is higher when growth needs are great, as in infancy and prepuberty, and it decreases slightly during the late teens. By about age 25, it starts to slow down by approximately 0.5 percent a year. It is because of this decrease that, by age 35, weight control becomes a challenge: fat accumulates even though we don't eat any more than we did in our twenties.

While both sexes experience a decrease in basal metabolic rate, the challenge to keep off excess fat is greater for women over 35 than it is for men of the same age, for reasons that have nothing to do with willpower, weakness, or self-indulgence. It is because male hormones program men to maintain their muscles, a process that burns energy (calories), while female hormones program a woman's body to have babies, whether she chooses to have them or not. In order to ovulate, at least 17 percent of a woman's body weight needs to be fat, thus ensuring enough energy reserves to support a fetus. When a woman does become pregnant, additional fat stores accumulate around the hips and buttocks to sustain the mother and provide extra energy for the ordeal of birth. This is the fat that remains in the weeks following delivery, and for some women (particularly those who breast-feed), it may come off fairly quickly. For others, however, losing this weight seems to take forever.

Pregnant or not, a woman's body is always gearing up for childbearing, at least during the fertile years of her menstrual cycle. In this regard, the now-documented premenstrual syndrome (PMS) actually influences her choice of foods. Seven to ten days before the onset of her period, a woman's appetite predictably increases, with some women craving sweets and others salty foods, with added calories in either case. The exact cause of these cravings hasn't fully been determined; but the presence of a raised level of insulin in the blood in the days prior to menstruation may explain this increased hunger.

Fluid retention is another complication faced by women. Have you ever heard a man describe himself as feeling bloated? Hardly. With their mantle of muscle, men tend to have a nearly equal distribution of total body water within their cells. But bloating is a fairly common complaint among women, because water is distributed both inside of and in between the cells. This extracellular space accounts for bloat. When a person grows fatter, fluid retention tends to increase; but for women, water-retention problems are also a real part of premenstrual syndrome. (Coping with PMS is covered in Chapter 15.)

Further safeguarding a woman's biological role as nurturer, Nature sees to it that she burns fat at a slower rate than men, thus starting her out in life with a BMR about 10 percent lower than a man's. Many women on weight-loss diets complain bitterly that their husbands can give up a few beers and desserts and lose 20 pounds in a month or two, whereas they gave up all those treats long ago and still can't lose a pound. The slower rate of metabolism is the reason this is so. Even athletic women whose weight is normal will have a higher percentage of fat stores than do their male counterparts—again to ensure ovulation.

This is not to say that there aren't other factors besides hormones that affect basal metabolism—in both sexes. Climate is one, for whenever the difference between body temperature and external temperature increases, BMR increases; as a general rule, people in cold climates need more energy to function than do those in warm climates. Illness also increases BMR. Depending on the disease, or extent of damage and loss of heat by fever, extra energy is required as the body works to make repairs. Though not as well defined, emotional or physical stress may also increase BMR. These factors notwithstanding, women simply have greater genetic and biological hurdles to contend with than men do in keeping to their optimum weight —especially after the age of 35.

Why Bother Losing Weight?

There are several good reasons for keeping to your optimum weight. Beyond cosmetic issues, we know that extreme variations in optimum weight can alter a woman's health prospects. If there are danger signals—lipid problems (high blood cholesterol), elevated blood pressure (hypertension), elevated blood sugar (early diabetes)—she should definitely get her weight into her optimum range.

The development of high blood sugar or even borderline blood sugar— that is, a situation moving toward a diabetic state—is one danger signal. Diabetes is actually a spectrum: it does not always present itself with a sudden, dramatically elevated blood-sugar level and all the symptoms of diabetes. Some women and men begin with a blood sugar that is not dramatically elevated but isn't normal, either—a fasting blood sugar of 160, for instance, would certainly dictate a weight-loss program if the patient is overweight.

In women who have developed mild high blood pressure, studies have shown that even a moderate reduction in body weight helps correct the problem, as it will for women with cholesterol problems, although there is not always a direct correlation between cholesterol and weight—we have seen some very obese patients who have quite low cholesterol levels.

There is another area in which weight impinges directly on health, and this involves arthritis in weight-bearing joints: the ankles, knees, and hips. Even if she has only mild arthritis, we suggest a 10 percent reduction of weight in a woman who is significantly overweight, since it lessens the load on (and subsequent deterioration of) problematic joints.

Still another area—albeit nonmedical—involves self-image. If you think about your weight day and night, it leaves little room for more productive thought. Setting reasonable limits for optimum weight and sticking to them can free you to truly enjoy other, more important areas of your life.

In spite of all these variables, *if a woman can medically rule out the big-three danger signals just mentioned, as well as joint problems, there is no medical evidence whatsoever to prove that being 10 percent (even 20 or 30 pounds) over the Metropolitan Life weight tables is inherently dangerous to the health of the average-framed person.* Moreover, a little padding actually can be beneficial, since superslim women have no reserves—either in terms of fat tissue or muscle—should they become significantly ill. Illness tends to be a catabolic process—using up calories—so that if someone has absolutely no reserves or is actually underweight, she has very little caloric cushion, in medical terms, to see her through the illness.

This is not to say a woman has free rein to eat all the wrong foods and stay very fat, but it does put some perspective on the preoccupation with slimness that is so prevalent today. Aiming for a realistic weight is the goal.

How Much Should You Lose?

Putting away standard weight tables, your successful weight loss should be based on a 10 to 15 percent loss of body weight over a two- to four-month period. Thus a 150-pound woman who aims to lose from 15 to 23 pounds would do so during that defined period, but it could take longer. Exercise safely speeds the process—curbing appetite and helping to burn calories— but depending on the basal metabolic rate, which is predetermined by genes and slows down with age, the pounds that take one woman two months to lose may take another four months or more.

Rebound Weight and the Yo-Yo Syndrome

The truth is, trying to lose amounts beyond 10 to 15 percent of present body weight may be testing the impossible. The 160-pound woman who tries to cut back to a size 10 may have to lose 40 or 50 pounds; and if she succeeds, there's a risk of what we call rebound weight gain—that is, she may gain back more than she loses. It may startle you to know that when we want someone to gain weight, we put them on a weight-loss diet, knowing that when they go off it, they'll gain weight at a faster rate. It all has to do with the response of the body after a fast (such as Oprah Winfrey's) or an extremely low-calorie diet, when refeeding is associated with a supranormal tissue response to nutrients. This response is characterized by increased fat formation—in fat tissue and the liver. In the fat cells, there is a faster production of triglycerides and carbon dioxide drawn from the glucose in the blood. This rapid conversion of glucose into triglycerides (fat in the form of free fatty acids) is triggered in part by increased insulin levels and greater tissue insulin sensitivity. This usually leads to lower blood-glucose levels, which further increases hunger.

According to the set point theory, this frustrating rebound can be even more acute if fat cells fall much below their normal size. Many times, obese people succeed at lowering their weight to the point where their fat cells are at the lower limits of normal size, but to go any further—to the point that fat cell size falls *below* normal—may trigger significantly more refeeding to compensate. When this happens, the person frequently regains all the weight that's been lost. This is another reason why more than a 10 to 15 percent total weight loss may defeat your overall objectives.

Yo-yo dieting also makes it progressively more difficult for anyone—but especially the 35-plus woman—to lose weight. In 1986, researchers at the University of Pennsylvania School of Medicine found that 14 wrestlers who, to compete in their weight classification, dieted no less than ten times over a two-year period, had a resting metabolism rate that was 14 percent lower than that of 13 noncycling wrestlers. When BMR falls, food efficiency increases—that is, you gain weight faster on less food. That is why Phase Three (see page 30) is so important for maintenance in the 35-plus diet, and another reason why the 160-pound woman is better off staying within her optimum range, aiming for a loss of no more than 10 to 15 percent of her present weight. This weight loss *must* be accompanied by regular exercise to keep the metabolic rate up and tone muscles.

JEAN SPODNIK'S 35-PLUS MEAL PLANS FOR PERMANENT WEIGHT REDUCTION

Look in the mirror. Let's say you have determined that you would be much better off losing that 10 to 15 percent of your present weight, and that the loss would put you within your optimum weight range. You're ready to lose the pounds, starting right now. How are you going to do it? How are you going to really make a change this time, even if you have tried and failed in the past? And if you lose with a so-called diet, how are you going to phase off dieting without regaining weight?

That's easy. If you really want to lose weight and keep it off, use the three-phase meal plans that follow, in tandem with the exchange lists in Chapter 22.

Using meal plans to achieve optimum weight has many advantages. First, because the foods included on them are what you normally eat anyway (adjusted to reasonable-size portions), you never really feel as if you are "on a diet." Second, my weight-loss meal plans are geared to normal changes in your metabolism. They utilize complex carbohydrates, high fiber, low cholesterol, low saturated fat, high potassium and calcium—in short, the same nourishing foods proved to be a winning combination for altering basal metabolism in the middle years, as demonstrated in studies from which my first book, *The 35-Plus Diet for Women*, evolved.

The 35-Plus Diet Works When Others Don't

My meal-plan approach to weight control was initially documented in a controlled test of women ranging in age from 40 to 60, 20 to 50 pounds overweight, and with sedentary life-styles. Over the course of seven weeks, those testing the 35-plus diet lost an average of 11.8 pounds in six weeks, while those in the control group lost 3.8 pounds.

For *both* groups, approximately 900 to 950 calories were consumed, which is close to most women's basal metabolic rate, but the 35-plus diet was composed of 37 percent carbohydrate, 34 percent protein, and 29 percent fat, with a "jump start" phase of 27 percent carbohydrate and 40 percent protein. The control diet was composed of 50 percent carbohydrate, 20 percent protein, and 30 percent fat. What the 35-plus formula effectively demonstrated was that it's not just *how many* calories, but *where they come from* that determines how readily you'll lose weight. Not only are the food exchange lists critical to the success of the meal plans, but so are the portion, or serving, sizes.

Follow the three-phase sequence exactly; it's the balance between proteins and carbohydrates in each sequence that makes this metabolism diet so effective. In Phase One, the ratio of protein to carbohydrate is intended to bring the dieter to the *brink* of ketosis (but not *into* ketosis) in order to release stores of excess water between cells. In ketosis there is an incomplete combustion of fatty acids that occurs when you are getting too little food or, specifically, too few carbohydrates. True ketosis, which can occur on high-protein high-fat fad diets, can be dangerous because it puts excessive demands on the excretory system (the kidneys) and can cause potentially serious electrolyte imbalances. Phase One provides just enough carbohydrate to prevent this, while forcing your body to release excess fluids. If you lose five pounds or more in the first week, you are ready to go on to Phase Two. If you lose less than two pounds in the first week, you may continue with Phase One for a second week—but *that's all*, as two weeks is the maximum safe duration for a diet that's severely restricted in necessary carbohydrates.

Note that throughout the diet, you may eat as many fresh, low-starch vegetables as you like (see the vegetable exchange list, page 299)—ensuring a good supply of fiber, vitamins, and other important nutrients as you lose weight.

Phase Two increases food intake; while it may not seem dramatically different from Phase One, it has been carefully orchestrated to provide just the right balance of lean protein and complex carbohydrate to foster the loss of fat and prevent a recurrence of water retention. Here again, stick to the portions and proportions of each type of food suggested, as it is the *ratio* of protein to carbohydrate that prevents water weight gain.

Following the first two meal plans, you will find a 35-Plus Vegetarian Weight Loss Diet—the same effective 35-plus diet specifically tailored for lacto- or ovolactovegetarians.

Phase One: Meal Plan 1 (Use for 1 to 2 weeks)*
Used for initial weight reduction—to "jump start" your weight loss—this first meal plan consists of 27 percent starch, 40 percent protein, and 33 percent fat. Note that in Phase One and Phase Two there are no *added* fats in the diet: the fat occurs naturally in the protein and dairy foods you'll be eating.

	VEGETABLES	STARCH	PROTEIN	FRUIT	MILK
Breakfast	0	1	1	1	½
Lunch	as desired	1	3	1	0
Dinner	as desired	0	5	0	0
Snack	as desired	0	1	1	½

* Note: Use a multivitamin and mineral supplement daily.

Phase Two: Meal Plan 2 (Use until optimum weight is reached)
Used to level off to optimum weight, this second meal plan adds one serving of starch and consists of 37 percent starch, 34 percent protein, and 29 percent fat.

	VEGETABLES	STARCH	PROTEIN	FRUIT	MILK
Breakfast	0	1	1	1	½
Lunch	as desired	1	3	1	0
Dinner	as desired	1	5	0	0
Snack	as desired	0	1	1	½

Phase Three, or Phase-off: Maintenance of Optimum Weight

Meal Plan 2 continues in this third phase, adding three servings of either polyunsaturated or monounsaturated fat a day (see exchange lists, Chapter 22) as phase-off considerations begin. Once you have achieved your weight-loss goal, use the guidelines for behavior modification (see Chapter 4, pages 38–40), and pick one day of the week to go off the diet. The following week, pick another day to go off. Most women find they can go off the diet comfortably two to three days a week without weight gain.

The 35-Plus Diet for Vegetarians

Here are the meal plans for the 35-Plus Vegetarian Weight Loss Diet. For more details on vegetarianism, turn to pages 280–282.

Although you are allowed one tablespoon of peanut butter a day, you must eliminate all other nuts and seeds from Phases One and Two of the diet to lose weight. A half cup of nuts has 16 grams of protein, 12 grams of carbohydrate, and 32 grams of fat, for a total of 400 calories; ½ cup of hulled seeds has 30.5 grams of protein, 23.3 grams of carbohydrate, and 59.7 grams of fat, or 752 calories. Except when used in small quantities with other foods to form a complementary protein (see page 281), seeds and nuts are not good protein sources because they contain too many calories for the amount of protein they provide.

Your intake of legumes is also limited—to one serving a day, at lunch. Protein foods for breakfast, dinner, and snacks must come from low-fat cheeses on the list, eggs, egg whites, or egg substitutes (no more than two whole eggs per week). One serving of legumes, as given on the low-fat protein exchange list for vegetarians (page 297), counts as 2 servings of protein. Take your starch exchange at lunch in the form of rice, whole-wheat bread or crackers, corn or cornmeal products to make the complementary protein. A bowl of bean soup and an old-fashioned unsweetened corn muffin at a vegetarian restaurant is good when you're eating out. Bean soups at nonvegetarian restaurants are usually made with meat or meat stock.

Phase One: Vegetarian Meal Plan 1 (Use for 1 to 2 weeks)*

	VEGETABLES	STARCH	PROTEIN	FRUIT	MILK
Breakfast	0	1 (whole-grain)	1	1	½
Lunch	as desired	1 (whole-grain)	2	0	0
Afternoon snack	as desired	0	1	1	0
Dinner	as desired	0	4	0	0
Snack	as desired	0 ·	2	1	½

* Note: Use a multivitamin and mineral supplement daily.

Phase Two: Vegetarian Meal Plan 2 (Use until optimum weight is reached)

	VEGETABLES	STARCH	PROTEIN	FRUIT	MILK
Breakfast	0	1 (whole-grain)	1	1	½
Lunch	as desired	1 (whole-grain)	2	0	0
Afternoon snack	as desired	0	1	1	0
Dinner	as desired	1 (whole-grain)	4	0	0
Snack	as desired	0	2	1	½

Phase Three, or Phase-off: Maintenance of Optimum Weight

Meal Plan 2 continues in this third phase, adding three servings of either polyunsaturated or monounsaturated fat a day as phase-off considerations begin. These are the same for vegetarians as for nonvegetarians. Once you have achieved your weight-loss goal, use behavior modification (Chapter 4, pages 38–40), and pick one day of the week to go off the diet. The following week, pick another day to go off. Most women find they can go off the diet comfortably two to three days a week without weight gain.

THE EXCHANGE SYSTEM

The food exchange system (see lists, pages 295–303) gives you enormous freedom in using these meal plans, letting you tailor them to your own budget, food preferences, and even special considerations, such as entertaining and enjoying special holiday foods.

How the Food Exchange System Works

The exchange system groups foods into six general categories: (1) protein, (2) starches, (3) vegetables, (4) fruits, (5) milk, and (6) fats.

Meat, poultry, fish, and cheese are listed as protein because that is their major component, or nutrient.

Though they contain a good deal of protein, milk and plain yogurt are in a separate group because they also contain carbohydrates and may or may not contain fat.

Fruits are a self-contained group based on their nutrient composition, which is quite different from vegetables. Although both of these categories are high in water and fiber content, fruit is higher in natural sugar (fructose), whereas vegetables are higher in starch. Some vegetables, such as potatoes, peas, corn, and beans, are so much higher that they move to the starch category.

The starch group also includes grains, pastas, cereals, breads, crackers, and combinations (as in soup) that are mostly carbohydrates.

In addition to these six categories, the exchange system categorizes fats, free foods (those permitted in unlimited amounts), and foods to avoid because they are high in sugar and fat—that is, those foods that have empty or too concentrated calories for people trying to lose weight.

The exchange system not only categorizes foods but also presents them in serving portions, as required in the meal plans. This need not be a tedious business of weighing and measuring. Since you probably use the same glasses and dishes every day at home, once you establish the portion size—that is, that a certain glass holds 4 ounces—you no longer have to continue using a measuring cup for your orange juice in the morning. You just pour it out. The same goes for ½ cup of fruit. If you use the same dessert dish each time, you will know what ½ cup looks like in the dish.

This easy, visual method of measuring portions applies equally well to all the food groups in the plan. Here are some additional tips for gauging portions:

4 ounces of lean, raw, boneless meat = 3 ounces cooked (you lose an ounce in the cooking)

5 to 6 ounces of lean, raw meat with a bone = 3 ounces cooked

8 to 9 ounces of raw, boneless fish = 6 ounces cooked (fish shrinks more than meat because it contains more water and connective tissue)

1 skinless chicken leg, medium size = 3 ounces cooked (always remove chicken skin, the only source of chicken fat)

1 skinless chicken thigh, medium size = 3 ounces cooked

½ skinless chicken breast, small = 3 ounces cooked

In addition, if you buy cheese in a ½-pound piece and score the piece eight times, each piece will be an ounce. If you measure ⅓ cup of cottage cheese once and see what it looks like in a small bowl or cup, you will use that same amount at meals.

Here's how the exchange list works to give you freedom in planning breakfasts, for example:

1. You have 1 serving of fruit, which means you can have ¾ cup strawberries on Monday, in addition to your protein and starch exchanges.

2. On Tuesday, you don't have time to prepare strawberries, so you choose ½ cup orange juice instead.

3. As the week progresses, you may decide you do not have time to eat

at home, so you grab a piece of fruit to have with the rest of your breakfast at work.

You can count on this kind of flexibility to help you succeed with every meal.

Food Preparation Tips

Many otherwise reasonable people seem unintentionally to ignore not only the portion size but also how the preparation of a food affects its calorie content. We've seen this happen with a professional cook, who claimed she could never lose weight even though she never ate a single whole meal; she was oblivious of sampling "a little of this and that" buttery dish all day long. Another woman meticulously removed all the fat from chicken breasts before she poached them in wine—and then ate three of them! Still another woman ate an exact 6-ounce portion of fish each week, breaded and deep-fried.

So to make sure you don't consume more calories than the foods already contain, avoid frying meat, fish, or poultry and avoid breading or batter-coating foods as well; these cooking methods add (sometimes double) the calories. Broiling (including pan broiling in a nonstick skillet), roasting, boiling, steaming, or cooking foods on a barbecue grill are the preferred cooking processes, using vegetable cooking spray on the pan, if desired, but adding no fats. (Also see Cooking Tips in Chapter 22.)

Seasoning makes food more interesting—for example, you can cook your vegetables with salt*, pepper, bouillon*, consomme*, or fat-free broth. You can season a variety of foods with any of the following without loading on a lot of calories:

Lemon juice	Vinegar
Mustard*	Horseradish*
Herbs	Spices
Artificial sweeteners	Unsweetened cocoa powder

You can also use any of the following:

Coffee, regular or decaffeinated (black or sweetened with artificial sweetener)
Gelatin (plain, unflavored, or artificially sweetened)
Tea, regular or decaffeinated, herb tea (plain or with lemon and/or artificial sweetener)
Soft drinks (sugar-free or artificially sweetened)

---

* These products are high in sodium.

Unsweetened powdered drink mixes
Water, mineral water, seltzer

Provided you are under no diet restriction for sodium, you can use the following condiments in the specified amounts.

Catsup, barbecue sauce,* or chili sauce*—1
    tablespoon
Relish—1 tablespoon
Soy sauce—2 tablespoons
Steak sauce—2 tablespoons

If you choose to drink some of the sugar-free products that contain milk, like the hot cocoa drinks, subtract them from your daily milk allowances. Cereal beverages like Postum may be used, but limit them to 1 tablespoon per day.

If you are on the weight-reduction diet, don't have any alcoholic beverages for the first two weeks; thereafter, you may have one drink a day (1 ounce of liquor, 4 ounces semi-dry wine, or 12 ounces of lite beer) if you wish, but no more. Alcoholic beverages simply add calories to your diet and nothing more. Also, after two weeks on the diet, you will find that your body chemistry has changed—one drink will have the effect of two.

Food Choices and Labeling

Guidelines for choosing foods wisely are given throughout this book, and in depth in Chapters 21, 22, and 23. Here we want to point out a few things to be aware of regarding portion or serving sizes:

- Look at the fine print on packaged snack foods that give calorie counts, especially "health food" snacks, paying special attention to the *serving size* and *servings per container* specified. Very often what's packaged to look like one serving is really two, and if you eat the whole package, you'll be taking on double the calories listed.
- Look at calorie counts and serving sizes for beverages. The calorie count shown on a 12-ounce can or bottle may be for a 6-ounce serving.
- Frozen fruit bars that advertise "17 calories per fluid ounce" are relatively low in calories at 68 calories per bar—just don't overlook the fact that each bar is 4 fluid ounces.
- Many "all natural" cereals (especially granola) are deceptively high in calories. The boxes list them for a serving size of ¼ cup; that's a rather puny 4 level tablespoons of cereal, or five or six bites!

* These products are high in sodium.

Eating Out

There is no reason why you can't eat out when you are on a diet, so long as the menu offered is fairly diverse or you can choose what you want from a cafeteria or buffet-type setting.

Breakfast could be dry toast, egg or egg substitute, and fruit or fruit juice. Or it could be smoked fish, half a bagel, and fruit or juice. Still another choice would be Canadian bacon, cereal, low-fat milk, and fruit or juice. Beverage (tea or coffee) of your choice is permitted in each case. But when ordering fruit, if it is canned, do not drink the juice.

Lunch could be an open-faced sandwich (one slice of bread or half a bun), with turkey, extra-lean ham, roast beef, or extra-lean corned beef. Or it could be 1 cup of cottage cheese and fruit (no bread), with extra fruit substituting for bread. If available, a small pita bread, which is the calorie equivalent of 1 slice of ordinary bread, can be used for a sandwich and you can always have a vegetable salad on the side.

Dinner—excluding fried foods, sauces, or gravies—can include roast beef, filet mignon, broiled fish, or roast chicken with the skin removed. With the meat, you could have half a large baked potato (skip the butter and sour cream) with a vegetable side dish and salad (avoid rich salad dressings).

Wherever possible, make a polite request that as little fat as possible be used in preparing your order.

Frequently Asked Questions

Many answers to questions people ask about the 35-Plus Meal Plans and metabolism diet have been incorporated into this chapter. Here are a few others:

Q: *Do I have to drink eight glasses of water a day if I follow this diet?*
A: With many other diets, drinking large amounts of calorie-free water is usually recommended to make the dieter feel full and presumably to reduce the temptation to eat more food. People following low-calorie diets do need water to eliminate the metabolic by-products of fat as they lose weight. But with the 35-plus diet, you'll be getting a lot of water from the vegetables you eat—water is 80 percent of fruits and vegetables and even meat is nearly half water. Drink four to six 8-ounce glasses of water a day, but keep in mind that fruit juices, milk, and decaffeinated coffee, tea, and colas contribute to your total intake of water as well. (Regular coffee, tea, colas, and alcoholic beverages, however, can be counterproductive because of their diuretic effect.)

Q: *Should a petite woman make any adjustments in the meal plans?*
A: Women under five feet tall should reduce their intake of protein and starch by 10 percent.

Q: *Will I reach a plateau with this approach to weight loss?*
A: How much you lose each week can fluctuate, and there may come a period when you're only losing ½ to 1 pound a week, when prior to that it was more. This can trigger a loss of motivation.

To avoid losing motivation:

- Increase the amount of exercise you have been doing or add on a new activity.
- Introduce a new food allowed on the diet, such as berries out of season. You may think they cost too much, but chances are you'd easily have spent that much on a sweet treat in the past.
- Reward yourself every two weeks instead of once a month; buy a new book, some cologne, a scarf; or go to a movie or have another (non-food!) treat.
- When an important weekend is coming up, go on the maintenance diet, allotting those two days as "days off." My patients are always surprised when they go off the diet but do not gain weight. They let their behavior modification take over and only have one scoop of ice cream, for instance, instead of several.

Q: *How does exercise benefit weight loss?*
A: Exercise limits the accumulation of body fat. Researchers have observed that even if caloric intake increases to compensate for calories burned in exercise, the body maintains a lower fat mass and body weight as long as the exercise is regular. If exercise is stopped, weight and fat levels return to normal.

Exercise guidelines are provided in Chapter 24. Remember that in order to lose fat, your body needs aerobic exercise. During exercise, the body initially draws energy from carbohydrates, in the form of glycogen, then as exercise continues, the body switches to drawing energy from fat stores, in the form of free fatty acids. Thus, while various forms of anaerobic exercise are good for toning muscles, it is aerobic exercise that accounts for weight loss.

CHAPTER 4

Beyond Diet

As THOUSANDS OF WOMEN have discovered, the meal plans and food exchange lists in this book provide a satisfying alternative to dieting and a tool for adjusting to the metabolic changes that occur at midlife. As you reassess your target zone for optimum weight, it is important to realize that while food intake is a big factor, it is not the only element in achieving your goals, as demonstrated by one woman who recently went on one of the new liquid-protein diets.

All summer she reported dramatic weight loss to a friend: first 10 pounds, then 20, then 50. Excitedly they made a date for the end of the summer so she could show off her new body and celebrate her first "real meal" at a restaurant. On the scheduled date, the dieter's friend was so excited she waited outside the restaurant in anticipation. Sure enough, there was the dieter heading down the block and looking svelte in spectacular clothes and a new hairstyle. But as she got closer, smiling and excited, it became terribly obvious that in losing all the weight she seemed to have aged ten years; the skin around her cheeks and chin sagged, and there were wrinkles etched deeply around her mouth and forehead. It was all her friend could do to hide her shock and try to muster some enthusiasm about the weight loss.

A week after that lunch, depressed in acknowledging how much older she looked, the liquid-protein dieter called to say she was contemplating cosmetic surgery if exercise did not tone up her muscles and improve her looks. Not quite a year later, she had regained most of the weight she had lost on the diet.

This is not an unusual story. Many people have a difficult time keeping excess weight off, even with the "miracle" liquid-protein diets that have recently become so popular. Spin-offs of the liquid-protein diets that have been around for many years, these modified fasting diets must be used with close, rigorous medical supervision, including having your blood chemistry checked weekly, especially for electrolyte disturbances such as low potassium, which can be dangerous. Moreover, they were never intended for everyone, but rather, for those who are morbidly obese and who are unable to succeed with normal diets.

Whereas the 35-plus diet makes it easy to shift into a lifelong maintenance diet, such a transition from a liquid-protein diet is not only difficult but in some cases almost impossible. The "shock system" approach to dieting can produce significant weight loss, but if basic behavioral or psychological problems are left unattended, even the best diet program ultimately does not have much chance to succeed. Where will the people who use these quick weight-loss diets be in five years?

This is the big question, and it's also where behavior modification—changing your eating habits—comes in. Current behavior therapy for obesity is quite different from the self-monitored, stimulus-controlled behavior modification programs of the past. There is greater emphasis on exercise, nutrition, and social support from family and friends to help you stay with your new eating habits, making this approach far more effective than in the past.

To help people grappling with the yo-yo syndrome of weight on–weight off, we offer the following:

35-PLUS STRATEGIES FOR CHANGING YOUR EATING HABITS (A BAKER'S DOZEN)

1. *Sit down and analyze your eating schedule.* If you crave food at 4:00 P.M., or in particular situations, try to arrange your activities so you can't eat during this time. The impulse to eat at a specific time may be a conditioned response that will gradually disappear if you stop reinforcing the cue with food. You must be sure the activity you choose is truly enjoyable, so that it can compete with the urge to eat.

2. *Wait to satisfy your hunger.* Make a bargain with yourself that you will eat only after twenty minutes have passed from the time you feel hunger pangs, which usually last only about twenty minutes. Usually your hunger will fade if you ignore it or delay eating. Many of our patients find this suggestion enormously effective in staving off the tendency to snack.

3. *When you eat, make it your only activity.* That is, do not eat and also read, watch television, or drive a car. Concentrate on every bite. It will help you appreciate the taste and texture of food, rather than the quantity.

4. *Reward yourself for losing weight.* Choose a present that you'd really like and set your sights on it before you begin your weight-loss program. Save all the money you ordinarily spend on sweets from the candy machine or other snacks, and put it in a jar to use for something more worthwhile— something more lasting than a chocolate bar eaten in a few minutes and then forgotten.

5. *Identify the emotions connected with your eating.* Do you eat when you are bored, nervous, or angry? Or do you eat when you are happy and excited? Emotions often play a role in overeating, directly or indirectly, and eating may be a conditioned response to a certain emotion. Once you have identified this emotion, put suggestion 2, given earlier, into play.

6. *Out of sight, out of mind.* Put food in opaque containers in the kitchen and refrigerator, and remove all candy and nut dishes from your office or living room. Acknowledge that eating is a premeditated act, and that you fill the dishes with goodies because you intend to eat them. Then replace junk food with low-calorie snacks, such as carrots and celery. In the time it takes to find a sinful snack, ask yourself, "Do I really want it?"

7. *Buy fresh vegetables that you enjoy eating raw.* Stock up on carrots, bell peppers, radishes, celery, broccoli, and so on. Prepare them as soon as you get home. Trim, wash, and cut them into snack-size pieces; refrigerate them in a Ziploc bag where they'll keep well for up to a week. (This does not apply to tomatoes and cucumbers, which tend to get mushy or dry out once they're cut.) This way, you'll have something on hand when you feel the urge to snack.

Most salad greens will also keep well if they're washed, spun in a salad spinner, and refrigerated in a Ziploc bag immediately after they're brought home. This makes salads less of a chore to prepare at mealtime. Two suggestions: If you don't have a salad spinner, get one. It's the easiest way to wash and dry leafy greens, especially those sandy ones that need soaking in cold water first. Secondly, if you have children, enlist their help when preparing vegetables in advance. Gear the tasks involved to each child's age and ability; let the little ones do the rinsing while the older ones use the scraper or knife. And, of course, let them sample as they work!

8. *Avoid situations that are obviously tempting.* The sight and smell of food are powerful stimuli. If you buy cookies for the children's lunch and keep them on the kitchen counter, you are purposely setting yourself up to eat those cookies. If you know you can't pass a bakery without the smell of fresh-baked goods inviting you in, take a different route or cross the street.

9. *Fix your plate at the stove or counter and bring it to the table.* That way, you eliminate serving dishes, a visual cue to eating more than one adequate portion of food.

10. *Choose a special place to eat.* At work, go to the lunchroom or, if you eat at your desk, use a placemat or paper towel so that you know you are eating. At home, eat all your meals or snacks in an attractive, comfortable location; if you wish, change it with the seasons. This way, you will avoid eating as you walk around the house or watch television.

11. *Eat slowly.* It takes twenty minutes for food to be absorbed and for your stomach to signal your brain that you've eaten enough. By eating slowly, you allow time for your body to respond to the food you've eaten. You will feel fuller on less food. Extend your enjoyment of what you eat. If you eat a meal in ten minutes, take fifteen, then twenty minutes to eat it.

12. *Make exercise a new force in your life.* Just as you would not think of skipping a meal, make time to exercise at least three times a week for thirty to forty minutes each time.

13. *If none of these suggestions significantly improves your eating habits, try a support group such as Weight Watchers or Overeaters Anonymous.* Keep trying different types of support systems until you find the right group for you—where you feel comfortable and fit right in. Keep an open mind.

Today's "State-of-the-Art" Weight-Loss Alternatives

While the meal plans and behavior-modification tips can provide the motivation most people need to stay within their normal weight range, many women who reach middle age are willing to consider other routes to losing weight.

In the past, girdles were used to contour the body, even with the risk of promoting indigestion and dyspepsia. Today there is a new array of options geared to helping people control their eating habits. Yoga techniques, hypnosis, and even acupuncture have proved effective; certainly these are less controversial than the more radical weight-loss treatments that have evolved. Because radical treatments are becoming more diverse and readily available to wider numbers of people, we feel it is important to assess them here.

Liquid-Protein Diets

Liquid diets are not for everyone. They are not recommended for anyone who has recently experienced a heart attack, has cerebrovascular disease, kidney or liver disease, cancer, insulin-dependent diabetes, or psychiatric problems, nor are they good for pregnant or nursing women.

The modified fasting diets (very low calorie formula diets of 800 calories or less) referred to in the beginning of this chapter are generally recommended only for adults who are at least 30 percent overweight or who are at high medical risk because of their obesity. These formulas have certain advantages: The dieter is spared any anxiety-producing decisions about what to eat. The diet suppresses appetite well, and consistent rapid weight loss is a positive reinforcement for staying on it. The formula is easy to prepare and, except for carbohydrates, should be nutritionally complete.

The disadvantages are several. Formula diets are monotonous. They don't promote changes in normal eating or exercise habits, which can become a serious problem once the dieter goes off the diet. Modified fasting dieters may experience cold intolerance, constipation, dizziness, dry skin, and even hair loss, although the latter is temporary. Because these diets may create electrolyte imbalances, the dieter must be kept under medical supervision with weekly blood chemistry tests, especially for low potassium.

Diet Pills

Promoted years ago as the way to "quick loss," diet pills have not fulfilled their promise. Traditional diet pills such as dextroamphetamine have an amphetamine, or "speed," base that works by speeding up the metabolism. The basic amphetamine component in many diet pills is in fact addictive, as are all amphetamines if taken over the long term, and they pose potentially serious cardiovascular risks. Over-the-counter diet pills do not contain amphetamines but many do have chemical components such as phenylpropanolamine, also found in many allergy medications, that can cause acute emotional imbalance with symptoms ranging from hyper or "manic" emotional states to acute depressive feelings. Although you might lose a few pounds taking diet pills, the effects usually last only as long as the pills are taken—hence the road to pill dependency.

Thyroid Pills

These generally are prescribed by physicians either as the original animal thyroid (what was called Thyroid U.S.P.) or as L-thyroxine, which is the modern synthetic form. Some diet clinics give out low-dose thyroid on the assumption that everyone is minimally hypothyroid or just because they think it's a good idea to speed up the metabolism, since the thyroid hormone is one of the basic determinants of metabolic rate. The person who has an overactive thyroid—known as hyperthyroidism—has a fast metabolism, and one of the medical hallmarks of this condition is unexpected weight loss even with a voracious appetite. Hypothyroidism is the opposite.

Clearly, assessment of a person who is particularly overweight should include thyroid testing, and it is perfectly correct to use thyroid medication if the person is hypo-, or low, thyroid. However, the use of thyroid to supplement weight reduction for any other reason is nonsense, even though some claim that the tests won't pick up hypothyroidism. The latest test, called the TSH, is extremely sensitive to low thyroid. Moreover, if someone has a normal thyroid, the extra thyroid wouldn't do much to begin with. But while a deliberately induced hyperthyroid state might result in weight loss, it is very dangerous, causing a fast heart rate and possibly precipitating heart problems.

Diet Surgery

There are several kinds of diet surgeries available.

Liposuction is when fat cells are literally sucked out from beneath the skin, usually around the hips and thighs. Of the various radical procedures available, this is relatively safe, although the treated area may be uneven in appearance and there is risk of infection and/or bleeding under the skin.

In a gastric bypass, the upper stomach is made into a small pouch by connecting it to the second part of the small intestine (the jejunum). This leads to rapid filling of the stomach, giving a sense of fullness and slow emptying of the contents. It is safer than an intestinal bypass, whereby the end of the jejunum is connected to the end of the ileum (the third part of the small intestine), which leads to less nutrient absorption even with the same intake. We advise *neither!* Nor can gastric stapling to limit stomach size—and thus increase early filling and early sense of fullness—be advised. These operations are expensive, fraught-with-danger, "high-tech" attempts to solve problems that are essentially behavioral or hormonal.

Your approach to weight loss and lifetime weight control, like so many other areas of health and wellness, involves personal choice. The most rewarding decision you can make is to adopt a strategy that deals with food and food-related behaviors in a balanced and reasonable way—a program that can be sustained for a lifetime, not just for a few weeks or months. If you have spent most of your life trying one diet after another, this is your chance to free yourself, once and for all, from eating habits that make you feel guilty and defeated. Crash diets, diet pills, and other quick "fixes" tend to become part of an endless cycle in which weight is lost only to be regained. Nutritional and behaviorial consistency is the only thing that will work over the long haul. By setting reasonable goals, committing yourself to regular exercise, and adopting the sound nutritional programs presented here, you can maintain your optimum weight for the rest of your life.

CHAPTER 5

The Skin at Midlife

WITH A FEW EXCEPTIONS, THE skin's most critical functions stay in perfect working order throughout our lives, but it's the way the skin looks that concerns most women in midlife. The millions of dollars that leading manufacturers spend annually on advertising are a pretty strong indication of how large and eager a market there is for skin-care products that promise more youthful-looking skin.

Some current ad campaigns have shifted from a focus on coping with wrinkles caused by age to protecting the skin from a hostile environment. A recent Estée Lauder ad proclaimed that only 20 percent of the fine lines you see on your face before you are 50 or 60 are caused by aging; the rest are the result of the irritants, oxidants, and ultraviolet (UV) light in today's polluted, ozone-endangered environment. Lauder's copy urges readers to take action "before your skin takes the abuse of another day," by using its Skin Defender. The packaging of other products emphasizes that theme, with labels designed to resemble those on cigarette packs, warning against the dangers of chemical carcinogens, sunlight, tobacco smoke, ozone, and other "free radicals" that supposedly destroy skin cells.

Less Than Skin Deep

According to Elaine Brumberg, a cosmetics consumer advocate and author of *Take Care of Your Face*, approximately 8,000 chemicals are currently being used in cosmetic products. A number of these are touted as scientific breakthroughs available only in expensive moisturizers and creams—products that claim either to protect the skin from the foregoing hostile attacks or to forestall or even reverse the aging process—making wrinkles disappear; preventing new ones; speeding up cell renewal; adding vitamins and elements like collagen or elastin that are lost by aging skin.

Most of us approach these claims with a degree of skepticism, but that doesn't prevent us from falling for particularly seductive ads. If reputable companies make these claims, and charge $50 for a jar of the stuff, and people are buying it—well, surely there's something behind it?

One of the pertinent questions here is whether or not the vitamin E or the collagen or the secret ingredient is actually able to penetrate the skin to a level that will have anything other than a superficial effect. It's true that vitamin E is a nutrient that's good for your skin, and it's also true that collagen and elastin are major components of the skin and that these deteriorate as you age. But the molecules of vitamin E, collagen, and elastin are quite simply too large to be absorbed by the cells of the skin. These substances may be effective in moisturizing the skin's surface, but rubbing them on is not going to replenish your skin's natural stores. Unfortunately, most of the ingredients in cosmetic preparations available right now don't go any deeper than the very outer layer of the skin—and that's not where the really important things are going on.

The good news is that whether any of these products help or not, there are many ways you can prevent premature aging of the skin and at the same time improve the condition of your whole body: by eating nourishing foods; by exercising to increase circulation, feeding skin cells with oxygen and nutrients and improving skin tone and texture; by quitting smoking, which constricts the capillaries and cuts off blood flow to the skin; by staying off drugs and reducing consumption of alcoholic beverages; by getting enough sleep; and by protecting your skin from the elements with sunscreens, moisturizers, and, if you like, even with Skin Defender. Although genes have a lot to do with how your skin ages, nothing mirrors what kind of attention you pay to your total health more clearly than your skin.

The Skin as a Functioning Organ

The skin is your body's largest organ and the first line of defense against many infectious agents. When either the outer dermal layer or the inner mucosa (the skin that lines the mouth and the vagina, for example) are broken, the risk of invasion becomes much greater, as with viruses (including the AIDS retrovirus) and staph and strep infections.

While certain chemicals such as insecticides can be absorbed through the skin, the skin is also an effective barrier against many of the chemicals and toxins we're exposed to. Within an ordinary range of temperatures, the skin also acts as a sensory detector and supplements the regulatory work of the body's nervous system. When we are too warm, sweat glands in the skin help cool the body, and blood vessels in the skin become dilated so that body heat can be thrown off at a faster rate. When we need to conserve body heat, the vessels in the skin constrict, saving heat for the body core and in the process giving us goose bumps.

Like the cells of a healthy liver, skin cells reproduce rapidly after an injury, forming new skin in the case of minor injuries or, in protective response to more severe damage, forming a scar. This rapid response to injury is not found in other organs such as the brain, where cells reproduce neither as well nor as rapidly, and damage is often permanent. Though the skin's critical functions—protecting against infection, interfacing with the environment, acting as a sensory and heat-mediating organ—remain intact, its remarkable healing and renewing processes do, unfortunately, slow down with age.

The Effects of Aging

The upper layer of your skin—the part you see—is the *epidermis*. Beneath that lies a thicker layer, the *dermis*, which is where the sebaceous (oil) glands are. The dermis is composed primarily of collagen and elastin— about 70 percent collagen. It is the outermost layer of the epidermis that forms the skin's surface. New epidermal cells are formed at the bottom layer of the epidermis, and are pushed toward the top as the cells of the uppermost layer are sloughed off. Thus the epidermis is in a constant state of renewal, with the very top layers (the stratum corneum) sloughed off and replaced every three weeks or so. It follows that the cells on the surface of your skin are older than those underneath. As you age, the rate of cell renewal in your skin gradually decreases, so that by the time you're 80 it may take four to six weeks to replace the outer layer of epidermal cells, whereas it took two weeks when you were 20. When a product promises to speed up cell renewal, the idea is to decrease this epidermal turnover time. Exfoliation is another method for showing a "younger" skin—either by mild physical abrasion (scrubbing off the old, dead cells on top) or by mildly irritating the skin with chemicals so that the skin responds by repairing the injury.

Properly done (that is, not overdone), exfoliation or other means of speeding up cell renewal in the epidermis may well give you a clearer color and more polished-looking skin, but the significant furrows and wrinkles that start to become features on our faces as we age are in the dermis, and no speedy epidermal renewal or exfoliation is going to get rid of those.

What does affect the dermis? Two things have a calculable impact: smoking and overexposure to the sun. For the moment we'll forgo discussing the other serious health issues involved and appeal to your vanity. Both habits—smoking and sunbathing—destroy collagen, the major component of the dermis. Some dermatologists believe that taking vitamin C can help combat these effects, but nothing will save your face from the premature aging caused by these habits except to quit them. Among the complicated changes that take place in the skin as a natural result of aging are a thinning of the dermis, with a decrease in the soluble collagen content and loss of elasticity, and a decreased circulation in the small blood vessels that feed that skin. Sun exposure dries out the skin and reduces elasticity. Smoking, with its impact on both collagen and circulation, is a double whammy.

Another visible effect of aging is a decrease in the production of sebum (oil), which gradually declines after adolescence and drops more precipitously after menopause, when estrogen production drops. This means that your skin will be less and less able to hold moisture. Those women who suffered from oily skin as adolescents may count themselves lucky at 35-plus, since dry skin may not have become a problem yet, but they should not assume that they're going to be an oily or even a "normal" skin type forever.

TAKING CARE OF 35-PLUS SKIN

There are two primary goals in caring for 35-plus skin: nourishment from within and protection from damage. It should be clear that two of the most important choices you can make in limiting damage to the skin are avoiding sun exposure and cigarette smoking. If you have no problem living without cigarettes and suntans, you're ahead of the game in keeping your skin youthful. But if you're a smoker still struggling to quit, you're not alone. Cigarettes are an addiction tough to give up, but according to the latest surgeon general's report, over half of all Americans who smoked when the first report came out twenty-five years ago have succeeded in permanently quitting. Chances are you can do it, too. And the good effect this will have on your skin will become apparent in a month, with improved color and improved skin tone—and continuing improvement over the months to come.

As for a tropical tan, it can make you look great, at least if you keep it up, but that's another addiction that can do a lot of damage. If you're caught in the cycle of keeping up a tan, sooner or later you will have to confront its serious effects.

Sun Damage Goes Deeper Than What You Can See

Not only does prolonged sunbathing "age" the skin with a decrease in elasticity and increase in dryness, but it also sets the stage for skin blemishes and, in some cases, even skin cancer. In trying to block the skin's surface from exposure to UV rays, the tanning cells also build up a layer that interferes with the release of oils and dirt from the pores—a condition that can encourage the appearance of "adult acne" and other surface blemishes that sunlovers seem to put up with.

Sun exposure also increases the risk of basal cell and squamous cell carcinoma and melanoma—the major skin cancers. If diagnosed reasonably early, the first two conditions are curable with local treatment. Melanoma, the final and most dangerous form of skin cancer, can be life threatening, and the prognosis for cure depends on how invasive it is at the time of diagnosis. At the extreme, cancer on a susceptible place like the nose can result in such extensive damage that the nose has to be partly rebuilt with plastic surgery.

Interestingly, new evidence suggests that not only is cumulative sun exposure a factor with melanoma, but the number and severity of sunburns is another, adding even more risk to the process of getting a tan. "Flash" sunburns—characteristic of northerners who go to Florida for a week, for example—appear to be linked to the subsequent development, many years later, of melanoma.

Does this mean you should stay out of the sun completely? Of course not. But it means you must take extra care when you're exposed to it, especially during the peak hours of 10 to 2, when the sun's rays are most direct. Short of keeping the skin covered, your best protection is to use a sunscreen.

Sunscreens and UV Light

Sunscreens were once an added plus in cosmetics for the skin; now they are touted as a main ingredient. While of some benefit, most cosmetics include minimal amounts that offer mild protection at best. Outside of a relatively sheltered situation, most dermatologists recommend routinely providing extra protection against the sun's ultraviolet rays. Noted dermatologist Dr. Albert Kligman once advised a roomful of people that every day of their lives they should use their deodorant, finish their morning grooming, and then put on their sunscreen.

Choosing an Effective Sunscreen

Skin type—more specifically, the quantity of melanin your skin produces —determines the degree of protectiveness, measured in number, that you need in a sunscreen. The darker your complexion, the more melanin you have. A fair-skinned show of freckles coupled with a tendency to burn puts you in the category of people with the least natural protection—about 15 percent of all Americans—who have the greatest need for a sunscreen.

Most available products now screen out both types of ultraviolet light, since both UVA and UVB rays have been implicated in skin damage. The degree of protection from UV rays is indicated on the label of any given product by its sun-protection factor (SPF), with the number ranging from 2 (the least protection), to 39 (the most). These numbers are determined by the U.S. Food and Drug Administration, and when a sampling involving one-third of the available products was put to the test by Consumers Union (as reported in the June 1988 *Consumer Reports*), the numbers were confirmed accurate in all cases—provided that a *full ounce* of the product, whether it be gel, mousse, cream, or lotion, was applied. If you use too little of an SPF-15 sunscreen, for example, the protection value may drop to that of an SPF-8.

Those products that claimed to be "waterproof" (effective through four 20-minute swims) and those described as "water-resistant" (effective through two 20-minute swims) passed muster in this area as well.

In their final analysis, *Consumer Reports* found that since the sunscreens they tested were about equally effective in the SPF range indicated, once you match up your skin type with the appropriate SPF, the choice really comes down to how much money you want to pay for the product. By using the required 1 ounce on a maximally exposed body (that is, when you're wearing only a swimsuit), you can run up a fat pharmacy bill using the more expensive brands.

Whatever your choice, if you have children, be sure to buy enough to protect them as well. This is an important consideration, since most youngsters are out in the sun three times longer than adults are. They can use the same products you use. Some babies develop skin irritations from the sunscreen ingredient PABA, so choose a product based on a different chemical if irritation becomes a factor.

Inner Lines of Defense

Good Nutrition

Some people think that by eating special foods, taking vitamins, or using special vitamin-enriched cosmetics they will improve their chances of revitalizing their skin. None of these things has been proved to offer any special advantages, but a balanced, nutritious diet—and vitamin supplements if indicated—can make a significant difference in the appearance and condition of your skin. High-fat diets will not, by the way, help replace oils that are lost in the skin, and it's important to stay away from them for other reasons.

A healthy skin requires full nutrition (see Chapter 21). Poor nutrition will leave you with sallow skin and less than healthy-looking hair. Patients with subclinical cases of malnutrition (not full-blown but marginal cases, which may show up in women on extreme low-calorie diets) may exhibit complex skin lesions—raw fissures on the skin. Hair will lack luster and be easily pluckable. Often in subclinical cases of vitamin A and B-complex deficiencies people exhibit rough, dry skin on various parts of the body. *Chelitis* is a swelling and chapping of the lips often accompanied by crusting and flaking. While physical causes or a recent fever can cause chelitis, it can also be brought about by a deficiency in riboflavin. A deficiency of vitamin C can lead to *perifollicular hemorrhages*, or small red dots on the skin. This is the first distinctive physical sign of scurvy.

But read the section on vitamins (pages 282–287) before you rush out and buy a supply of them; with vitamins, a little goes a long way. For a number of reasons, a well-balanced diet that includes plenty of vegetables, fruits, and protein, plus six glasses of water a day, is an absolute must for a good healthy skin.

Exercise

Regular aerobic exercise will do more for your skin than you may imagine. It helps the skin indirectly by maintaining muscle tone and directly by increasing the circulation of blood to the outermost branches of the cardiovascular line—the small arteries (capillaries) that supply the skin with oxygen and nutrients. This has a toning and tightening effect on the pores and improves sallow skin color. Consistent exercise over a period of time may actually help to stimulate blood-vessel growth and cell repair. For smokers, starting an aerobics program when they quit smoking will give the skin a double boost (and aerobic exercise, by the way, will usually reduce the craving for cigarettes).

Alcoholic Beverages

Drinking immoderately causes repeated dilation of the blood vessels, which accounts for an unhealthy, blotchy complexion but also, in chronic drinkers, the appearance of tiny broken vessels on the skin—"spider veins" (pages 55 and 97) that pop up on the face, especially on and around the nose and cheekbones, as well as on the chest and abdomen. While they can occur in people who don't drink, they are more common and more proliferative on people who are chronic drinkers.

Weight Fluctuations

Weight gain and rapid weight loss also affect the appearance of the skin; the stretch marks or striae that often result from rapid weight gain commonly appear after pregnancy as well. These are permanent, and no cosmetic or topical vitamin treatment will remove them. Rapid weight loss can also cause flab and skin folds that present a special challenge to get rid of; only long-term exercise can help return underlying muscle tone and a pleasing shape. Ideally, of course, weight loss should be gradual *and* be accompanied by exercise; the skin does have a natural elasticity and it can contract to fit your new shape, given time.

Cleansing and Moisturizing

Before getting into a discussion of moisturizers, there are some common-sense steps in combatting dry skin that are worth mentioning.

Avoid harsh soaps on the body and face. Wear rubber gloves when using detergents and cotton gloves when gardening; detergents and garden soil both can dry out your hands and nails. In general, bathe less, especially in winter in northern climates. Unless you're involved in strenuous daily activity that works up a sweat, there is no biological reason to shower or bathe daily, and it clearly dries the skin to do so. There are only three areas of the body that produce odor—the underarms, the anal-genital area, and the feet. Give yourself an old-fashioned sponge bath: wash these areas, and your hands and face every day; for the rest, bathing two or three times a week is sufficient. Be cautious with bath oils. Many of our patients have reported falls because they make the tub slippery; better to use them out of the tub.

Apply moisturizer immediately after washing or bathing. Putting moisturizers on after you are bone-dry defeats the main purpose of using these products, which is to keep existing moisture in. Include this treatment for dry, cracked, or brittle nails, which can develop with age, owing again to general dehydration. Many women are quick to assume that dry nails are the result of a vitamin or mineral deficiency, when often all they need is this simple moisturizing treatment. (However, if there has been no chronic problem with the nails, and dryness is suddenly noticeable, a test to rule out a low thyroid should be done.) In bitter weather, consider applying a thin layer of petroleum jelly on the extra-thin skin near the eyes. It does a good job of protecting this delicate area from wind or snow.

If this general plan doesn't help prevent chronic dryness or itchy skin that has no specific cause, the various cortisone creams or ointments can be used. Always start with a low potency such as hydrocortisone 1 percent and work up. Some of the higher potency cortisones can lead to skin thinning (atrophy) and must be used with great caution, especially on the face. If dry skin–eczema problems or dermatitis remain hard to treat, allergies, or contact dermatitis, may be the cause, and you should consult a dermatologist.

Choosing Moisturizers

Moisturizers for dry skin—and just about all of us have dry skin on some part of our bodies—do help keep the skin hydrated, locking in moisture and helping to keep the upper layers of cells plumped up and moist looking. How do you go about choosing one? Just as the contents of a can of soup are listed on the label, so are the ingredients in cosmetic preparations, in descending order according to how much of each substance is present. This is not to say that they're listed in descending order of importance; the first ingredient in most cosmetics is water. Most moisturizers are a mix of water, emollients, humectants, and emulsifiers—the latter making the mixture of oil and water possible. In addition to these, cosmetics manufacturers may add sunscreens, color, fragrance, and any number of other ingredients from proteins to vitamins to aloe and other plant extracts.

Emollients are occluding agents—oils and waxes. These form a barrier that helps trap moisture and keeps it from evaporating from your skin. Petroleum jelly is a pure emollient. In addition to petrolatum, other familiar emollients found in moisturizing creams are lanolin and mineral and vegetable oils. In previous generations, face creams tended to be water-in-oil suspensions—heavier preparations with more emollient than water. The labels on heavier creams usually show an oil or emollient as the first ingredient. The preponderance of moisturizers offered by the cosmetics industry today are oil-in-water suspensions, which are lighter and provide more of the "moisture" in the moisturizer, but which may form a more fragile barrier against evaporation. Creams for very dry skin and for "all night," as opposed to daytime, moisturizing tend to be heavier in emollients.

Humectants can usually help attract moisture to the skin. These include propylene glycol and other glycerine derivatives. Natural substances found in the skin, such as urea and lactic acids, act similarly in helping to bind moisture to the skin. Interestingly, if the surrounding atmosphere is extremely dry, an effective humectant like propylene glycol can actually work in reverse: if it can't draw moisture from the air, it will draw it from your skin.

Under most circumstances, however, humectants are very effective moisturizers that can make a difference in lighter preparations. Some occluding agents, especially in heavy amounts, tend to block pores and encourage comedones (blackheads), especially if they are also slightly allergenic. Lanolin and cocoa butter are among these. (Curiously, in lighter preparations, forms of petrolatum don't seem to be too bad in this regard.) If your skin is susceptible, or if you suddenly discover it's breaking out after you've tried a new cosmetic, you may be reacting to an ingredient in the cream. Stop using it and look for a moisturizer that is advertised as "non-comedogenic." Of course you should avoid products that contain ingredients you know you're allergic to. While a product advertised as "hypo-allergenic" may be a bit better in this regard than its ordinary counterpart (most are free of fragrances, which tend to be irritating), it's not going to be entirely free of possible allergens. The cost of the product is no guarantee, either; even very expensive cosmetics can cause skin eruptions if they aren't right for your skin type. If you pay a lot for a cream and it makes you break out, take it back to the store and tell them so. Most reputable department stores will give you a refund. If possible, ask for a sample to try at home before you invest in any new creams or cosmetics. Many lines, especially if they've got a new product, will make samples available. Better yet, think twice before purchasing expensive creams that make big scientific-sounding claims for rejuvenating your skin.

The truth is, the FDA makes a careful distinction between *cosmetics* and *drugs*. Anything that actually has a direct impact on a biological structure or process comes under much more stringent FDA regulations, requiring tests both for safety and effectiveness, than do cosmetics. Cosmetics may not contain ingredients that have been shown to be harmful (with the exception of coal-tar dyes), but they may very well contain ingredients that are not effective. The tip-off here is in the careful phrasing of advertising copy: a manufacturer may say that a product "helps" to do something or gives you a younger-*looking* skin without having to prove much; stronger claims come under FDA scrutiny and must be substantiated, although the FDA can be slow to move in this regard. Another tip-off in any over-the-counter preparation is the term "active ingredient" on the product label. These are ingredients that have been shown to be effective in doing what they're supposed to do. You'll see the active ingredient listed on fluoride toothpastes and dandruff shampoos. In cosmetic preparations, antibacterial substances and sunscreens may be listed as active ingredients.

Fountains of Youth in a Jar

We've talked about the skin's permeability in this chapter. It's clear that the skin is a fairly effective barrier to a lot of substances that would be toxic if ingested, and equally, a barrier to most substances thought to be beneficial. Nineteenth-century snake-oil cures—lotions and liniments which promised miraculous relief from all sorts of external and internal problems—have long since been properly recognized as frauds, and as we've seen, there's little evidence to support the idea that the scientific-sounding ingredients in today's cosmetics are going to do much to alter or rejuvenate the skin, or replenish what your skin has lost in the aging process.

But experience over the last couple of decades has made it apparent that the skin can absorb more than we may have thought. In some instances we simply stumbled over the evidence. Bitter experience with Agent Orange and certain insecticides has shown us that certain highly toxic substances can be absorbed all too readily by the skin. Other chemicals that provide some benefits to the skin itself were discovered to be toxic because they were getting past the skin barrier and into the body. Hexachlorophene, a popular additive in many good soaps and cleansers like Dial and pHisoHex up through the 1970s, was taken out of them and banished from other over-the-counter products when it was discovered that it could cause neurological damage in infants. The amount of hormones in skin creams was regulated by the FDA when it was discovered that sufficient exposure to creams containing estrogen or progesterone could create hormonal imbalances within the body.

There's a positive side to this picture, however. Researchers have developed topical applications of certain medications that release them into the body gradually and avoid some drawbacks of taking them orally or by injection. Skin patches for the slow release of estrogen in estrogen-replacement therapy and nitroglycerin patches for patients with heart disease are two of the more current ways to administer these medications through the skin. As for the skin itself, cortisone creams, minoxidil, and Retin-A are topical treatments that appear to do more than merely soothe or moisturize the skin or give a cosmetic effect.

The Rush for Retin-A

Retin-A is a prescription drug for acne, topically applied, that came on the market in the 1970s. Many dermatologists found it to be a significant advance over other topical treatments for acne, to the extent that in some cases patients could be taken off orally administered antibiotics. In the late 1980s, when users discovered that it seemed to decrease wrinkling as well, Retin-A became a hot item. Right now it is only approved as an acne medication, however, and not all dermatologists are equally sanguine about its antiwrinkle properties. It doesn't do much for deep furrows and wrinkles, and the results last only as long as you continue the medication. Vitamin-derived, it can be harsh on the skin, with some patients exhibiting irritation or intolerance. It must be used with a strong sunscreen, and as a prescription drug it can only be used under the supervision of your doctor. Nevertheless, some current research suggests that it *may* help to reverse the effects of sun damage (although it actually increases the skin's susceptibility to subsequent exposure). Advocates of Retin-A claim that it accelerates cell turnover, stimulates blood-vessel growth, and boosts production of collagen and elastin. These effects, insofar as they are borne out by research, are more than cosmetic. Even if Retin-A is not the kind of cure-all its proponents say it is, it and developments like it suggest that in time we may discover ways that will slow down the effects of natural aging on the skin.

Cosmetic Safety

We've given some basic information here on moisturizers, but a thorough evaluation of cosmetics and skin-care products isn't within the scope of this book. This topic has been commendably covered by other books, including Elaine Brumberg's excellent *Take Care of Your Skin* and Paula Begoun's bestselling *Blue Eyeshadow Should Be Illegal* and her updated *Blue Eyeshadow Still Should Be Illegal*. Look in your bookstore for these and other titles that can guide you toward wise choices in purchasing cosmetics and skin-care products.

We will, however, mention here a few additional things to be aware of in cosmetic safety:

CERTIFIED COAL-TAR COLORS. Identifiable with D&C or FD&C preceding the color name and number, these are permitted only in cosmetics not used around the eye. This includes the area up to the brow and the skin immediately below and on either side of the eye. Certain coal-tar colors can cause serious eye injury and even blindness. Don't use cosmetics like blushes around the eye that were not intended for use there. Remember that these cosmetics won't necessarily stay where you put them; your own skin oils, not to mention any moisturizers you may use, may cause colors to run, and swimming and showering may well bring these chemicals into direct contact with your eyes.

MASCARA. A couple of caveats about mascara. Be careful of waterproof brands that promise to wear all day and all night without ever smudging or running. All of these are going to require a special remover, since they simply won't come off by ordinary means, and you're going to lose some lashes if you try tugging the stuff off. If you have trouble with mascara smudging during the day, try a brand that is water soluble. Most "conditioning" and water-resistant mascaras are removed with oil. Here again, the oils on your skin may cause them to leave tracks on the skin directly above or below the eye. Being able to swim, weep, or stand bareheaded out in the rain without your mascara running is an advantage you won't need during the ordinary working day. You can select a water-soluble mascara by looking at the directions for removal; if the package says to remove it with soap and water, you're on the right track. Finally, if you wear contacts, don't use lash-lengthening mascaras that contain fibers. These can get lodged under a lens and irritate or, worse, scratch the cornea.

TANNING PILLS. These are not, in the strict sense of the word, cosmetics, but since patients ask about them a word here is in order. They are said to tan the skin without exposure to the sun, but of course they don't really tan your skin; they color it. Most of the so-called tanning pills contain canthaxanthin, a food color. Some also contain beta-carotene, a natural food color and precursor of vitamin A. High doses of either substance dye the blood and, consequently, the skin. The color of beta-carotene is more orange than tan, and may even be mistaken for jaundice. We know of no scientific studies evaluating either the safety or efficacy of tanning pills. *Think twice* before trying them.

SPECIAL MEDICAL CONCERNS INVOLVING MIDLIFE SKIN

Many noncancerous skin growths can accumulate in time and should be discussed with a dermatologist. These include:

SEBORRHEIC KERATOSES. These are oily, flaky brown or black growths that are often unsightly or a nuisance (as on a belt or bra line); they can be frozen with liquid nitrogen or burned off with electrodesiccation, or removed surgically.

ACTINIC KERATOSES. These are similar to seborrheic keratoses, but are usually flatter and reddened, not brown or black. They should be seen by a dermatologist and removed, since they are precancerous.

SPIDER VEINS (Telangiectases). These are broken superficial capillaries that can easily be removed in a dermatologist's office by electrodesiccation or by the new pulsed-laser treatments, the latter being less painful but more expensive.

CHERRY SPOTS (Angiomas). These tiny, raised red spots are benign overgrowths of capillaries, known to increase with age. While they can be safely ignored, if they become cosmetically bothersome, cherry spots can be treated the same way as seborrheic keratoses, with liquid nitrogen or electrodesiccation, keeping in mind the possibility of a small scar forming.

SKIN TAGS. These are little flaps of skin that can sprout out of no-where, especially after pregnancy. These, too, can safely be ignored, but if they cause a cosmetic problem, they can easily be removed by a dermatologist. (The linea nigra, or vertical line of darkened pigment on the abdomen that appears in many women during pregnancy, may appear to be permanent, but by some law of nature it miraculously sloughs off in the weeks after birth.)

MOLES (Nevi). These are usually only a nuisance, but because they can occasionally lead to melanoma, any change in size, color, or border should be evaluated promptly by a dermatologist.

WARTS. Caused by viruses, these are rare in 35-plus women. If they appear, they can be ignored—since in most cases, warts run a cycle of two to three years and will disappear on their own—or they can be treated effectively with liquid nitrogen.

CYSTS. The most common kind of cyst seen on the face or scalp is a sebaceous cyst—basically, those that form in the sebaceous glands in the deeper skin layer. They can range from pea to marble size and even occasionally to walnut size, as seen every so often on a woman's back, and are filled with a puslike substance, though quite unlike the substance in a boil. Cysts are benign—consequently the reason for removing them is purely cosmetic. This would normally be the province of a dermatologist or surgeon. If the cyst has been present for many years and is quite large, it will almost always leave a slight-to-significant depression in the skin after removal.

AGE SPOTS.   Changes in pigmentation due to sun exposure can occur in the middle years, resulting in "age spots," or "liver spots," the technical name, *senile letigines,* translating as "freckles of old age." Bleaching creams used for age spots will reduce coloration by 50 percent at most, and are more effective on light spots than dark ones. Changes are only temporary; once the skin is exposed to the sun, the melanin will darken again unless sunscreens are used or areas with spots are covered.

COSMETIC SURGERY

Skin health is not simply a "pure" medical issue (if anything is), but involves major social and psychological components. While the general population is increasingly an older one, society remains set in preserving the appearance of youth; it is no surprise that cosmetic issues loom large.

From face-lifts to trendy liposuction that removes fat, cosmetic surgery usually falls exclusively into the province of plastic surgeons; in most cases, barring specific medical contraindications, neither major medical nor dermatology issues come into play. Most cosmetic surgery provides relatively temporary improvement, since no procedure (except a "nose job") is going to change a person's looks forever. Some procedures—liposuction, for example—seem especially problematic if there isn't a strenuous commitment to the diet and exercise that help sustain the results of this surgery. But let's look at the various available procedures by degree of change involved. While not surgical, the first two treatments are included here because, when used as described, they are meant to achieve the same purpose: a more youthful appearance.

COLLAGEN INJECTIONS.   These are primarily used for deep furrows (frown lines) and pitted scars. Collagen is a proteinaceous solution in liquid form that is injected via syringe into the second, or dermal, layer of the skin. The goal is to "plump up the skin," lifting the floor of the defect—in this case, the crease or scar. Sometimes a series of injections are needed to get the desired effect, which, although not permanent, may last for several years.

DERMABRASION.   This is a technique that is very much described by the word; that is, it's a sanding procedure in which the dermatologist or, in some cases, plastic surgeon uses a rotary motor with what looks like a tiny rubber tire at the end to level or sand down the outer portions of the dermis that are sticking up around a scar, in the case of pitted acne. The difficulty lies in getting enough of the dermis down to bring it into sync with the lower portion, and thus to get a good cosmetic result without going too far, causing more scarring. Dermabrasion and chemical peels are also used to reduce surface wrinkles.

With dermabrasion, there is usually one treatment and a recovery period of several weeks; after that the procedure presumably can be repeated if necessary.

FACE-LIFTS. These are surgical procedures done usually by a cosmetic or plastic surgeon. The typical face-lift involves cutting a long line along the hairline; the skin is then trimmed—a small rim of tissue is actually cut away—and the remaining facial skin is pulled up and back, then sewn back together. If a face-lift is done properly, it should not cause any visible scar because the cut will have been made just outside or slightly behind the hairline. Recovery from associated swelling and bruising usually takes between two and four weeks.

Over the short term (usually two to five years), a good face-lift can be a remarkable temporary cosmetic improvement, if that is what is desired. The rest of the body, of course, is going to continue to age; and unlike a nose job, in which there is removal of cartilage and a resetting of bone and cartilage, in a face-lift the remaining skin eventually begins the natural sagging process again. It all depends on the individual as to when results will be noticeable.

LIPOSUCTION. This has replaced the body-tuck procedure (similar to a face-lift) of the past, though both are intended to give the same results. With liposuction, small incisions are made in fatty areas, and the fat is literally sucked out. The traditional areas for this procedure are the hips and abdomen, where fat tends to accumulate. When liposuction is done in women who are in their middle years, because of the skin's resiliency, it usually pulls back to give a good cosmetic look, although this can take a full year. It's purely cosmetic in objective, but many good dermatologists do not see liposuction as a quack procedure, although it is a costly one with potential for some hematoma (blood under the skin), infection, and unevenness.

The Normal Signs of Aging

This chapter has emphasized good skin care and prevention of premature aging; if your skin is in reasonably good condition now and you use this approach, there is no reason you can't keep it looking its fresh and healthy best. But even normal skin will in time show signs of age—some more than others. In time, more than any skin treatment or skin-care program, your attitude about yourself will influence how you look and feel. Like most 35-

plus women today, you will eventually find your own path in sorting out how to approach your changing appearance, putting the whole matter into a healthy perspective. The most sensible approach, of course, is to start with the gentlest treatment possible, and most often that involves nothing more than continuing to use a moisturizer daily. As time progresses, you may want to move on to consider other options—or you may not. The median age for cosmetic surgery is 55, and even then only a relatively small number of women go ahead with it, despite what the media might have you believe. Proceeding with cosmetic surgery is certainly not in the same league as deciding whether or not to color your hair. It involves a degree of pain, a high degree of discomfort, and lots of money—in some cases many thousands of dollars. Nor is cosmetic surgery usually covered by medical insurance, except in cases involving accidental injuries and birth defects. And although having a reputable and skilled cosmetic surgeon is crucial, even then there's no guarantee you'll be completely satisfied with the results.

Aside from these issues, far more factual information than what's provided in this book is required if you are seriously considering cosmetic surgery, including—most important—researching the reputation and ability of the cosmetic surgeon. Notwithstanding all these caveats, if you really feel your face looks far older than your years, or if you have scars or other skin traumas that you find hard to live with, don't be timid about investigating cosmetic surgery. If your professional work requires "on camera" appearances and high visibility, that's certainly a factor to consider. A good face-lift is subtle; it will not make you look like you're wearing a too-tight ponytail, and there are no social stigmas attached.

We know that when it comes to the skin's normal aging process, there is really no such thing as "normal." Each woman's skin is the product of many individual factors—her genetic heritage and skin type, environment, life-style, and childbearing experiences; her health habits, diet, and much more—each contributing to hasten or delay the visible signs of aging. We also know that many negative effects imposed on the body are cumulative. But by caring for your skin early on, you stand an excellent chance of looking young for a long time to come.

CHAPTER 6

Hair and Nails

COLOR, CONDITION, texture, and style—cosmetic care and continued good grooming are the focus when assessing your 35-plus hair and nails. Let's begin with hair, particularly hair color, since this is a major concern for most women at midlife.

Hair Color

Most women will remember the time they discovered their first gray hair—probably with a mixture of dismay and fascination. But just as a touch or more of gray in a man's hair is often thought to look distinguished, so can it look distinctive and flattering on a woman. The cult of youth no longer dominates our culture the way it did twenty years ago, and we certainly are more enlightened about the role of appearance in the grand scheme of living. Despite all this, for some of us gray hair remains a symbol of fading youth, a harbinger of old age, and the first ones often get yanked out.

Thoughts about mortality may be prompted by their arrival, but gray hairs are no more dead than the hair you were born with. All hair is composed of dead skin cells that are filled with keratin, a fibrous, tough protein material which is also the main constituent of the nails. The color or pigment of the hair is determined by the amount of melanin each strand contains. Gray is just a new phase in the life (perhaps better termed, *existence*) of each hair strand that occurs when the melanin pigment is depleted. The average woman has about 125,000 strands of hair on her head at various stages of growth, defoliation, and in the middle years of her life, gradually turning gray. *When* this happens, it has nothing to do with diet, the level of stress you encounter, or whatever else you may have heard; like baldness in men, it is determined simply by your genes.

Just as the appearance of skin wrinkles is unavoidable, eventually nearly everyone's hair is going to turn gray or white; it's merely a matter of time. If you find this inevitability mildly alarming, there are ways to cope with it, and you may even find some humor in the process as well.

"Does she or doesn't she?" is no longer a heavily cloaked secret, at least among friends. Comparing notes with other women, finding out how *they* are coping, can put this particular rite of passage into perspective. One 35-plus woman tells the story of how she and a friend decided to color their hair at home together, feeling like a couple of teenagers working on their hairdos. One of them had a toddler, so they waited until nap time and then quickly got to work. Of course right in the middle of pouring the stuff on and wrapping their heads with plastic, the toddler woke up crying—only to become inconsolable when he couldn't positively identify his mother or understand why the stranger hovering behind her was laughing so uncontrollably.

You've got many choices in deciding what you want to do about the gray. If you confidently hold to the philosophy of "going with it" when the first round of gray appears, great! Many women look and feel marvelous when their hair is all gray or snow-white; and, as the median age of the population increases, the range of tested hair products aimed at toning down yellow and keeping gray hair lustrous and shiny increases as well. If this is the way you want to go, just keep in mind how your hair color affects your hairstyle and the colors in your wardrobe—and change them, if need be.

If you find your determination wavering when a lot more gray appears, that's fine, too! This can happen when you realize your favorite wardrobe colors no longer suit you, or it suddenly seems as if most of your colleagues at work are twenty years younger, or you simply feel you are ready for a change.

More than 33 million American women dye their hair, three-quarters of them using permanent coloring agents. In the past, hair dyes and colorants contained potentially dangerous chemicals, but after eighteen years of tests focusing on hair-dye safety, these have been eliminated and the chemicals and dyes used now are considered safe and appear on the GRAS (Generally Regarded as Safe) list.

If you decide to experiment with coloring the gray, you'll probably want something close to your original shade or a bit lighter. (Too dark a shade can be harsh and unflattering and it will look dyed.) The more permanent the coloring agent, the better off you will be in the hands of a professional colorist, but some conservative experimenting at home with temporary coloring can be fun and relatively inexpensive. Be sure to follow the package instructions to the letter, especially when they ask you to do some testing first, to make sure you have no allergic reactions to the product. If your hair is fine, dry, or fragile, permanent colorings will affect the texture, occasionally making fine hair feel thicker but generally not doing much good for dry and fragile hair. In this regard, the closer the coloring is to your own shade, the safer you will be. It's generally the colorants with peroxide that are damaging. Colorants without it tend to be gentler. Henna is probably the gentlest colorant, and it comes in many subtle shades now, not just red.

Recognizing the ever-growing market for their hair-coloring products, cosmetic companies compete each season to introduce new and improved shades, treatments, and coloring techniques to the consumer. Be creative, but also be cautious about taking any big plunges. Upkeep can be expensive, and you need to decide how much time and money you're willing to spend on it. Sometimes the nicest route is highlighting, a technique best entrusted to a professional, that lifts the color a little and blends in the gray. Because this process doesn't change overall color, new hair growth is less conspicuous and you can go a bit longer between touch-ups. Another option is to use a shampoo-in hair-coloring product that gradually rinses out after a number of shampoos. There is also permanent color, but if you choose this option, maintaining the color must be part of the deal; there's nothing more unattractive than a distinct inch of gray growing in at the scalp.

If you have your hair cut and restyled at the same time as you color it, chances are you will gain the satisfaction of a whole new "look" that greatly improves your appearance and your self-image, and the new cut and style may be enough of a distraction that no one will particularly notice you've (subtly) changed the color. We do not, by the way, recommend hair treatments applied over a period of time to "gradually tone away the gray." These products affect overall color—not just the gray—and the result is usually sooty looking and unattractive.

General Hair Health and Condition

Regardless of age or the prevalence of gray, the growth and nourishment of your head of hair is controlled by hormone secretions and the general state of your health; when you are healthy, no vitamins or minerals are going to affect its thickness or texture. You can, however, damage and dry out your hair with permanents; colorants containing peroxide; blow-drying or curling irons; not to mention exposure to sun, saltwater, or chlorinated water in pools. Experiment with moisturizing and conditioning treatments for the hair, and otherwise protect it from abuse.

In many instances, benefits in texture and hair appearance can certainly be achieved from nothing more than simple grooming. Gently brushing from the roots with a natural-bristle brush distributes oils from the scalp along the length of the hair strand. Making this a daily ritual can improve hair appearance and texture, particularly if it seems increasingly dull and dry. This can occur in the years around menopause when hormone levels are shifting, although some women never experience any noticeable change. The proverbial hundred strokes a day, however, is too much of a good thing. Do use a brush with smooth bristles, rounded at the tips, and give your hair 20 to 25 firm-but-gentle strokes in the morning and again at night.

Styling and Texture

However curly or straight your hair in its natural color has been, the texture surely changes when it starts to come in gray. It seems to have a life of its own—springy and curly and determined to behave as it pleases. If you keep going with the gray, this is manageable if you work with, and not against it, styling in loose, easy lengths rather than pulling it straight back, which tends to give the shorter, incoming gray hairs an antennalike appearance as they pop free from the rest. When color is added to gray hair, even with something as mild as henna, the texture will improve for some women, but not always for others.

Hair conditioners—primarily to reduce tangles and promote shine— have been on the market for years. The newest entry that aims at improving manageability is hair mousse (French, for "foam"—a styling and conditioning product made from synthetic resins that coat the hair shaft in order to make it more manageable without becoming sticky. Some mousse products also contain other ingredients geared to add moisture or prevent static; some are free of alcohol, and since alcohol is associated with dryness, supposedly this is a plus. The October 1988 issue of *Consumer Reports* included a beautician's evaluation of 39 brands of hair mousse used by 24 women (a total of over a thousand comparisons). Consumer's Union reported that all of these products do in fact improve hair manageability, and that differences among them were not dramatic. In the survey, mousses were said to "work wonders" on short, limp hair; highest ratings for improving body were given to Estée Lauder Swiss Styling Mousse, Brylcreem Men's Grooming Mousse (Extra Control), and Styling Mousse de Pantene Extra-Firm. A rundown of other new styling and conditioning products accompanied the article. Gels ranked high in popularity among teenagers and were described as the most versatile product, able to achieve either a plastered-down look or an airy, expansive one; hair texture that is slightly wavy and full bodied gets the best results, while gels tend to decrease body in fine hair and pack down thick, coarse hair. Styling lotions and "glazes" were pegged as a top choice among many young professional women who want a perfect, well-behaved look, adding body to thin hair, helping to "fight frizz," as well as creating a "wet look." Sprays—now containing none of the ozone-destroying propellants that were banned in the 1970s—are back in vogue, with a new array of products to be used in tandem with the styling products mentioned, supposedly to hold the hairstyle until the next shampoo.

Hair Loss

Overall hair loss, or alopecia, is a condition that is also determined by genes, and no dermatologist or product can arrest it. This is not the "cold-turkey" hair loss in one spot that many middle-aged men are plagued with, but rather, a diffuse, all over thinning of the hair that may have been occurring over time but that isn't noticed until the middle years. (Note: Just because you are in the 35-plus bracket, do not assume this will happen!)

In the never-ending quest to arrest baldness in men, the newest treatment involves topical applications of the drug minoxidil, which, as a side effect to treating hypertension, was discovered to promote new hair growth. The topical preparation of minoxidil used for baldness is marketed by Upjohn as Rogaine.

Rogaine often does produce new hair growth in younger men with certain male-pattern baldness—in this case, bald spots that appear on the crown of the head. It doesn't seem to do much for men who have been balding for years or whose baldness is advanced. It usually takes several months to get results, and these last only as long as the preparation—which is expensive—is used. Since it seems to be effective primarily for male-pattern baldness, there's little reason to think it would help women with a diffuse thinning condition.

As with nail problems, it is reasonable to rule out a low-thyroid problem if you become aware of hair loss, but good nutrition and gentle hair care are about the only palliatives available. Excessive hair treatments—certain permanents and straightening procedures—can cause hair to fall out, but in these cases it will grow back, as will the hair that falls out in the weeks after a pregnancy. Many women are concerned with post-partum hair loss when they see more hair than usual collected in their hairbrush, but the situation is perfectly normal. The hormones of pregnancy cause the gradual defoliation process to cease altogether; in other words, hair simply stays put for the nine months of pregnancy, and then it begins to fall out again after the baby is born. The rate of hair loss is no different from what it was before the pregnancy, but the length of the accumulating hairs probably is, and when you see them in your brush, the loss appears to be more.

From a purely cosmetic standpoint, to give a fuller look to the hair, there are hairpieces that can be woven discreetly into the hair and actually stay in place through one or two shampoos. You run the risk of losing more of your own hair, however, unless these are used correctly. Periodically (not permanently) wearing a wig is an alternative, provided it is made from good-quality, porous materials that allow the scalp to breathe.

Hair plugs, or transplants—whereby small disks of scalp and hair (including the hair follicles) are cut out from one location on the scalp and moved to another—are an act of desperation. This costly technique involves many painful procedures in the hands of a skilled physician, often with dubious results; infection and other complications are a real risk. It's far better to use the money that would be spent on this approach on regular visits to a professional hair salon instead, where expert styling can safely minimize the look of thinning hair, usually to your satisfaction.

Facial Hair

In contrast to hair loss, some women note an increase in hair around the chin, upper lip, and sometimes sprouting from the earlobe—a phenomenon referred to as hirsutism. Adrenal problems may be a cause: If suddenly hairs seem to start sprouting out of nowhere, see an internist or dematologist to see if you have this or another hormonal imbalance. There may not be an endocrine problem at all but consultation with a professional will determine what route to take and whether hormonal tests should be done.

If increased facial hair is gradual, it may simply be a genetic trait passed along from one's mother or grandmother, so that a woman who has a bit of down on her face when she is young may see it increase as she ages. A sharp eye and grooming with a tweezer may be all that's needed: if the problem increases or becomes a nuisance, then waxing, depilatories (but not on the face), or permanent removal with electrolysis may be a viable, albeit expensive, alternative.

There is, however, a new home-electrolysis implement on the market that may be worth investigating. It plugs into an ordinary outlet and uses radiofrequency waves. It uses a sort of tweezers rather than a needle, so it should be easier to use than the old-style home devices. Made by the Selvac corporation, it sells for about $100, which is significantly less than you'd pay for a series of electrolysis treatments at a salon. Whether or not it's effective remains to be seen.

Hair that grows from a mole is in a different category altogether and should never be tweezed or treated without medical consultation, since complications, specifically bleeding, can result. See a dermatologist for safe removal of both the mole and the hair.

FINGERNAILS, TOENAILS, AND FEET

Like your hair, your fingernails and toenails are composed of keratin. Both hair and nails seem to grow faster in warm climates, but new nail growth—pushing upward from the softer living matrix of the nail below the cuticle

—occurs at a much slower rate than hair growth, with a half-inch of new nail growth for every three inches of hair.

Topical applications may help the cosmetic aspect of your nails, and creams may keep them from drying, but as with your hair, your genes, overall health status, and total nutrition ultimately determine their health and appearance.

Healthy nails are clear, pink, and lustrous. Take note if they appear otherwise, since variations can be a clue to minor disorders as well as more serious ones. A bluish cast usually indicates a change in the rate of circulation or respiration; most likely it can be countered with nothing more than getting up and moving around if you've been sitting in one place or holding the same position for too long. But if a bluish cast persists, it may indicate more serious disorders that should be brought to your doctor's attention. Arthritis in the finger joints can affect the nails, causing them to split or become deformed, but sometimes faulty diet can account for these, too. If you injure a nail and it comes off, it may not always grow back exactly the same as before, but here again good nutrition helps encourage healthy new growth. If you have the kind of nails that chip or break easily, protect them by wearing rubber gloves whenever your hands are exposed to detergents or chemicals.

Much as the advertisers would like to persuade you otherwise, you will not strengthen or improve your nails by drinking gelatin. Gelatin comes from animal collagen; it is not what we call a "complete protein" that can support life but must be added to other proteins to make it complete. Gelatin is perfectly useful in salads and desserts, and some people also drink it before a meal because it is low in calories and the satisfying texture makes them feel they will eat less, but don't depend on it to strengthen your nails.

Grooming Your Fingernails

For most women, form usually follows function when it comes to fingernail shape and appearance: short nails for an active, indoor-outdoor life-style in which hands are used to garden, push swings, care for pets, cook, clean, and so on: long nails for women whose hands are not subjected to rough work and whose nail length won't interfere with manual dexterity. Overuse of polishes and removers dries out nails; moisturizers help keep unpolished nails glossy. Hangnails should be removed carefully and promptly with a cuticle clipper or small scissors.

If the special attention involved in more elaborate nail care provides a calm break from stress, this is good enough reason to indulge in it, and a professional manicure every couple of weeks is a relatively inexpensive luxury.

Toenail and Foot Care

Toenails should be treated with the same basic grooming care and hygiene as for fingernails, but always kept short and clipped straight across. Do use an emery board on your toenails after trimming; they'll look better and it will help prevent runs in your pantyhose.

Grooming is a simple routine for most 35-plus women, but in some cases—particularly if you are diabetic or have very poor vision—toenail clipping either by a podiatrist or in a salon that specializes in pedicures can be a great help in avoiding unnecessary infections and related problems that result from imprecise grooming.

Fashion may cast a benign influence over the health of the fingernails, but toenails can be adversely affected when tight, pointed-toe, or high-heeled shoes are worn. In time these can encourage ingrown toenails and subsequent infection, as well as corns and calluses. (See Chapters 12 and 24 for information on other foot problems and injuries.)

A callus is a local area of thickened outer skin (epidermis) caused by chronic irritation and wear. A corn is a thickened, enlarged and tender buildup of a callus. If a corn is painful, you can usually get relief by trimming it or by treating it with medicated plasters. Corns should be protected from pressure with plasters that provide padding *around* the area. Both the medicated and unmedicated pads are readily available at most drugstores. Some persistent corns, especially on the bottom of the foot, can be caused by bone abnormalities or spurs within the foot. In these cases especially, treatments prescribed by a podiatrist are the best route for long-term improvement and prevention. (Once again, if you are diabetic you must pay special attention to possible callus or corn formation and schedule regular podiatric care for their treatment.) Since most corns and calluses are caused by pressure and irritation from your footwear, however, wearing comfortable, well-fitting shoes is the first order of business in taking care of your feet.

One 35-plus change you may have noticed with dismay is that your toenails have gradually thickened and become slightly yellowish in color. This is probably normal. The only way to improve their appearance—besides keeping them scrubbed and the cuticles pushed back—is to polish them. Use a nail brush regularly. A leisurely, soaking bath is a good opportunity to give your toenails a scrub and it will soften the cuticles so that it is easy to push them back. Follow with a moisturizer rubbed into the nails and cuticles as you would with your fingernails.

If a thickening or yellow cast to your toenails is new, it could represent a fungal infection. If this is the case, there may be nothing much you can do about it until the affected area of the nail grows out since toenail fungal infections commonly do not respond at all to topical applications and respond fairly poorly even to long-term antifungal pills. Some patients can be cured of fungal toenails by prolonged (more than six months) daily antifungal medication, but the outcome is uncertain. Still, it would be wise to get a firm diagnosis of the condition by a dermatologist or podiatrist before chalking up the situation to the normal process of aging. Such a visit is particularly advised if the nail becomes too big or "heaps up," a common condition with fungal nails that is termed onychomycosis and that benefits from trimming—but *only* by a podiatrist.

CHAPTER 7

Teeth and Gums

IF YOU GREW UP HOLDING your breath in the dentist's office while he looked into your mouth to count up new cavities, you will be relieved to know that, over a lifetime, the incidence of tooth decay definitely declines —even when decay owing to soft enamel "runs in the family." If you are a parent, you've probably discovered that your children have fewer problems than you did as a child. Thanks to fluoride treatments and fluoridation, the era of rampant tooth decay in young children, except among the very poor, is pretty much over.

Of course genes have something to do with how susceptible you are to cavities at any age, but in general, the focus in dental care during the middle years shifts from tooth decay to extending the good health of the periodontal tissue, or gum area surrounding each tooth.

PERIODONTAL DISEASE

Periodontal disease is the primary cause of tooth loss in American adults over age 35. More than 90 million people suffer from periodontal diseases, ranging in degree from mild gum irritations to loosening of the teeth and tooth loss.

If, up until now, you have focused most of your attention on your teeth, a basic understanding of periodontal disease is in order, particularly as a preface to the program of dental health and hygiene that follows.

Whatever its origins, the phrase "long in the tooth" rather neatly describes the visible effect of periodontal disease. Bacteria build up in the invisible, sticky substance known as plaque, which coats the teeth, causing irritation at the gum line and, without routine removal with a toothbrush and dental floss, in time causing the gums to recede and the normally hidden roots to become exposed.

Without attention, problems only progress. The exposed roots have no protective enamel and are thus especially prone to further bacterial destruction and decay. As the gums recede, the chance of bacterial invasion below the gum line increases, leading to the eventual deterioration of soft tissue and, ultimately, to the destruction of the jawbone itself.

Treatment of Peridontal Disease

Rapid advances in dentistry are currently underway that offer new hope for advanced periodontal disease. Certain synthetic materials that resemble the mineral crystals in our bones—two of them, hydroxyapatite and beta-tricalcium phosphate, long endorsed by the American Dental Association as materials for anchoring dentures—are now being used experimentally for repairing jawbone defects, and are even being used in bone grafts.

As dentists and their patients wait to assess whether these synthetic substances can successfully adhere to soft tissue and natural bone over the long term, the synthetic HTR (hard tissue replacement) is competing for a place in jawbone reconstruction in periodontal disease, and is rapidly gaining favor. Patented by Dr. Paul Bruins, a polymer chemist, and Dr. Arthur Ashman, a New York City dentist and associate clinical professor in the biomaterials department at the N.Y.U. College of Dentistry, HTR is promoted to be an excellent material for repairing bones throughout the body, and in the jaw may even encourage formation of new natural bone. This has yet to be proved, but when it was used on 50 patients with periodontal disease, new natural bone appeared to form, rather than just fill in. A survey of 64 dentists who used HTR to treat periodontal disease in 647 patients reported, albeit subjectively, that it proved successful in 90 percent of the cases.

In addition, periodontal disease is the focus of research underway in the fields of molecular biology and genetics, specifically to try to determine what substances and developments in the body account for the regeneration of the alveolar bone that anchors the tooth and periodontal ligament that holds the tooth to the bone.

The new restoration techniques and research hold hope for those in danger of losing teeth from advanced periodontal disease, but clearly it's better to prevent such damage in the first place.

Preventing Periodontal Disease

Healthy teeth and gums are the reward of cumulative years of good dental care and oral hygiene. Although dentures are better and more natural now than in the past, they are no substitute for the real thing. Avoiding your dentist's office, even as you faithfully take your children there, may postpone pain, but if you eventually lose your teeth because of it, the result could have a tremendous impact on the shape of your face, making you look far older than your years, as well as on what you can eat (Poli-Grip ads notwithstanding).

Conversely, if you have supplied your body with the basic daily nutrients and have gotten into the habit of careful brushing and daily flossing to remove plaque, and visiting your dentist every six months, you have every chance of making it to a ripe old age with all your teeth accounted for, and no limit on what you can chew.

NUTRITION AND TEETH

While the merits of brushing, flossing, and regular checkups are self-evident, many people are unaware of the unseen role of nutrition in dental health. It is a vital one. Like nails or hair, teeth appear to be relatively inanimate parts of our body, but in fact the tooth pulp is composed of living cells. Seen in cross section by way of X-ray, tooth roots are anchored deeply in the jawbone, tapping into the same arteries and veins that transport nutrients to all parts of the body and capillaries that carry those nutrients right up into the center of each tooth. Good nutrition, then, can extend the health of the teeth and gums at any age.

Gums and teeth are affected by food even before a person is born. Of course a baby has nothing to do with it at this stage of life, but his or her mother surely does. Her genes, but also her diet, ultimately determine the good health of her unborn baby. Cells that will become teeth and gum tissue, as well as the glands that produce saliva, are formed before birth. These elements have just as critical a need for nutrients as the rest of the developing fetus. While we now know much more about these vital, prenatal connections than we did in the past, unfortunately much of what we know is from negative evidence. We know, for example, that a mother who takes the antibiotic tetracycline during pregnancy risks problems years later when her child's permanent teeth come in badly discolored. Certainly we can theorize that when teeth are not as strong, straight, or big as they should be, it might well be the result of poor diet during gestation.

But even if you inherited soft, cavity-prone enamel or came into the world with less than the ideal formation of tooth or jaw, it does not automatically follow that you are destined to experience lifetime problems. There are other factors that significantly influence the good health of your mouth.

We know, for instance, that calcium and fluoride are important in maintaining strong enamel. Phosphorus is another important nutrient, since an adequate calcium-to-phosphorus ratio helps form the jaw and mineralize the teeth. These nutrients also help the gum tissue resist disease and maintain the flow of saliva.

Vitamin C is also extremely important in the healthy development of gum tissue; in fact, bleeding gums are one of the earliest signs of scurvy or vitamin C deficiency. If your gums bleed despite good dental care and hygiene, you may not be getting enough vitamin C. Other necessary nutrients include protein for healthy tissue growth, vitamin A for epithelial cells, and folate for healthy blood.

The incidence of cavities may decline in the middle years, but the risk is still present. The sweets and candies of youth are no less forbidden now than before, and the chance of gum disease definitely increases. Good nutrition, keeping teeth clean, and getting problems taken care of *early* by your dentist are still the primary means of maintaining healthy teeth and gums. The basic strategies haven't changed much over the years; at midlife, they include:

1. *Keeping the teeth clean.* While there is no adequate replacement for daily use of a toothbrush and dental floss (preferably after each meal), we recommend your diet include the so-called detergent foods: crunchy raw vegetables or hard fruits like apples that have a naturally abrasive texture which helps clean the teeth. Beware of chewing gum that is advertised as "cleaning" the teeth or purported to be "no-stick," especially if you have a mouthful of crowns and fillings. Even this type of gum can pull them out.

2. *Paying special attention to plaque.* Periodontal disease begins when the gums come in contact with an irritant. In nonsmokers, the most common of these is plaque, a bacteria-laden substance that interacts with food particles to form destructive acids and yet more bacteria. Without frequent and thorough cleaning, plaque builds up in the cracks and crevices where teeth and gums meet—the perfect media for decay around and below the gum line. The longer it remains, the more chance there is for plaque to harden and form mineral deposits, or calculus (from the Latin for "stone"), on the tooth surface, continuing to act with the bacteria to inflame the gums. This inflammation, or gingivitis, can irritate periodontal membranes under the surface, causing periodontitis, which in turn can injure the alveolar bone in which the teeth are anchored.

Periodontal disease can be almost entirely avoided by removing plaque with routine daily flossing, brushing, and periodic appointments (ideally, once every six months but depending on your dentist's recommendations) for a routine scaling procedure done with professional equipment by your dentist or hygienist.

According to the American Academy of Dentistry, some mouthwashes may kill mouth bacteria but only temporarily; the natural environment of the mouth soon takes over again. Plax, a rinse made to help loosen plaque before brushing, can help if you follow directions on the bottle.

But—and we emphasize—nothing replaces brushing and flossing. Brushing methods should be aimed at cleaning the teeth well without doing harm to the teeth or gums; your dentist or dental hygienist can advise you on technique. Most recommend a soft toothbrush, but any toothbrush should be replaced when it shows signs of wear. Dental floss is the most effective way of removing bacterial plaque from the hard-to-reach surfaces between the teeth. Although water irrigation devices (such as Water Pik) can supplement cleaning techniques in these areas by dislodging food particles, they will not remove plaque.

Regardless of the toothbrush you use and the meticulous attention you pay to your own dental hygiene, you will not be able to completely remove all bacterial plaque, particularly at the gum line, which is why those twice-a-year trips to your dentist for a professional cleaning are so important.

3. *Maintaining ample saliva production.* Teeth that are not rinsed by saliva develop plaque and cavities very quickly. Make it a habit to become aware of the amount of saliva in your mouth and whether it feels dry, particularly after eating. Plain water, sipped frequently, may help the saliva glands make more saliva, while at the same time rinsing the mouth. Protein foods can help stimulate saliva production and keep the pH of the saliva near or above neutral. Fat, which has a neutral pH, is another food that may affect the pH of saliva, although its full role is not yet clear.

While saliva production normally drops during sleep, it can also decrease in the presence of certain drugs, such as the anti–high blood pressure medicine catapres (Clonidine), as well as the anti-depresssants amitriptyline (Elavil), doxepin (Sinequan), and others; certain medical treatments, such as head or neck radiation treatments when the mandible salivary glands under the lower jaw are included; or even with certain illnesses, such as arthritis, when dryness or sicca syndromes can occur. In this case extra water, sugarless gum, or sugarless mints can help.

4. *Controlling your intake of certain acidic and bacteria-promoting foods.* Everybody knows sugar causes cavities, but there's more to preventing cavities than simply avoiding sugar: the presence of acid in the mouth is something most people are unaware of. Two agents are needed to make acid: bacteria and the food substances that can be broken down or fermented into acid. The most highly fermentable foods are the carbohydrates, especially simple sugar or sticky carbohydrate foods which, in the process of being chewed, are broken down by enzymes in the saliva. Bacteria in the mouth use these carbohydrates to make more acid, causing the pH in the saliva—normally a little above neutral, or around 7 to 8—to drop quickly to around 5 or 5.5. In other words, when the bacteria in your mouth increase, so does acidity—and the risk of decay.

5. *Minimizing snacking.* . . . or at least monitoring it closely. Bacteria begin producing acid within twenty seconds of their first contact with food. This production of acid lasts for 20 to 30 minutes after initial contact, during which time the tooth is subject to acid eating away at its protective surface. If the same food is eaten again in a short time, the whole process begins anew. Thus constant snacking puts your teeth at a much higher risk of decay than if the sweets were spaced several hours apart or, better yet, taken with meals. If you can't brush after each meal, at least rinse out your mouth with water.

Snack foods high on the list of those that can cause cavities include cookies, pies, cakes, and sweet rolls, all of which are high in sugar (sometimes as much as 3 tablespoons per serving of cake, for example) and adhere to the surface of the teeth. Also avoid the following foods:

- *Those that obviously stick to the teeth*, including candy apples, cotton candy, caramel popcorn, dried fruit (including raisins), honey, "natural" fruit rolls, toffee, caramels and similar candy, and peanut butters with sugar.
- *Those that are sucked, sipped, or chewed over an extended time period* (that is, for more than a minute or two), including chewy candy, gum, hard candy, regular soda pop, and other sugared drinks.
- *Highly acidic foods*, including chewable vitamin C tablets and "sour" type hard candies containing citric acid.

Good alternative snack foods include fresh fruit, raw vegetables, protein foods, low-fat cheeses, lean meats such as thin-sliced turkey, plain yogurt, nuts, sugarless gum and mints, whole-grain crackers or bread, and natural peanut butter.

6. *Using fluoride.* Fluoride has done more to prevent tooth decay in the general population than any other advance in dental health. It is found in toothpaste, mouthwash, and most water supplies, where it either occurs naturally or is added. Epidemiological studies done in the towns and cities where fluoridation occurs naturally have documented that inhabitants have a lower risk of cavity production than comparable populations elsewhere, thus putting the squash on earlier notions that fluoridation was probably a conspiracy and would lead, among other things, to mushy brains. As it turned out, the areas with natural fluoridation had no differences in terms of IQ level or behavioral problems from any other part of the country. As a result, adding fluoride to the water in other areas of the country became the norm, usually at an effective rate of one part per million, or 0.5 milli-

gram per quart. Since the RDA of fluoride is 1.5 to 2.5 milligrams, there is no danger of fluoride toxicity, even if you consume several quarts of water every day.

Shorter-term studies involving smaller groups of people have shown that fluoride, either in toothpaste or in direct application, also decreases the risk of decay. In addition to fluoride, adequate levels of calcium and phosphorus in the diet (see also page 155 regarding osteoporosis) will benefit the teeth and jaw.

7. *Attending to gum disorders promptly.* Sore spots, extrasensitivity, particularly along the gum line, visibly receding gums—in short, any abnormal condition of the gums warrants immediate attention. As with the teeth, problems with the gums only increase when they are ignored.

8. *Quitting smoking.* The chemicals and poisons in cigarettes are gum irritants that encourage gingivitis and subsequent periodontal disease.

9. *Keeping up with state-of-the-art dental techniques.* Although orthodontia is preferable as early in life as possible, it is not too late in the middle years to have your teeth straightened. This may significantly increase your chances of saving teeth when they are misaligned, and the newer "invisible" braces are barely detectable.

New bonding materials and techniques, which allow the surface of a tooth to be evened out, whitened, or made stronger, can not only dramatically improve appearance but also significantly extend the life of a tooth that otherwise would be pulled. Restorative periodontal work, highlighted at the beginning of this chapter, allows many women who would have lost their teeth in the past to keep all of them well into their seventies. Discuss these techniques with your dentist.

Sometimes, despite all efforts to avoid it, pulling a tooth becomes inevitable. You must be confident in your dentist's judgment in this regard, even if it involves getting a second opinion. Do not hesitate to get one. If a tooth simply must come out, unless it's a wisdom tooth, it should be replaced so that proper spacing and tooth function can be retained. In the hands of a good dentist, replacement techniques today are so refined that a good porcelain tooth is virtually impossible to distinguish from a real one.

10. *Periodically assessing your professional care.* Last but not least, midlife is the time to reevaluate your dental care. If you feel the procedures are particularly painful, or that some aspect of your dentist's treatment of your mouth could be improved, by all means discuss it openly with him or her. Feel free to ask questions, if you have them, about procedures that concern you. Fillings, caps, and tooth replacements should be comfortable and stay in place; if they don't, go back to your dentist until she or he gets it right, or get a new dentist. You should be as willing to insist on good value for these services as you are for any other service you pay for. If you have

"grown up" with your dentist and feel that perhaps he's behind the times with current techniques and procedures that you may benefit from, get an outside opinion. Ask your dentist if he or she has a philosophy about long-term preservation of teeth, and again be prepared to change dentists if you are not satisfied with the response.

One woman described how she never thought to do this until suddenly, when she turned 65 and got her first hint of periodontal problems, her dentist announced matter-of-factly that, per the normal procedure in his office, it was time to schedule another appointment—to begin pulling out all her teeth!

The woman jumped out of the chair and fled. While another dentist was able to save those teeth the first dentist had neglected (she never questioning his treatment and he glad to save her a lot of bother over teeth he'd soon be pulling out), the mistake cost her a big chunk of money she'd saved for her retirement.

That she kicks herself for not discussing her dentist's long-range plans for her teeth goes without saying. Let it be an example that midlife is no time to let loyalty stand in the way of maintaining your mouth.

PART THREE

Taking Care of What You Don't See—Vital Organs and Body Functions

WHILE EACH VITAL ORGAN and system in your body requires care and protection, certain parts may seem more vulnerable than others. In the early 1900s, pneumonia, tuberculosis, diarrhea, and enteritis were the leading causes of death; today heart disease, cancer, and diabetes lead the list. If you have special concerns, you may want to go right to the two-pronged medical and nutritional "mini-programs" we've provided for preventing or coping with particular conditions, and then go back for a more systematic review of the body.

However you approach it, using the information in this part of the book will not only help put you in peak condition now, it can greatly simplify your life after you turn 60. The advice you will find here is the same advice we give thousands of 35-plus women to head off some of the primary health risks that have their beginnings in midlife. By understanding some of the common health problems that may not manifest themselves until you're over 60—hypertension, diverticulosis, osteoporosis, for example—you stand an excellent chance of either preventing them or greatly reducing their impact on your overall health. It's no fluke that we have a much larger, healthier group of "seniors" in our culture than ever before. If strength, stamina, and mobility do predictably decrease in women (and men) over 75, we know that any decrease in vigor earlier than that is determined primarily by life-style choices made in the middle years.

When real problems arise, medical support and technical advances make illness or dysfunction more manageable than ever before, as you will see with the routine treatments and coping strategies that are outlined all through this section of the book. But most of the signs of aging we encounter at 35-plus are relatively benign. No matter how you feel about them when they first occur, consider this: in a very real sense, they are nature's way of gently prodding you toward readjusting your health goals. Physical changes have a way of creeping up slowly, but at 35-plus, good health more and more becomes a matter of making sound choices that, for the vast majority of us, are well within reach.

CHAPTER 8

Blood Circulation and the Heart

THE VICTORIANS PERCEIVED the heart to be the site of feeling and emotions, giving rise to the notion that it was "fragile," especially in women. Nothing could be further from the truth. Stress, smoking, alcohol, and drug use may have increased the incidence of heart disease in women, but you still stand a better chance of avoiding serious heart problems than does the average American man. Moreover, new and astonishing evidence of the heart's strength and resilience comes to light with every surgical advance made in repairing it. These include complicated cardiac-bypass operations, whereby heart and lung machines take over circulatory functions and the heart is literally stopped so that arterial obstructions can be circumvented by grafting procedures, and other operations whereby pacemakers, new valves, and other such "hardware" are successfully introduced. That such radically invasive procedures work as well as they do proves that we are only just beginning to comprehend and appreciate the miraculous vigor and tenacity of the beating heart.

The Healthy Heart

Divided into four chambers and about the size of a large fist, the heart propels the body's blood supply (about four to five quarts in most American women) through a high-speed, one-way circulatory system carrying fuel and oxygen to all the cells of the body.

Dr. Jonathan Miller, author of *The Body in Question*, uses a visual analogy to explain the efficient pumping action of the heart: If you cup your hands underwater and squeeze them together quickly, you will squirt a little jet of water into the air. Your heart, however, would blow that jet nearly six feet high. Each beat pumps out about a cupful of blood, pushing it through an intricate network of branching arteries, picking up oxygen from the lungs and carrying it, along with food, to the one-cell-thick arterial capillaries for delivery to the body's cells. At the same time, vein capillaries pick up waste matter and carbon dioxide from the surrounding cells, and bring the blood back to the lungs for reoxygenation before it's returned to the heart for recirculation.

By the time we reach the middle years, the heart has amassed an extraordinary record of achievement. Other muscles relax and recuperate while we sleep, but the heart, which is nearly all muscle, works day and night, circulating the body's total blood supply about 150 times every twenty-four hours. It pumps at about 70 beats a minute, about 100,000 times a day, and well over 30 million times a year. By the time you are 75, the average number of beats can be calculated at over 2 billion.

"Protecting" the heart defies the image of fragility, too. As with all the muscles in the body, the healthy heart thrives on strenuous exercise; in fact, it depends on this activity to keep it in peak condition. In following a regular program of exercise that specifically includes a cardiovascular workout, women well past their middle years show no sign that their "prime time" is over. However, fitness heroics have nothing to do with keeping the heart healthy; consistency does. While the 40-year-old women who win marathons are great for inspiration (and their numbers are increasing), you can keep your heart in good condition with a far less ambitious exercise program (see Part Seven).

Here, our objective is to focus on medical conditions and nutritional guidelines, exploring the problems and risks that can increase with age. They should concern every 35-plus woman. If you are on a path that can lead to heart problems, perhaps even unaware this is the case, this chapter will show you how to change course.

The health of the heart is contingent on life-style and diet; with no other vital organ is this more true. Medical research and studies in the field of nutrition have uncovered valuable information about how these factors combine to influence all aspects of the heart—not just how to keep it healthy and prevent problems but also how to manage problems successfully when they occur.

HIGH BLOOD PRESSURE

If you understand why high blood pressure is such an important health topic, you're one step ahead of the game, because most Americans—even those who have it—don't. Despite a constant flow of facts and statistics from the medical profession to the general public, most people are confident such sweeping figures don't apply to them. They blithely ignore their doctor's warnings or brush off what they hear about this silent but deadly disease which affects 60 million men, women, and children in this country.

Make no mistake. When present and left unchecked, high blood pressure is a major contributing factor in debilitating, if not fatal, strokes, heart attacks, and kidney failure. Since it affects the whole vascular supply, peripheral vascular disease and impaired vision can also result. You may not see or feel any symptoms, but what you don't see or feel can indeed hurt you, because the health risks to the heart very definitely increase with age. The risk of dying before age 65 is one and a half times as great in a person with so-called mild hypertension, and three times as great in a person with moderately severe hypertension, than it is for someone with normal blood pressure. When it is detected and controlled, however, high blood pressure can be managed quite successfully, and the risk of adverse effects dramatically reduced.

Diagnosing High Blood Pressure

High blood pressure, or hypertension, occurs when the heart is forced to pump harder than usual to circulate the body's blood supply. In about one in ten cases, hypertension may have a special "secondary" cause relating to hormones or blood vessels, but for most, the cause is ruled simply as "essential"—which is a nice way of saying that we don't know the exact cause.

Of course, some pressure is necessary to move blood through the circulatory system. It's highest when the blood is being forced ahead through the arteries by the pumping action of the heart (the systolic pressure), and lowest between beats, when the heart momentarily relaxes during the filling phase (the diastolic pressure). In a normal 35-plus woman—and in most people under age 50—the recommended standard is an upper number (systolic pressure) no higher than 140, though some "creep up" is allowed in the later decades of life, with an upper limit around 150. There may be exceptions, as in cases when the systolic is 160 and the diastolic is low—for example, when an older woman's reading is 160 over 80. However, the lower number (diastolic) generally should be 90 or below for any age, with the ideal diastolic pressure being less than 80. Normal blood pressure would range from 100 over 70 at the low end, to 140 over 90 at the high end.

When the number is borderline or only modestly elevated, multiple "casual" checks should be made, by the same observer, and preferably in a normal office setting. In other words, if you are late for a job interview and have just missed your bus, getting a free blood-pressure reading at the mobile unit stationed near the bus stop is not going to be very reliable— although it might give you a shock. In fact, everyone's heart rate and blood pressure normally fluctuates, sometimes a bit higher and sometimes a bit lower than usual throughout the day. The arteries are built to withstand occasional elevations of pressure that result from momentary stress as well as occasional overindulgences in food or alcohol. Even the elevations that occur during the course of a nine-month pregnancy, when a woman's blood volume increases by about 30 percent, are considered "momentary" if the mother is healthy in all other respects (although her obstetrician would watch those elevations closely). In these instances, the heart, arterial walls, veins, and kidneys work together to accommodate the higher pressure (which explains why certain veins become very noticeable during pregnancy), but return to normal once the elevation passes.

But problems come when blood pressure remains constantly high, and the body's ability to adjust runs out. Like a garden hose that's left under pressure, gradually the arterial walls weaken and bulge, creating pockets where fats and waste tend to accumulate and eventually cause a block. The heart, working harder and harder, gradually enlarges, weakening as it does so. And the kidneys work overtime.

Since there is a normal, gradual thickening of the heart tissue as we age, it's obvious that avoiding extra problems connected with high blood pressure should be a top midlife priority. When repeated readings show that your blood pressure is consistently above 140/90, then it is time to discuss the situation with your doctor, and work out a monitoring or maintenance plan that will bring your blood pressure back into the normal range. Most physicians will want baseline blood tests, a urine check, and probably a baseline chest X-ray and electrocardiogram (EKG) as they begin treatment.

The good news is that while it cannot be "cured," high blood pressure can be controlled as soon as it is detected, through adjustments in life-style and nutrition, as well as with medication, though the latter may not be necessary. In as many as 90 percent of those cases of high blood pressure termed "essential" hypertension, a diet heavy in fats and salty foods, an overweight condition, habitual smoking, excessive alcohol consumption, and constant stress are contributing factors that a doctor-patient team can work to eliminate or control.

Lifesaving Strategies for Control and Prevention

Life-Style
Treatment for high blood pressure usually begins with considerations that relate to life-style, although often these are the hardest to come to grips with. Stress at home or at work is an issue that must be resolved once high blood pressure comes into the picture.

"Workaholic" habits, schedules, and attitudes must be readjusted to give you the much-needed outlets of regular, moderate exercise (such as walking), relaxed social activities with family and friends, and quiet time by yourself—health essentials so often lacking in the Type A life-style. Pencil in "appointments" in your date book that will ensure a well-rounded schedule of work, rest, and play; and don't let anything interfere with them. Not only will your heart benefit but so will your outlook, and most likely your work as well. Midlife is a time many people reassess the way they spend their time—and for good reason. Day by day, how are your days spent?

A Six-Point Nutritional Plan for Controlling High Blood Pressure
The link between nutrition and high blood pressure is a crucial one, and there are basic strategies you can adopt that by themselves may be sufficient to deal with hypertension.

1. *Cut down on (better yet, cut out) alcohol.* If your blood pressure is normal, an occasional drink should not be a problem, but if your blood pressure is high, you'd be wise to avoid alcohol altogether.

Beer, wine, liquor—all stimulate blood pressure; in too many patients we see that it is an obstacle to keeping blood pressure under control. Even the social drinker, who perceives her consumption of alcohol to be light to moderate, should discuss her habits plainly and specifically with her doctor, who can confirm the necessary guidelines to ensure control.

2. *Maintain normal weight.* Studies published in the *New England Journal of Medicine* have shown that in patients who are obese, weight reduction alone improves blood pressure control. Even if you are satisfied with your present weight, if it exceeds your optimum range, a loss of 10 to 20 pounds will probably lower your blood pressure.

3. *Use the low-sodium food lists on pages 318–320 for guidelines, and reduce salt.* "But I never use salt" is the typical reaction we hear, at least until daily diet is scrutinized. This is how one of our patients described her "no salt" diet: "For breakfast, bacon (but I boil it first and then microwave it), toast with regular margarine, orange juice, and coffee; for lunch, a ham and turkey sandwich (turkey is low in fat, isn't it?), dill pickles, and diet soda; for an afternoon snack, peanut-butter crackers out of a vending machine and then before dinner, a couple of chips with the children; for dinner (at a Chinese restaurant), wonton soup, egg rolls, chicken chow mein, fried rice, almond cookie, and tea."

No doubt you've spotted some of the culprits here: bacon, ham, processed turkey, salted margarine, chips, and salty peanut butter crackers are the obvious ones, but pickles and most Chinese food are high in salt too, especially when the latter is prepared or dressed with soy sauce. Even if this patient never shook a single grain of salt on her food at the table, with this daily diet she takes in at least double the quota of salt recommended by health-care experts—and far more than if she had prepared fresh foods at home and added a little salt for flavor.

Sodium is the troublesome component. Salt consists of 40 percent sodium and 60 percent chloride, and 1 teaspoon of salt has 2 grams of sodium.

The Food and Nutrition Board of the National Academy of Science believes that an adequate and safe daily level of sodium is 1.1 to 3.3 grams. Americans consume an average of between 2.3 and 6.9 grams of salt daily. At the high end, that's the equivalent of 3½ teaspoons of salt each day! Salt is a necessary part of life, but we get an adequate amount from the naturally occurring sodium in a well-rounded diet.

While certain people may be more sensitive to sodium than others, the strategy of salt reduction is valid for people looking to lower their blood pressure, particularly since over time the blood pressure increases slightly anyway. A low-sodium diet may help lower the amount of fluids that the body holds, and this in turn can mean less pressure in the bloodstream. Additionally, sodium control seems to help medication for high blood pressure work more effectively.

If you gradually reduce the amount of salt you cook with at home, you should have no problem adjusting, and you may even discover flavors that were previously hidden by salt. If some foods seem bland, use herbs, spices, and lemon juice to flavor them. Alternate bites of different foods and try simply chewing more thoroughly. This actually increases the number of molecules that interact with taste receptors.

Salt substitutes may help if they are not contraindicated for medical reasons, which include renal complications and the type of drug therapy used. See page 320 for a list of salt substitutes and their sodium and potassium content. Salt substitutes are usually potassium chloride and do contain some sodium as well.

4. *Avoid foods with substances that contain hidden sodium.* Don't rely on your taste buds for salt content; check the label. Certain foods that do not *taste* salty may have been processed with substances that are high in sodium —monosodium glutamate (MSG), sodium nitrate, sodium phosphate, brine, and soda are all high in sodium. Meals that come from a can—chili con carne, hash, soups, and even canned vegetables are generally high in salt and fresh or homemade versions should be used instead.

Labels can help you choose acceptable foods, too. Many food manufacturers list the sodium content of their products on the labels; in fact, foods labeled "salt free," "sodium free," "low salt," or "low sodium" *must* provide this information. For others, if sodium is one of the first three ingredients listed, you know it is high in sodium. (See pages 318–320 for low-sodium foods.)

Avoid drinking "soft" water, as a high amount of sodium is used in the softening treatment.

5. *Order carefully when you eat out.* Some restaurants will prepare low-sodium meals if you request it. When this is not an option, order fruit and fruit juice for appetizers; avoid soups, broths, bouillons, and vegetable juices.

When ordering meat, fish, or poultry, select the broiled or grilled dishes and ask that no salt, garlic salt, or MSG be added in the cooking processes. If you order roast beef, lamb, pork, or veal, ask for an inside cut and trim off the outer edge, which has been salted.

While it's best to skip gravies and sauces, you're always safe with a plain baked potato or one seasoned with a bit of plain yogurt and chopped chives. When in doubt, substitute a plain green vegetable or fruit salad.

6. Since most fast foods are high in sodium, make trips to the salad bar when you eat in fast-food restaurants. Skip the bacon bits, canned bean salads, and croutons. Instead, choose toppings that don't come from a can, jar, or package—they usually pass the low-sodium test. Bottled salad dressings are also usually high in sodium; substitute lemon juice, oil, vinegar, herbs, and pepper.

Medications

While in many instances hypertension can be controlled by life-style changes, it is important to realize that high blood pressure is affected by a combination of many factors affecting heart rate, volume, and peripheral resistance. Some factors are hormonal; some have to do with the nervous system or structural anatomy. These elements all play a part in considerations made by your doctor when recommending medications for lowering blood pressure.

For years, *diuretics* (water pills) have been the first step in treating high blood pressure. While still useful for many patients, their effects are considered a mixed blessing, in that they pull sodium and water out of the blood system but, in some people, also cause imbalances in varying degrees —depleting potassium, for example, or raising blood sugar, uric acid, or cholesterol. Dosages used today are much lower than they were even five years ago, and imbalances are monitored more closely, with periodic blood tests to check blood potassium levels.

Beta blockers, which are widely used, refer to a category of medications that affect the beta-adrenergic receptor sites. These are the main receptors of the sympathetic nervous system for epinephrine (also called adrenaline). Beta blockers act literally as a blockade at these sites, decreasing the amount of adrenaline reaching the heart and effecting a decrease in heart output— the main determinant of any blood pressure, normal or high. They also blockade the kidney beta-adrenergic receptors, inhibiting the release of renin, one of the hormones that plays a part in high blood pressure. Propranolol (Inderal) was the first beta blocker introduced in this country in the mid-1970s; it is also used to prevent migraine headaches and even to reduce performance anxiety. Since then, many kinds of beta blockers have become available, all metabolized in different ways.

Beta blockers can have side effects—among these are fatigue and depression—but with close monitoring of dosage, these can be minimized or avoided. Improvements in this category of drug treatment are continually being made so that some of the new beta blockers have significantly fewer side effects than their precursors.

ACE (angiotensin converting enzyme) inhibitors basically have their effect by interfering with the release of angiotensin II, the hormone produced by the kidney that can lead to high blood pressure. The first ACE inhibitor was captopril (Capoten). They are excellent first-line medications with few side effects.

First developed for heart pain (angina), *calcium channel blockers* (for example, nifedipine, or Procardia) work on the calcium metabolism of the myocardial cell of the heart. They are basically classified as vasodilators, helping in coronary artery disease to expand or dilate the artery, and in hypertension they probably provide some metabolic effect as well. These have been particularly effective in dealing with hard-to-treat high blood pressure, although not all are FDA approved for this as yet.

With this variety of options for drug treatment, a program of appropriate medications for those who need them can almost certainly be tailored to suit individual needs and tolerance. While no physician can promise zero side effects with medications, frank discussions about them will help you arrive at an effective and reasonably tolerated program that ensures good control.

Medical Follow-ups

If your blood pressure reads high, your doctor will want to check it frequently to monitor your condition all through the treatment phase. Once blood pressure has been lowered and stabilized, office visits can be cut down to about once every three or four months. Home monitoring, as with home glucose monitoring for diabetic patients, can be very helpful; your doctor can give you guidelines.

CORONARY ARTERY DISEASE

For most people, "heart trouble" is synonymous with coronary artery disease: blockage of the blood vessels that supply the heart. This form of heart disease is the most frequent cause of heart attacks, and it is the issue behind the current national concern with high cholesterol, one of the major elements that contributes to fatty plaque deposits inside the arteries. In 1987, the total estimated number of U.S. citizens who had coronary artery disease was 4.7 million, a figure that included those who were clinically diagnosed to have angina and those who actually had a heart attack. The prediction for 1988 was that 1.4 million men and women would have a heart attack, and 500,000 of them would die from it.

Coronary artery disease, like high blood pressure, is progressive; that is, it gradually builds up until finally an "attack" occurs. The statistics on those who die suddenly from heart disease, either from heart attack (infarction) or arrhythmia (irregular heartbeat), include people with previously diagnosed coronary artery disease, as well as those who showed no previous signs of pain or heart problems.

In men, the incidence of coronary artery disease starts to rise in the fifth decade (age 40) and continues steadily upward. In women, the statistical increase doesn't begin for another ten years, coinciding with the onset of menopause. All other health factors being equal, the presence of estrogen in a woman's body protects her from coronary artery disease and is the main reason why women live longer than men in this country. Even so, today's widespread concern about coronary disease is shared by women, especially those reaping the well-deserved benefits of higher salaries, new careers, and job equality. Ironically, this is the group most likely to experience overwork and chronic high stress—prime risk factors in heart disease. Women who smoke and drink also significantly increase their risks.

There are other factors as well, including a family history of heart blockage at an earlier age than expected; diabetes that is poorly controlled; a sedentary life-style; and high blood pressure left unchecked. Elevated cholesterol is also high on the list, and though it remains to be proved, some health professionals theorize that high blood pressure actually forces fat into the arterial walls.

Although cholesterol is the most highly publicized current risk factor, worrying about it makes little sense unless all the factors just mentioned are dealt with in a complete program of prevention.

Diagnosis

For most women and men, chest pain—more specifically, sensations of pressure or aching—is what sends them to the doctor for a diagnosis. When the arteries become blocked, it is harder for blood to get through and feed the heart muscle. This is not always a problem (at least early on) at rest, but with exercise, when the heart muscle signals for more fuel and strains to get it, pain (angina) may be felt. Those who experience angina describe it as a dull pain or pressure, usually under the breastbone; sharp, shooting pains that last a few seconds rarely represent coronary artery blockage. Do not depend on self-diagnosis, however. Any recurrent feeling of pressure in the chest warrants review with a physician.

Pain can provide a clue, but critical blockage may be present without overt pain. Firm diagnosis of coronary artery blockage is made with a stress test or an angiogram.

A *stress test* is an exercise cardiogram—a somewhat more elaborate version of a resting cardiogram, in this case involving a treadmill to assess the heart's performance. Both a technician and a physician are present to monitor blood pressure and to watch the cardiogram screen. The patient walks on the treadmill, with increases in speed and grade at three minute intervals, all done in a continuous fashion. The objective is to arrive at the maximum predicted heart rate (or at least 85 percent of the maximum heart rate), an age-derived value of 220 minus the person's age. Usually after nine to twelve minutes of progressive exercise, the patient spends about four to six more minutes in a "recovery period," walking at about 1 to 1.2 miles an hour at no grade. This allows the heart rate and blood pressure, both of which will have risen during the test, to fall back toward the baseline.

The stress test is widely used as a safe, noninvasive, indirect test (that is, it looks at function rather than anatomy) for signs of heart disease. If there are blockages, usually there will be predictable changes on the electrocardiographic record printed out every 2 to 3 minutes. Inexpensive and easy to administer, the stress test is very good for people who have heart-disease symptoms (chest pressure, for instance) or significant risk factors (smoking, hypertension, and so on) and who perhaps want to start a new exercise program. However, it is not used as a screening test for healthy people. Also, for reasons that are unknown, women tend to have more false-positives on this test than do men.

For most people, the stress test precedes an *angiogram*, which is a more direct test. Dye is injected through a catheter into the heart arteries so they can be looked at. The angiogram, by definition, is more invasive and thus more risky and expensive. It is, however, the definitive test.

If either of these tests—particularly the angiogram—indicates a problem, the next step is to consult a cardiologist, if this has not already been done. It is vital that your own doctor, knowing your individual situation, be part of that consultation process. Barring instances where severe coronary artery disease is evident—for example, where marked blockage of all three arteries warrants an immediate triple bypass or where there is significant blockage of the left main artery—medical treatment is likely to involve oral medication and changes in diet and life-style. Clearly, this is the optimum path of treatment *before* coronary artery disease has become so advanced that surgery is necessary.

Medical Treatment

The medications used to treat coronary artery disease include the various forms of *nitrates* (the classic being nitroglycerin), which help both to temporarily dilate or "open up" the heart vessels and to reduce the blood flow to the heart, as well as medications also used to treat high blood pressure: the *beta blockers* that decrease heart work and oxygen use and the *calcium channel blockers* that expand the artery. The calcium channel blockers have added remarkably to the medical management of angina, stabilizing patients who in previous years would have required surgery.

Certain kinds of blockages are being treated by cardiologists with an in-between route called *angioplasty*, whereby a balloon catheter placed into the affected artery opens up a localized blockage. Skills in this technique are increasingly being perfected, and in time this procedure will doubtless save many people from the necessity of heart surgery.

Prevention Through Nutrition

Even with the new medications and technologies, intervention and damage control hold a poor second to prevention of coronary artery disease. Not even surgical and medical interventions provide a cure if they are not followed with positive adjustments in life-style, health practices, and eating habits. For some, the issues of smoking, poor aerobic fitness, blood pressure control, and diabetes must all be tackled. For many others, the overriding issue is lowering cholesterol.

A Crash Course in Cholesterol

Cholesterol is a white powdery substance that cannot be seen or tasted. It is found only in animal products, since animals—including humans—are the only creatures who manufacture it (in the liver) and use it in making cell walls and hormones. However, sticking to plant sources for shortening and oils—even choosing products labeled "no cholesterol"—is no guarantee of safety. Just as with animal fats, certain vegetable oils and solid fats encourage the body to make cholesterol.

Many people are unaware that there are actually two types of blood cholesterol: the "good" type (HDL, or high-density lipoprotein) and the "bad" type (LDL, or low-density lipoprotein). The high-density lipoproteins carry cholesterol from cells to the liver for processing or excretion, and contain a great amount of protein and a small amount of cholesterol. Researchers have noted that persons with high HDL levels have less heart disease than people with low HDL levels, so we call this the "good cholesterol."

Low-density lipoproteins carry cholesterol from the liver to the cells and arteries and contain a large amount of cholesterol and a small amount of protein. These lipoproteins may be responsible for depositing cholesterol in artery walls, so they are known as "bad cholesterol."

The general rule is the higher the HDL and the lower the LDL, the better.

In obese people—those 20 to 30 percent over their optimum weight—LDL levels are usually higher and HDL levels are usually lower than in individuals who are in their appropriate weight range. Calorie restriction and weight loss can balance these levels out. This is why the American Heart Association urges people to maintain their optimum weight.

Blood cholesterol is influenced by the food you eat and by your inherited body chemistry, both of which account for your body's individual response to diet and the amount of cholesterol it manufactures. This fact is central to an understanding of why some people build up more cholesterol in their bodies than others, and why they will benefit not only from an ongoing low-cholesterol, low-saturated-fat diet but in some cases need cholesterol-reducing medication as well (see pages 95–96).

For most 35-plus women, the ideal goal for LDL would be less than 130, with a total serum cholesterol count ideally below 200, and certainly no higher than 240.

Putting What You Know into Practice

Although medication can play a role in cholesterol reduction, we are convinced, after seeing the results of our nutritional programs, that diet is the primary route to lower cholesterol levels.

Perhaps no other nutritional topic has received more attention in the scientific and lay press than the role of cholesterol and lipids (fats) in causing disease. Thirty years ago, most people, including dietitians, had never heard the word *cholesterol*. But after years of research, under the auspices of the National Institutes of Health, a panel of experts concluded "beyond reasonable doubt that lowering definitely elevated cholesterol will reduce the risk of heart attacks. . . ." It made perfect sense. When fats and cholesterol circulating in the blood are deposited on the inner walls of the arteries, over the years scar tissue and other debris build up as more fat and cholesterol accumulate at these sites. In this process, known as arteriosclerosis, the arteries become seriously narrowed. If a clot becomes stuck at the site of a narrowing, a heart attack results.

While the message rang out loud and clear, most people still don't know how to apply the information to their eating habits. They eat bacon for breakfast, but don't eat eggs and use corn-oil margarine on their toast. They choose chicken for protein, but of the fast-food variety—deep-fried. They order "fat-free" luncheon meats, erroneously thinking that bologna passes the test because it has no "white spots" of fat.

But consumer awareness in this area is rapidly growing, bringing with it a new wave of pressure on the food industry to take the cholesterol-producing fats and oils out of their products. Some of this pressure is paying off. Last year, an eye-catching, full-page ad funded by Phil Sokolof, an advocate of the nonprofit National Heart Savers Association of Omaha, was published in various major newspapers across the country. It angrily criticized the food industry for its use of palm, palm kernel, and coconut oils—highly saturated fats found in cereals, baked goods, cookies, and other products that, along with beef tallow and lard, raise cholesterol levels in the body. There was a definite response from the food industry. Kellogg's, for example, reformulated its Cracklin' Oat Bran to replace coconut oil with a vegetable oil low in saturated fat. The switch from saturated to unsaturated fats is occurring as quickly as the big food companies can make the substitutions. To date, General Mills has removed the saturated fat from Bisquick; Sunshine has removed palm oil from its Hydrox Creme Filled Chocolate Cookies. Nabisco claims that of twenty-four new products introduced in 1987, only two are made with tropical oils. And Pepperidge Farm, while working intensively to reformulate its cookies, now uses 100 percent soybean oil in its bread. While the oils in these products "are relatively minor contributors of saturated fats to the American diet," according to Dr. F. Edward Scarbrough, the deputy director of the FDA's Office of Nutrition and Food Sciences, the trend to cut them out of staple foods is encouraging. With the food industry working on the side of the consumer to help lower cholesterol, there is a good chance we will see substantial changes on the supermarket shelves.

The low-cholesterol, low-saturated-fat diet on pages 306–308 will give you a detailed list of food choices to lower your cholesterol. The following tips will also help you make healthy choices in the supermarket.

Cholesterol-Wise Shopping

1. *Gear your purchases to a preplanned, cholesterol-wise menu for the day (better yet, the week).* The American Heart Association suggests you take in *less than 300 milligrams* of cholesterol per day in their Dietary Guidelines. We think you can do even better than that. We'll show you how most 35-plus women can meet the goal of a total cholesterol under 240 milligrams, with an optimal goal of less than 200 milligrams. All it takes is picking wisely from among the foods you ordinarily use.

As an example of how you can drastically lower cholesterol, compare the elements of a day's typical high-cholesterol diet with the elements of a cholesterol-conscious diet:

Typical Diet

	mg/CHOLESTEROL
Breakfast	
1 whole egg	220
Lunch	
2 ounces Swiss cheese	61
Dinner	
6 ounces veal	240
Total cholesterol	521

Cholesterol-Conscious Diet

	mg/CHOLESTEROL
Breakfast	
¼ cup egg substitute, or 2 egg whites	0
Lunch	
1 cup low-fat cottage cheese	15
Dinner	
6 ounces lean beef	150
Total cholesterol	165

Of course, this comparison highlights only the elements of a day's diet that have a direct affect on cholesterol levels. But you can see that you would be well below the recommended 300 mg a day, even if you added one serving of low-fat milk or low-fat yogurt. The low-cholesterol diet on pages 306–308 will help you plan your menus. If you have an elevated cholesterol and wish to lose weight, you can very easily do so by planning and choosing the right combinations of lean protein foods.

If you have inherited your elevated cholesterol, you can either eliminate red meat from your diet and eat poultry and fish—4 to 6 ounces a day —or you can shop as an ovolactovegetarian, using complementary proteins in grains and vegetables and selecting low-fat dairy products and egg whites.

2. *Choose fats wisely.* For years, health professionals have known that polyunsaturated fatty acids are effective in reducing elevated blood-cholesterol levels when substituted for saturated fatty acids. This is the cornerstone of diet therapy for prevention and treatment of coronary heart disease. According to the American Heart Association, fats should constitute no more than 30 percent of your diet, with 10 percent being saturated fats, 10 percent polyunsaturated fats, and 10 percent monounsaturated fats.

Saturated fat is usually solid at room temperature and is found primarily in meats, dairy products, coconut, cocoa butter, and palm oils. A diet rich in saturated fats will raise blood-cholesterol levels by causing the liver to make more cholesterol. This is why some of those "no cholesterol" labels on certain foods are misleading; they can contain no cholesterol, but will encourage your body to make more of it.

The two unsaturated fats—poly and mono—are usually soft or liquid at room temperature, and are found in vegetable products. Polyunsaturated fats lower all cholesterol—the good as well as the bad—whereas monounsaturated fats seem to reduce more bad cholesterol than good.

When shopping, then, your first choice should be monounsaturated fats: olive oil, peanut oil, or rapeseed (canola) oil. Your second choice should be polyunsaturated fats: safflower oil, sunflower oil, corn oil, or soybean-plus-cottonseed oil. You should avoid saturated fats: coconut oil, cocoa butter (found in chocolate), palm oil, butter, poultry fat, and fats from beef, lamb, veal, or other animals; also avoid lard, hydrogenated margarine, or solid vegetable shortening.

When buying margarine, the first ingredient should be liquid vegetable oil instead of hydrogenated vegetable oil. "Hydrogenated" means that hydrogen has been added to change the physical structure of the oil molecules so they become hard at room temperature and thus simulate butter. Here again watch out for "no cholesterol" claims. While there is no cholesterol in plants, hydrogenation results in a solid fat that encourages production of cholesterol by the body.

3. *Shop cholesterol-wise for other staple foods, too—read all labels.* Many foods you'd never guess were linked to cholesterol—cookies, crackers, and so on—may actually be high on the list of things to avoid. That's why reading labels is important.

Look closely at a product's long list of ingredients. When you see lard, coconut oil, palm oil, or cocoa butter early on in the list of ingredients, steer clear. Instead, particularly when buying baked goods, look for "allowable" vegetable oils. Alas, even homemade baked goods from local bakeries are suspect because of the shortening they are likely to contain. We recommend that people who want cookies and cakes make them from scratch at home.

Assuming weight or other dietary restrictions pose no problems, you can choose sweets in moderation, including fruit ices (made with juices); frozen desserts made with skim milk and no other saturated fats or egg yolks; pudding made with skim milk; gelatin; fruit whips, junkets, and frozen yogurt made with skim milk; also "allowable" cookies (made with polyunsaturated margarine or oil); Tofutti (but in small amounts, as its fat content—even though unsaturated—is very high); angel food cake (mix or homemade) and other homemade cakes, cookies, and pies made with allowed fats, skim milk, and no egg yolks; frostings made with allowed fat; and cocoa (not solid chocolate) in cakes, cookies, and frosting. Sweets can include hard candies, jams, jellies, honeys, sugar, syrup (nonfat), and molasses. Avoid other candy, coconut, and solid chocolate.

4. *Think twice before stopping to buy beer or liquor.* You may not know it, but alcohol is actually a type of fat—the kind your liver will turn into cholesterol. This is why the American Heart Association recommends restricting alcohol to no more than 50 milliliters a day—less than two drinks. Better yet, we recommend only an occasional drink or none at all for people with normal cholesterol levels, and no alcohol for people whose levels are elevated.

CHOLESTEROL-LOWERING COME-ONS

Misconception 1

Fish oil reduces heart disease. No, fish oil does not reduce heart disease: in fact, it may even raise cholesterol.

A hot issue right now are fish oils or, more exactly, omega-3 fatty acids. The evidence that fish oils may offer some protection against coronary heart disease comes from studies of Greenland Eskimos, who consume diets primarily of fatty fish yet who have a very low incidence of coronary heart disease. Claims have been made that these fish oils not only offer a protective effect against coronary heart disease but also lower blood cholesterol and even improve hypertension and arthritis. As a result, over-the-counter fish-oil capsules have become widely available. Beware. Some of these are actually *high* in cholesterol because they are extracts of fish liver oil, and because liver is a source of cholesterol, they actually add cholesterol to your diet.

While people would love to believe that Eskimos know the secret of preventing heart disease, fish oil by itself has not been tested in a clinical trial of heart disease prevention, and neither the American Heart Association nor the National Heart, Lung, and Blood Institute recommend it. Though studies show there is a correlation between the presence of fish or marine animals in the diet and a decreased rate of vascular disease, it's possible that some other component of fish besides its oil may actually be the protective element. Further testing will tell; for now, we do know that making fish (the varieties low in cholesterol) a regular item on your menus is a good idea.

Misconception 2

Lecithin lowers cholesterol. We are constantly asked about the benefits of lecithin. You eat lecithin every day. It is found naturally in peanuts, pecans, peanut butter, soybeans, wheat germ, wheat flour, cornmeal, spinach, potatoes, lettuce, and carrots, as well as cheese, eggs, milk, liver, ham, lamb chops, and beef round.

Lecithin is a complex, fatlike substance belonging to a group of compounds known as phospholipids. Because it is an effective emulsifier, making foods more palatable by dispersing or blending ingredients evenly, lecithin is added to many foods, including ice cream, cooking-oil sprays, chocolate, and margarine. The human body uses it to form cell membranes and various important compounds.

The current focus is on one of lecithin's components—choline—which through research appears to be used as a vitamin for some animals. It is not a vitamin for humans, however, since the body can manufacture sufficient choline from protein. Even if it were proved that the choline from lecithin is beneficial to humans, the type of lecithin commonly sold in health-food stores usually contains little choline at all and only a small percentage of real lecithin. Generally, studies of lecithin's effect on lowering blood cholesterol have to date been inconclusive. If it does help, it may be because lecithin is composed largely of polyunsaturated fatty acids.

5. *For lower cholesterol, shop for complex carbohydrates.* The American Heart Association gives three good reasons for recommending that 50 to 55 percent of daily calories be made up of carbohydrates: (1) they have no cholesterol; (2) properly combined, they can supply part of your protein requirement and thus reduce the need for fatty protein from meat and dairy sources (see the Complementary Proteins list, page 304); (3) they contain not only insoluble fiber but also water-soluble fiber.

6. *Choose cholesterol-lowering soluble fiber, but set a limit on calories when you do.* The whole question of fiber in the diet is covered later, on pages 125–127. What is significant here is that soluble fiber may actually reduce blood-cholesterol levels by one or more mechanisms that affect cholesterol absorption. These mechanisms include serving as a physical barrier to absorption because of their high viscosity, working in the intestines to bind cholesterol into bile acids, and altering gastrointestinal activity.

Oat bran is a useful source of such soluble fiber, and it has become very popular. But when oat bran is used in baking (muffins, for example), you may be getting your soluble fiber in a high-calorie form. A new study points out that two large raw carrots a day can have an effect similar to oat bran. Our list of foods high in soluble fibers, given on pages 313–316, was prepared not only to offer variety but also to help keep calories down when you are looking for ways to add fiber to your diet. If you gradually increase fiber to an appropriate level of five to six servings a day over several weeks —from the kinds of wholesome foods on our list—you will reduce the possibility of side effects that come from suddenly eating more fiber all at once—namely, bloating, gas, and problems absorbing key minerals like calcium, iron, and zinc. Because of the possibility of these side effects, fiber supplements are not generally recommended.

Medication to Lower Cholesterol

Your doctor must be involved in a decision to take medication, but if cholesterol levels do not improve with diet alone, medications may be called for. One of these is *niacin* (nicotinic acid), which acts to lower the liver's production of cholesterol. It is inexpensive and usually effective. Sustained-release capsules, taken with food, can minimize the flushing or itching that at least one-third of the patients experience as a side effect. In some cases, taking niacin with one aspirin is helpful as well, but in all cases, *medical supervision is important*, with periodic checks of cholesterol levels and liver function, since these can occasionally become abnormal. Overdoses of niacin *can* cause liver damage.

Resins, such as cholestyramine, have proved to be a safe and effective medical option, albeit with common intestinal side effects of constipation and bloating. If tolerated, it usually works well, especially to lower LDL.

As an alternative, Metamucil, a bulk laxative, has recently been shown to be safe and effective in lowering cholesterol. In an article published in the *Archives of Internal Medicine* (February 1988), Anderson and colleagues reported a study from the University of Kentucky which showed a cholesterol reduction of 15 percent using a dose of 3.4 grams of Metamucil three times a day, without any negative effects on HDL. There was a good follow-up and few "dropouts," so this clearly is a practical approach. (Citrucel and other fiber laxatives based on insoluble fiber [cellulose] do not have this cholesterol-lowering effect.)

The new medication lovastatin (Mevacor) shows promise in lowering blood cholesterol by decreasing its production in the liver. Although it is usually used only when diet or the aforementioned medications are ineffective, once its safety is well established, lovastatin may well become the medication of choice, since there are few bad side effects and treatment with lovastatin often raises HDL.

Hopeful Thoughts on Coronary Artery Disease

While we know that rigorous management of risk factors, especially cholesterol level, can help to prevent coronary artery blockage, could such a program also reverse the disease? Years ago, those who said yes were scorned—but no more. Small, angiogram-controlled studies are showing some degrees of reversal, though the reports and numbers involved are modest thus far. The next ten years should tell the tale. But in the meantime, it is unreasonable to rely on high-tech solutions to save ourselves. We can't change our ancestors, but we can decide what we'll eat, if we'll smoke, and whether we'll exercise. Making smart heart choices, not next week or next year but day by day, is one of the keys to wellness for all 35-plus women.

PERIPHERAL VASCULAR DISEASE

Varicose Veins

Varicose veins are not in the same category as the serious heart and circulatory problems we've just discussed, but for many women nothing is more disheartening than to see these veins appear on otherwise good-looking legs. Genetics plays a big part in whether or not you develop them, but chances are you're going to see a few varicosities, or broken veins, in your thighs and lower legs after you turn 35, or after your first pregnancy, even if that occurs in your twenties.

Varicose veins—those bumpy, bluish protrusions that appear on the backs of a woman's calves and thighs—occur when veins become distended and the walls are weakened, or when a malfunction in the one-way valves permits a backflow, or pooling, of blood.

Why either condition occurs is hard to explain. Heredity and life-style, particularly when that life-style involves standing for long periods, are factors, as are pregnancy, when blood volume normally increases, and obesity. In some cases, varicose veins can lead to an aching or burning feeling in the legs, and can contribute to general fatigue. In extreme cases, they can lead to phlebitis (inflamed veins) and in some cases even to ulcerations; for this reason you should be sure your doctor evaluates the condition of your veins, particularly on the backs of your legs where you may not be able to see them, when you have your regular checkup.

If you are having problems with recurrent superficial phlebitis, or have had no success with conservative suggestions, such as those that follow, your primary physician might request an evaluation by a vascular surgeon. If surgery is warranted, procedures can include the traditional stripping, or removal of the vein, or ligation (tying off the veins), or one of the newer forms of sclerosing, or scarring treatments, done by injecting sclerosing substances into the veins and making them nonfunctional, with the blood diverted to deeper veins. In the majority of cases, because varicosities occur in superficial veins not essential to circulation, surgical treatment is not medically warranted, and the issue becomes a cosmetic one: keeping them from growing larger and more prominent.

Some ways to relieve the discomfort of varicose veins include:

- *Weight reduction.* If you are overweight, this is a top priority.
- *Support stockings.* Try over-the-counter support pantyhose for minor varicosities, and surgical support hose such as Jobst stockings, which require measurement and fittings, for more prominent ones.
- *Get off your feet.* If you must stand for long periods, elevating the legs whenever possible can provide symptomatic relief.
- *Move around.* If you must sit for long durations, periodically get up and move around, and be aware of the pressure you may put on your legs in the way you sit. Avoid crossing your legs at the knee.

Spider Veins

Spider veins—telangiectasias—are small broken capillaries that appear near the surface of the skin. Like varicose veins, these usually show up on the legs, but they present less of a problem in terms of medical complication and comfort than true varicosities. Still, they're not much more attractive, and if they become such a nuisance to you that you tend to keep your legs covered with long pants, you might want to try makeup preparations for the legs available at cosmetic counters in waterproof versions that won't rub off and offer very good coverage with a natural look, so long as you carefully match the shade with your skin tone.

Spider veins can also be safely removed without leaving a scar by a dermatologist using fine needle electrodesiccation, although this process can be tedious (and expensive) over a large area like the legs. The "zapped" spiders won't recur, but the treatment won't prevent new ones from occurring elsewhere—though more careful treatment of your legs will help.

Venous Insufficiency

This is another vein "disease," whereby the veins do not efficiently return blood from the lower extremity back to the heart. It frequently results in edema, or swelling, of the legs. On a long-term basis, management of this condition is similar to that for varicose veins, with the use of diuretics an occasional option. You and your doctor would need to discuss this route. If you experience *any* sudden, unexpected swelling in the legs, it's essential that you see your doctor to make sure the problem isn't a blood clot.

Leg Pains

Peripheral artery problems usually involve the legs and can include blockage of the arteries, similar to blockage of the heart vessels. With exercise such as walking, this condition can lead to leg pain called claudication. The problem is best evaluated by a vascular surgeon, although treatment is often medical rather than surgical: discontinue smoking and lower elevated cholesterol. Some medications, such as pentoxifylline (Trental), and exercise programs can be helpful and may delay the need for vascular surgery, which could include a bypass of a blocked artery with a graft or the newer use of balloon angioplasty.

Artery spasms from Raynaud's disease in the upper extremities may affect some 35-plus women. Symptoms include pain and temperature changes—usually coldness. See your doctor if you exhibit any of these. Although Raynaud's disease is difficult to treat, in some cases there has been success with calcium channel blockers, such as nifedipine (Procardia).

Poor Circulation

Cold hands and feet may be caused by anemia, low blood pressure, or an underactive thyroid. But poor circulation may even bother women with perfectly normal readings in each of these areas.

Here again, smoking is a big culprit. Nicotine reduces circulation by constricting the small arteries that feed the extremities.

It bears repeating that regular, aerobic exercise enhances circulation throughout the body. Even in restricted situations—at work or at home— you can warm up and wake up just by getting out of your chair and moving around a little.

In any case, if you suspect a real problem with circulation, see your doctor. He or she can put the problem into a broader health perspective and, most important, can provide sound guidance as to the best course to take.

ANEMIA AND THE 35-PLUS WOMAN

Anemia occurs when the body's red blood cells are reduced in number or are deficient in hemoglobin. Signs of anemia include pale skin, easy fatigue, shortness of breath, and even palpitation of the heart.

Women are particularly vulnerable to anemia because of blood loss during menstruation, particularly with the typically heavier menstrual flows that can occur as menopause approaches or with the use of IUDs (now in decline because of other risks). Nutritional deficiencies can occur for a number of reasons, including pregnancies, breast-feeding and the nutritional boost that requires, and poor diet.

Far more prevalent than any one of these factors is the iron deficiency anemia that results from blood loss coupled with an iron-poor diet and poor eating habits. The classic case is the woman who uses fad diets, skips meals, and omits green leafy vegetables and other iron-rich foods in favor of highly-refined, iron-poor foods like pastries and sweets. If she also has extremely heavy menstrual periods (menorrhagia), eventually she's going to use up her body stores of iron and become anemic as production of red blood cells falters because there is not enough iron to make them. Even with improvements in diet, when there is a very heavy menstrual flow, it may be a good idea to take an iron supplement (see pages 102–103) and even to get a blood count if fatigue levels are unusual or the menses seem to increase in frequency, duration, or intensity.

As we will show, every 35-plus woman can successfully treat nutritional anemia—better yet, prevent its occurrence. But first, an overview of the blood and its components will put this and other problems into context.

Your Blood Cells

Red blood cells, white blood cells, and platelets—the major components of the blood—are all produced in the bone marrow. The bone marrow's rate of production and renewal of each of these elements varies greatly, with red blood cells having a life span of about 120 days and white blood cells and platelets lasting less than twenty-four hours.

The quantities of these three components also vary greatly and are readily analyzed on the blood slip that comes when a doctor orders a CBC (complete blood count). This quantitative measurement provides an accurate picture of the relative condition, or "health status," of your blood.

The red cell component can be expressed either in terms of hemoglobin, which is preferred, or the derived value called the hematocrit—that is, the percentage of total blood volume composed of red blood cells (the other component being the blood serum). In a healthy 35-plus woman, the hematocrit should be 35 to 45 percent, with serum making up 55 to 65 percent of total blood volume.

A normal hemoglobin is usually between 12 and 14 grams/100 ml. In women who are menstruating heavily, it can be lower than 12, resulting in anemia.

White blood cells are described in terms of thousands per cubic millimeter with the normal average running between 5,000 and 12,000, as tallied on an automatic counting machine.

Platelets are counted in a similar fashion. Much smaller in size than white blood cells, their number is much larger, and an appropriate platelet count would usually be between 150,000 and 400,000. Previously, a platelet count would simply be labeled as adequate or not, but more sophisticated machines now give specific numerical counts.

As it circulates throughout the body, blood serum passes through a whole series of capillary-level filters called the glomeruli, located in the upper part of the kidneys called the cortex. The kidneys filter about eighteen gallons of blood, plus 60 percent of all fluid taken into the body, every hour. The red cells, white cells, and platelets stay behind in the blood vessel while the serum enters the glomeruli and is cleansed of toxins such as urea (which builds up in cases of kidney failure) and too-heavy concentrations of potassium, calcium, and salt, which the kidneys shunt to the bladder, and then the serum is filtered back into the blood vessel.

As described earlier, when discussing the function of the heart, the primary job of the red blood cells is picking up oxygen from the lungs and transporting it to body tissues, and returning carbon dioxide to the lungs, where it's exhaled. A slightly elevated red cell count may be seen in some smokers—the body's attempt to compensate for a decreased supply of oxygen.

The white blood cells act primarily in defense against bodily infections —bacterial, viral, or fungal. A defect in the body's immune system involving white blood cells is clearly a serious matter, as demonstrated most dramatically in cases of AIDS.

An elevated white count usually indicates the presence of an infection.

The main role of platelets is enhancing the body's clotting ability. An inadequate platelet count (below 50,000) may affect the blood's ability to make normal clots. The effects of this can be seen in people who bruise easily. (A different deficiency is found in hemophilia, which affects only the male population, although it is inherited through the mother.)

When the body loses blood, the bone marrow simply speeds up blood-cell production, becoming what is called hyperplastic as it works overtime. Under ordinary circumstances—with a cut or even with an average menstrual flow—blood cell quantities soon return to normal. But if there is heavy blood loss or a deficiency of raw materials to make the new cells—the most important of which is iron—the result can be a reduction in the size and total number of red blood cells, hence a low hemoglobin.

Diagnosing Anemia

If you suspect you are anemic, call your doctor and make an appointment for a blood test. The CBC, or complete blood count, will confirm whether the hemoglobin and the hematocrit are normal—the latter, once again, ranging between 35 and 45 percent of total volume.

Other than confirmation with a blood test, there is another, more important reason for bringing your doctor into the picture if you suspect anemia. Nutritional deficiencies are not the only reason for becoming anemic: Blood loss and red-blood-cell destruction caused by certain illnesses can also be a factor, as can ulcers, gastritis, cancers such as lymphoma, or bleeding from the colon caused by diverticulosis, polyps, or colon cancer. These anemias will *not* respond to nutritional therapy, but in fact must be confirmed and discussed with a physician *before* any program for building up red blood cells is undertaken.

Treatment of Nutritional Anemia

Most nutritional anemias are relative—that is, some red cells are being produced but not enough to meet the body's needs. The common response to most nutritional anemias is simply to increase the amount of iron in the diet. Sometimes there are other elements lacking as well—protein, vitamin B_{12}, folic acid, vitamin B_6, vitamin E, or copper—and we will take these into account.

IRON SUPPLEMENTS. Understandably, doctors who are rushed through a busy schedule of appointments too often neglect to take a careful diet history, and they treat anemia with medicinal iron preparations that can cause stomach upset and constipation. In addition, some of the over-the-counter multivitamins or iron supplements (Femiron, for example) simply do not have enough iron in them to significantly treat anemia, and prescription supplements such as ferrous gluconate or ferrous sulfate tablets would be more effective.

In making choices, it's beneficial to take a broad view of iron supplements in correcting anemia. There are many more options available now than in the past. When dramatic ongoing blood loss is not a factor, the traditional treatment has been iron tablets as directed. If constipation or cramps occur with the tablets, the liquid iron Feosol, taken as directed, often serves as a suitable alternate.

Occasionally we see women who have absolutely no intestinal tolerance for any oral supplement. They, too, have options, both in the long-standing route of intramuscular iron injections, involving a whole series of strategies for where and when to give the injections, and more recently, with iron supplements given intravenously. The latter has proved to be a tremendous source of elemental iron, circumventing the problem of low absorption rates of iron in pill form and providing a quick route to raise hemoglobin. In one patient, hemoglobin count was raised from 7 to 10 grams on the basis of a single day's intravenous infusion of 500 milligrams of elemental iron.

NUTRITIONAL THERAPY.   Once illness and acute anemia have been ruled out, in consultation with your doctor you may determine that a broader-based program of nutritional therapy is best to build up the red blood cells. The three most common nutritional deficiencies—in iron, vitamin B_{12}, and folic acid—can largely be eliminated by improving your diet.

Iron Requirements in the Daily Diet

The amount of iron the average American woman consumes daily falls almost a full 40 percent *below* the recommended dietary allowance, making this nutrient the most deficient in her diet. This is not always out of neglect, either. You can be fully aware of your special needs (blood loss, pregnancy, and so on), make an attempt to compensate for them by increasing your iron, and still end up anemic. The problem lies in the bioavailability of iron: only a small percentage of the iron you consume is actually absorbed by your body.

Granted, a large number of women can remain perfectly healthy on, say, 70 percent of the RDA, since there is such a wide margin of safety factored into the recommended daily allowances. But if intake and absorption are low enough, anemia can result.

To help get the full RDA for iron, women in the childbearing years need to consume 18 milligrams of iron a day. That's a tall order. In many cases it may mean you will need to take iron supplements or a multivitamin with iron. Although there are a few exceptions, most women seem to be able to tolerate vitamins with iron better than medicinal preparations of iron alone. Iron supplements also need vitamin C or other acids for good absorption. Remember, however, that once menopause is over and menstruation has ceased, the RDA goes down to about 10 milligrams a day.

There are four main steps you can take to encourage your body to absorb more of the iron in the foods you eat, or even in the supplements you take.

1. *Plan your diet with an awareness of the kind of iron you give your body.* There are actually two kinds of iron: heme iron from animal foods and

nonheme iron from plants. While the body is capable of assimilating as much as 40 percent of the heme iron carried in red meats, shellfish, and other animal foods, it absorbs less than 10 percent of the nonheme iron present in plants. (See page 288 for a list of nonheme foods containing iron.)

While there are many foods that are "enriched with iron," the iron added to processed foods is very much like nonheme iron in terms of its absorption. That is why eating a bowl of cereal from the package that states "fortified with 100 percent of your RDA for iron" probably will *not* meet your iron needs for the day. Don't jump to the conclusion that cereals, grains, and other plant foods are useless iron sources, however, and that you must now choose only animal foods over plant foods.

2. *Eat foods rich in ascorbic and other acids.* By increasing the acidity in the GI tract, you can help increase absorption of both nonheme and heme iron. For example, drink juice or eat a food that contains vitamin C at the same meal; orange juice, grapefruit, or tomatoes will enhance iron absorption. Something about the presence of acid makes the situation more conducive to absorbing both forms of iron.

This strategy is especially important if you limit your intake of animal foods, because it helps compensate for the decreased amount of heme iron you would have gotten from eating meat. Good to moderate iron absorption results when you eat carrots, potatoes, beets (not the greens), pumpkin, broccoli, cauliflower, cabbage, turnips, or sauerkraut, since all of these contain substantial amounts of malic, citric, or ascorbic acid.

On the other hand, the iron in foods high in phytates—wheat germ, butter beans, spinach, lentils, and beet greens, for example—is generally thought to be poorly absorbed, since phytates chelate iron, reducing absorption of the mineral. Some doubt has been cast on the importance of this effect, however, in tests that indicate both rats and anemic pigs seem to absorb iron equally well from phytate-rich and phytate-poor diets.

3. *Use combination foods.* Including heme iron in a meal further increases the absorption of nonheme iron. A bowl of red chili is a good example of how to make the most of a meal, at least where iron absorption is concerned. Most chili is made from beans (a nonheme iron source), chopped beef (a heme iron source) and tomatoes (a source of vitamin C). Once you catch on, you'll see how easy it is to find iron-rich combination foods.

4. *When the goal is to increase iron, avoid caffeine during the same meal.* The caffeine in tea, coffee, and soft drinks inhibits the absorption of iron. To benefit from the iron in foods, avoid caffeine for at least 30 to 45 minutes before and after a meal. Also limit tea intake, because the tannins in tea further lower iron absorption.

Vitamin B_{12} and Folic Acid Deficiencies

Other kinds of anemia involve shortages in B_{12} or folic acid, both of which are necessary for production of red blood cells. Years ago, B_{12}-*deficient anemia*—referred to as pernicious anemia—was far more common than it is today. It was usually caused by inadequate absorption of vitamin B_{12} through the stomach. *Folate anemia*, like B_{12}-deficient anemia, is often referred to as macrocytic anemia, with blood cells becoming larger rather than smaller, as with iron deficiency anemia.

Both anemias can occur not only in people who are malnourished or have certain stomach disorders but also in those who abuse alcohol. Alcohol uses up body stores of these and other important nutrients. Once identified, treatment of these anemias is extremely simple: for B_{12}-deficient anemia, a monthly injection of vitamin B_{12}; for folate anemia, a tablet that is easily absorbed. If B_{12}-deficient anemia is due to pernicious anemia, the vitamin B_{12} injections will be needed for a lifetime.

CHAPTER 9

Lungs and Respiratory Tract

TO ENSURE THE GOOD HEALTH of your 35-plus lungs and respiratory tract, your primary goal should be to protect them from damage. By way of the air you breathe, your lungs are your body's only internal organ directly exposed to the outside world. Because of this, they're designed with a remarkably intricate and efficient filtering system that is crucial in preserving their health and ability. The same environment that supplies vital oxygen also contains poisons from air pollutants, environmental hazards over which we have too little control. In smokers, additional toxins are deliberately introduced to the lungs. The lungs work to filter out toxic substances, and most of the time they succeed very well; but if the filtering system is overwhelmed, the lungs and the body are placed at serious risk.

The Cardiopulmonary Team

If the heart is the pump, the lungs are the bellows, sucking in air as the chest cavity expands and expelling it as the cavity contracts. Every breath supplies the body with the mother lode of oxygen that the red blood cells pick up in the cells in the lung and deliver, via the heart's pumping action, to all the tissues in the body. That's only on an intake of a breath. On an exhale, carbon dioxide, the waste product of the respiratory system, is carried back to the lungs by way of the vein capillaries and expelled.

The air we inhale, about fifteen breaths per minute through the nose or mouth from the moment after birth, is really just a big blast of raw material that the respiratory system, acting as a giant refinery, continuously processes for delivery to the circulatory system, filtering, warming, cleaning, and carrying off waste.

The refining process begins as tonsils and adenoids meet an incoming breath at the entrance of the throat, filtering out infectious agents. Mucus secreted from tiny gland cells all through the passage linings trap impurities from the air and add moisture to prevent the lungs from drying out. Hairlike cilia—millions of them in every square inch of the mucous membrane lining the respiratory tract—keep a fresh supply of mucus moving, systematically getting rid of trapped dirt and impurities by moving them up from the bottom of the lungs and out through the nasal passage, or throat. The millions of delicate cilia are vital; when damaged or slowed down by cigarette smoke and various gases in the air, they leave the way open for infection and disease.

Purified air reaches each lung by way of the bronchial tree, traveling through increasingly smaller subdivisions to the millions of bronchioles, or small airways, that lead to the alveoli. These small sacs (about 300 million of them) carry the oxygen to the blood vessels in the lungs and hence into the bloodstream, where the oxygen generates heat and other forms of energy for the body through chemical reactions.

That's what happens with every breath!

With their built-in protective mechanisms, healthy lungs will work efficiently for the rest of your life—provided they get optimum working conditions.

LUNG PROTECTION AT 35-PLUS

There are four ways to ensure optimum conditions for your lungs.

Choose a Nonsmoking Environment

If you smoke, you must stop now. Smoking cigarettes is a progressive risk. This means that if you are a smoker, by the time you are 35, your chances of getting sick increase with every cigarette you smoke. That's not just the risk of lung cancer, either. A two-pack-a-day smoker shortens her life by an average of eight years, but even the light smoker who smokes less than half a pack daily shortens her life expectancy by approximately four years, risking not only lung but heart disease and debilitating, irreversible emphysema.

Smoking is a compelling physical addiction. Some people can quit in one round, while other would-be nonsmokers need several attempts, each representing a step forward toward permanent quitting. And thanks to the surgeon general's antismoking campaign, one way or another literally millions of hardcore smokers have succeeded in permanently cutting cigarettes out of their lives.

Don't let the claims of lower tar or "light" touted in the commercials fool you. Every cigarette, even the lightest, most exotically filtered brand, contains over 200 identifiable poisons: tar and nicotine, but also arsenic, cyanide, formaldehyde, carbon dioxide, carbon monoxide, and phenol. All of them enter the body through the lungs.

Today, because more women smoke than in the past, a whole new body of health risks linked to smoking has come to light:

- In 1986, lung cancer surpassed breast cancer as the number-one killer of women.
- A 35-plus smoker who uses birth-control pills has ten times the normal risk of a heart attack and twenty times the risk of a cerebral hemorrhage.
- Smoking during pregnancy increases the chance of premature birth, miscarriage, and sudden-infant-death syndrome. Intrauterine pictures show with startling clarity the effects of smoking on an unborn baby's circulatory system. The mother inhales one or two puffs on a cigarette, and the delicate network of capillaries in the baby's fingers constrict, their blood supply decreasing and temporarily disappearing from view. If this is happening in the baby's fingers, might one ask what is happening in the baby's brain?
- Studies now link smoking to early menopause.

On and on, new facts and statistics on mortality are published. Next year there will probably be more of them. But one of the most tragic effects of smoking is emphysema—and we've known about that risk for years.

Emphysema, often called COPD, or chronic obstructive pulmonary disease, is a progressive disease of the lungs that occurs almost exclusively in smokers as a result of damage done by cigarette tars. For patients with severe emphysema, there can be some medical stabilization and nutritional support including special food supplements, but that's about it.

A one-pack-a-day smoker puts approximately one quart of tobacco tars into her lungs every year—sticky, chemical-laden tars that can destroy the walls of the delicate, grapelike clusters of tiny air sacs making up the lungs. As more and more of these tiny walls break down, damage that progresses with every pack of cigarettes smoked, the lungs eventually lose their elasticity and ability to function; they cannot shrink down and blow air out. As a result, the body gets too little oxygen and retains too much carbon dioxide. Thus emphysema slowly kills its victim by smothering her to death from a lack of oxygen. To repeat, the damage is irreversible, so while existing damage will always remain, the only "cure" is to arrest its further progress.

What is the option, then, for women who smoke today? To quit. It's that simple.

What about "passive" smoke inhalation? Fortunately, because of the growing evidence that sidestream smoke (smoke inhaled by nonsmokers) is a serious health risk, laws are going into effect that limit smoking in public places. This, coupled with the increasingly popular perception of smoking as downright socially unacceptable, puts new pressure on all smokers to quit—and encourages those who love them to *insist* they quit.

Eat Properly and Exercise Regularly

Keeping the body fit with good nourishment and exercise is one of the best routes to providing optimum conditions for the lungs. In addition to respiration, the lungs also perform important metabolic tasks, which include processing a wide variety of chemicals carried to them by the blood. One example of these is the formation of angiotensin II, one of the body's most powerful natural substances used in maintaining blood pressure.

Reduce the Spread of Germs

It is almost impossible to keep a cold from spreading among family members or colleagues at work; the germs are there before the symptoms give the tip-off. But there are commonsense ways that you can help slow the spread of germs.

- Cover all sneezes and coughs, and during "cold season" keep boxes of tissues around the house, readily available. Dispose of used tissues at once.
- If you have young school-age children, insist they wash their hands the moment they return from school. It's a good idea for everyone, especially commuters, to wash their hands when they first come home, and certainly before meals.
- Keep bathroom sink areas and the space where you prepare food in the kitchen extra clean. With small children sharing the bathroom, think of ways to provide alternatives to "communal" toothbrush holders, and give each child his or her own cup—or use paper cups.
- Unless they are kept scrupulously clean, humidifiers can actually grow germs and spread more infections into the atmosphere. If you use a humidifier, follow the instructions and be extra cautious in keeping it clean.

Get Prompt Medical Attention When Necessary

Don't neglect yourself. It is not uncommon for 35-plus women to take admirable care of their children's respiratory illnesses and then neglect their own, out of a sense of urgency involved in juggling jobs and living up to a hectic array of commitments. Your first responsibility is to yourself. Chest congestion (coughs that last more than four to five days), progressive shortness of breath, or coughs marked by yellow-green, gray, or blood-flecked sputum all warrant medical consultation. The most common bacterial infections can be eliminated far more effectively and quickly with antibiotics than by "waiting them out," which can lead to bronchitis, walking pneumonia, and worse.

David Cogan on Cold and Cough Medications

Treatments for coping with colds cover a wide spectrum. Whether the cold medicine is nonprescription or stronger (that is, stronger than what may be available in your medicine cabinet), it makes good sense to check with your doctor before taking any cold medications. (For treatment of sore throats, see page 116.)

Match Cough Medications to Cough Symptoms

When someone has a productive cough—meaning it brings up phlegm—it is important not to use a suppressant. Rather, you want to get the congestion up and out with an expectorant. In this case, use Robitussin plain—that is, Robitussin without any initials on the label—or its equivalent. If the cough becomes dry and unproductive—what is referred to as a hacking cough—then a mild over-the-counter suppressant such as Robitussin-DM might be used.

For coughs that are too harsh or too difficult to be handled by over-the-counter preparations, a mid-strength cough suppressant such as promethazine with or without codeine, elixir of terpin hydrate with or without codeine, or a prescription form of Robitussin (Robitussin DAC) may prove effective.

For the rare individual who needs an extremely strong cough suppressant, the stronger narcotic cough syrups such as Hycodan or Tussionex may be prescribed.

Match Allergy and Cold Products to Cause

Choose remedies for nasal congestion with the source of congestion in mind, and with an awareness that some remedies can cause drowsiness. For a clear-cut case of nasal congestion without allergy, pseudoephedrine, the most popular of which is Sudafed, is recommended. The generic product is just as effective and much cheaper than the brand name. Pseudoephedrine does not cause drowsiness, but in high doses it can act like caffeine.

When congestion occurs in the presence of an allergy, I usually recommend Dimetapp in tablet form, since it combines an antihistamine with a decongestant, as do Actifed or Drixoral. It should be noted that these combinations can cause drowsiness.

Read All Labels

Many over-the-counter cold and cough remedies have a surprisingly high alcohol base and should be avoided.

Avoid Multipurpose Cold Preparations

Most all-in-one cough-cold preparations—Vicks Formula 44, for example
—have at least six to eight medicines in them, including the problematic
decongestant phenylpropanolamine, a drug that can cause a high degree of
emotionality in some individuals. When there are adverse reactions to drugs
that combine so many medicines, it is impossible to pinpoint the source of
the problem.

A Word About Vitamin C

Though some people swear by it, evidence supporting the effectiveness of
vitamin C in treating or preventing colds and upper respiratory infections
isn't very consistent. Many studies lack proper controls; those that are scientifically sound usually suggest that the use of vitamin C leads to a slight
but not very significant difference in the number and duration of colds.

The best way to get vitamin C is to drink fruit juices and eat fruits and
vegetables daily. Also, there is evidence that smoking destroys vitamin C,
so if you are still trying to kick the habit, taking a supplement, in addition
to eating foods high in vitamin C, may be a good idea.

If you do decide to take supplements, you should be aware that there
may be side effects with large doses. Here again reports conflict, but various
studies show side effects beginning at 1,500 to 2,000 milligrams a day; these
can include diarrhea, kidney stones and urine samples that indicate a high
blood sugar when you don't have it (see Chapter 21 for more on megadoses).

ALLERGIES

While most of us don't suffer from chronic or acute allergic reactions, some
adults find their resistance to certain allergies progressively diminishes, particularly those caused by pollens. When that happens, high pollen counts
can indeed become their seasonal curse.

Allergies can be triggered by foods such as cow's milk or eggs, by plant
substances including pollen and plant molds, and even by household dust
or pet cats. (In the latter, suspected allergens are now thought to be in the
cat's saliva, not the fur.) With an allergic reaction, certain signals in the
body's immune system are mixed up in such a way that the body reacts to
ordinary, harmless elements as if they were invaders. The result is a chain
of events that is identical in all cases: the release of powerful chemical
substances (histamines) that trap the invaders (most commonly in the respiratory or intestinal tracts); at the same time, the histamines irritate
nearby body tissues, causing any number and degree of reactions including
hives, skin inflammations, asthma, or allergic rhinitis—the proverbial hay

fever—with its sneezing, runny nose, itchy eyes, and sinus irritation. Allergies to pollen tend to be both predictable and progressive; once someone becomes sensitized to the proteins in the local ragweed or autumn molds, the reaction only gets worse. If you were to view one of these prickly airborne irritants under a microscope, you would see immediately why it causes sneezes and tickles in the nose. Since many of them resemble burrs and miniature cacti, it's no wonder your body treats them like invaders.

Treatment of Allergies

It seems we are on the verge of big changes in the area of allergy treatment, based on a dramatic new discovery of what causes them.

Up until now, the main preventive treatment for allergies has been to use drugs that desensitize a person to the particular allergen involved, a process that can take many months and involve many allergy shots. But according to reports published in *Nature* in January 1989, and hailed as "a landmark accomplishment in allergy research," a team of scientists working out of the National Institutes of Health in Bethesda, Maryland, has now discovered the cell-surface receptor to which antibodies bind in a crucial early stage of an allergic reaction. The next step—finding inhibiting drugs either to block the cell receptor or to prevent the release of those powerful histamines—is apparently just on the horizon, with the potential for treating allergies earlier and with far more effectiveness than ever before.

In the meantime, the standard route for treating allergies involves proper identification of the allergen, usually by an allergist, so that an effective medication can be chosen and a program of desensitization can begin.

Specific treatments of allergies are determined by the severity of the allergic reaction. All but the most severe cases should focus on the least aggressive method, starting with avoidance of the substance known to cause the allergy. In those rare cases where all else fails and symptoms are unbearable, the next step is to move to allergy shots, but only when the exact cause of the allergy has been specified.

When you cannot avoid the cause of your allergy and the symptoms create real discomfort, certain drugs can help, and it is worthwhile to discuss them with your physician. These include antihistamines (not decongestants), of which there are literally dozens. Many of them are sold over the counter and tend to be remarkably similar variations on chlorpheniramine maleate (trade name Chlor-Trimeton). Most of these preparations cause drowsiness, but the new, fairly expensive mid-strength antihistamine terfenadine (Seldane), eliminates that side effect with great success.

SINUS TROUBLE

Sinus congestion and sinus infection (sinusitis) are common problems in 35-plus women who have seasonal allergies or prolonged upper-respiratory infections.

If sinus congestion is the only problem—stuffiness, clear mucus drainage—a combination of antihistamines and decongestants like pseudo-ephedrine (Sudafed) can be tried. If there are signs of sinus infection—tenderness to the touch over the sinuses and production of dark yellow, green, or brown mucus—antibiotic treatment may be needed. Sinusitis is hard to treat, and prolonged treatment of up to several weeks is sometimes needed.

Smoking is a major sinus irritant and should be stopped in the presence of sinus congestion or infection.

ASTHMA

Asthma involves reversible spasm—that is, constriction and contraction of the bronchial tubes that carry oxygen from the mouth and nose to the lungs. While the overall incidence decreases over a lifetime, asthma can be a problem for those 35-plus women with prolonged encounters with smoking, air pollutants, and various airborne irritants.

The first step for treating asthma—in tandem with stopping smoking, if that is involved—is usually to determine or rule out allergies. Thus an allergist can be invaluable in evaluation and treatment, which may include anti-allergy medication.

Recent years have brought steady advances in the medicinal treatment of asthma. The long-used aminophylline drugs that act to dilate, or open up, the airways continue to be a prime treatment, and they can be taken in pill form at home or given by vein in an emergency. We witnessed the effectiveness of this drug during hospital rounds, when we encountered a frightened, gasping woman in the throes of an acute asthma attack who literally could not breathe. As others nearby panicked, the attending physician spoke in calm, quiet tones, firmly urging the woman to breathe "slowly and deeply" as she received an infusion of aminophylline. His calming presence helped, and the medication worked in a very short time.

Other asthma medications can be given in spray form, as bronchodilators, to open up the airways. These include albuterol (Proventil), and for some patients with asthma this is the only treatment necessary. Primatene Mist, advertised on television, is a similar spray although a milder one, but very few serious asthmatics can get by on it alone.

In more serious situations, cortisone medications (steroids) are given, sometimes chronically—for months, years, or even a lifetime if that is the only option. These can be given in sprays, pill form, or intravenously.

Sometimes asthma "fades" with age, sometimes it does not, but if a patient works with her regular doctor, severe flare-ups of asthma can usually be avoided and hospitalization should be a rare event.

CHAPTER 10

The Digestive System

THE DIGESTIVE SYSTEM—or as it is also known, the gastrointestinal (GI) or alimentary tract—is the main pipeline of the body's fueling system. It processes all solid foods, liquids, and most oral medications for absorption into the bloodstream. By midlife, the digestive system has seen many rounds of action. For the average 35-year-old American woman who eats three meals a day, the GI tract has processed over 38,000 meals. Depending on your diet and life-style it is either running as smoothly as ever or showing signs of wear and tear. Gastrointestinal disorders can develop anywhere along the GI tract, with the most common complaints of 35-plus women centering either on pain in the upper or lower abdomen or on problems with bowel function, especially constipation.

Children tend to be amused and a bit mystified by all the attention adults seem to pay to digestion and "regularity." The number of ads for antacids and laxatives on television alone is a strong indication of our preoccupation with this topic. The ads would have you believe that the iron stomachs of youth grow up to become delicate, cranky, and tired, needing the support of stimulants, laxatives, magnesias, mineral oils, and softeners. This is pure sales pitch; in fact, it can be a dangerous line to pursue. Each of these works in a different way, but each can cause dependence, actually reducing the ability of your body to digest and eliminate food properly. The best way to get your digestive system into shape and keep it in working order is through diet. As specific problems crop up throughout this chapter, both diet and medical solutions will be suggested.

But first, we'll start at the top, since the GI tract begins at the mouth.

THE MOUTH, TEETH, AND THROAT

Good dental hygiene and care of the teeth (see Chapter 7) is important not merely for the sake of a beautiful smile but also to ensure good chewing, which is vital to preparing food for digestion. While your dentist is probably the first person you'd call with a "tooth problem," people often confuse medical problems of the mouth—lips, palate, tongue, and soft tissue, for example—with dental problems, and vice versa. Your personal doctor can really help in delineating any mouth problems by doing a thorough examination in the office and, if necessary, ordering the appropriate X-rays.

Furthermore, any unexplained soreness, swelling, or nonhealing problem with mouth, tongue, or lips that continues for as long as two weeks clearly warrrants a thorough examination by your physician, mainly to rule out other illnesses. This is especially true for those women who smoke cigarettes, where the rate of oral cancer is much higher than for others and unfortunately is rising.

Gum Disease

Gingivitis and other serious problems with the gums and alveolar (jaw) bone are properly treated by a periodontist (see Chapter 7), although some gingival conditions may be caused by poor nutrition and can be treated medically and nutritionally. Cigarette smoking is also a primary irritant to the gums and a factor in gingivitis. (Gingivitis sometimes appears in chronic alcoholics, but in these cases it is usually the result of global malnutrition and vitamin deficiency rather than of specific problems located in the mouth.) Bleeding gums are a sign of possible vitamin C deficiency.

Cold Sores

The lips—the entrance to the mouth—can be a source of discomfort when cold sores caused by a herpes virus (*Herpes labialis*), occur. The treatment for cold sores is largely symptomatic—that is, using nonprescription medications such as petroleum jelly. It is rare for a doctor to use antiviral treatments for this condition, but in cases of severe or recurrent oral herpes, the antiherpetic medicine acyclovir (Zovirax), which is the same medicine used for herpes simplex (see pages 237–238), may be prescribed.

Stomatitis

The mouth can also become inflamed, sometimes in a generalized way but more often in small, separate lesions or sores that can appear on the inside of the lips and sometimes scattered throughout the mouth. Stomatitis is the medical term for this condition, from the Greek *stoma* ("opening") and *itis* ("inflammation"), usually the result of a viral infection of the mouth. Warm saltwater gargles, occasionally combined with cortisone designed for mouth use (specifically the medication Kenalog in Orabase), can be very helpful, as can lidocaine, the topical anesthetic or painkiller in semiliquid form called Viscous Xylocaine.

Thrush

This fungal disease of the mucous membranes usually occurs in infants, but in adults it can herald uncontrolled diabetes or indicate depressed immunity, as with AIDS. The thrush itself is usually easily treated with antifungal lozenges (Mycelex Troches).

Throat Infections

Throat, or pharynx, infections can impede the process of digestion and should be attended to promptly. Such infections usually are viral, but they can also be caused by the streptococcus germ. Diagnosing a viral or strep throat is almost impossible with just an office exam, while a simple and inexpensive throat culture will make the delineation clear within twenty-four hours. If a person has a viral pharyngitis, there isn't a great deal that can be done except for symptomatic support: rest, drinking fluids, and taking aspirin or Tylenol (although the latter in many clinical cases has proved less effective when the pharyngitis includes soft-tissue inflammation). The old-fashioned route of drinking hot tea and lemon (specifically in place of coffee) can make a dramatic improvement with sore throats, as can saltwater gargles (½ teaspoon of salt in a glass of warm water) several times a day. (Fortunately, while it is relatively common in young people, the virus infection of mononucleosis, or "mono," rarely infects 35-plus women.)

If a throat culture comes back positive—indicating streptococcal sore throat (bacterial pharyngitis)—antibiotic treatment such as penicillin or erythromycin is recommended. The earlier strep is diagnosed the better, since complications can arise without treatment.

"Above the neck" infections of the digestive tract involving the lips, mouth, and throat generally are the exception rather than the rule. Cancers of the mouth and throat are risks for anyone using tobacco products, and these risks are enhanced when you drink and smoke at the same time. Positive health choices for 35-plus women—no smoking and limited alcohol intake—will keep problems of the mouth and pharynx to a minimum, at least reduced to the episodic infections that affect virtually everybody.

THE UPPER ABDOMEN—ESOPHAGUS AND STOMACH

A run-through of problems that can occur in the upper abdomen begins with the not-so-obvious issues of inadequate chewing and rapid swallowing —"eating on the run." For many 35-plus women, these are an accepted part of a life-style that sets a premium on being fast at everything. Good, *thorough* chewing provides three major mechanical benefits: it regulates the temperature of the food, breaks it into small morsels and mixes it with the first round of digestive juices contained in the saliva. Eating on the run accomplishes none of these, and often leads to belching, regurgitation, bad breath, stomach discomfort, and other "digestive problems." In fact, these usually have nothing to do with any underlying problem with the esophagus; rather, they are results of hasty eating habits that can easily be altered. Belching, for example, is evidence that air is being swallowed, either consciously (as with seltzer after a meal or in the hope of relieving stomach upset) or unconsciously (gulping air or eating rapidly).

So before jumping to conclusions that you suffer from digestive problems, pay attention to the way you eat. What your mother always told you —take modest bites of food, chew them thoroughly, and wait until you've swallowed one mouthful before taking another—wasn't just a lecture on manners.

The Esophagus

True problems with the esophagus—the food tube between the mouth and stomach—involve either trouble with swallowing (the sensation of food sticking in the upper chest) or pain in the midchest during or after eating. Either of these problems can point to *spasm of the esophageal muscle*—that is, a contraction not part of the expected peristaltic activity—or a spasm of the lower esophageal valve or sphincter, which is termed *achalasia*.

Either condition responds well to the same simple measures described for hasty eating: slower eating and smaller meals. Drinking water when the spasm occurs can help, too. However, if these simple measures don't alleviate the problem, then an exam of the esophagus may be necessary, probably including a barium X-ray (the patient swallows a chalky white substance that shows up on X-rays) and possibly further consultation with a gastroenterologist to determine if true achalasia is the problem. If so, dilation—or spreading apart the valve—might be needed and some persistent cases may call for surgery.

A spasm in the muscles of the esophagus is often relieved by slow and thorough eating and improved chewing habits. Drinking moderate amounts of water at room temperature (not ice water) also helps. Muscle relaxants designed specifically for smooth muscle, such as clidinium bromide, found in Librax, are often very successful in reducing spasm.

More common than either of these spasm complaints is *heartburn,* or what is often described to doctors and dietitians as a burning sensation beneath the sternum, or chest bone, that reaches up to the back of the throat and is accompanied by a sour taste in the mouth. These symptoms can represent gastric reflux, which occurs when the esophageal valve lies open, creating an acid-food backup (hydrochloric acid from the stomach moves back up through the valve opening and into the esophagus), or as the result of a hiatal hernia, when part of the stomach is pushed up through the muscle of the diaphragm where it does not belong, causing the contents of the esophagus to flow sideways around the bump.

Heartburn caused by the lazy-valve syndrome is usually worse after eating and when lying down, which allows the gastric juices to flow more easily into the esophagus. Sometimes, however, people will have the very same reflux problems in a standing position. Discomfort with hiatal hernia is more of a problem because it can damage the esophagus. Sufferers feel worse when they bend over, lie down after a meal, eat large meals, or eat or drink highly acidic foods. Because with hiatal hernia indigestion and heartburn often last for hours, some sufferers arrive in their doctor's office thinking they have symptoms of a heart attack.

Both conditions—gastric reflux and hiatal hernia—can often be relieved or eliminated with simple dietary changes, including weight loss if weight is a problem. In addition, the following have proved useful to 90 percent of our patients who complain about these conditions:

Coping with Heartburn or Hiatal Hernia

- Work to pinpoint and eliminate stress, which aggravates these conditions and makes it hard to get rid of them.
- Eat small, leisurely paced meals.
- Sip small amounts of water at meals, but don't drink too much. This will help prevent an overfull stomach. Drink fluids between meals to compensate.
- Cut out dairy products if they seem to cause heartburn, a sour taste in the mouth, or belching. While dairy products are traditionally thought of as good for the stomach, the opposite holds true for some people, especially those who are lactose-intolerant.
- Eliminate, or strongly decrease, all caffeine, alcoholic beverages, and citrus fruits if these appear to be implicated.
- Don't smoke. Smoking—more specifically nicotine—stimulates acid secretion.
- Prevent food in the stomach from flowing back up and causing dis-

comfort at night by not eating or drinking anything two to three hours before bedtime.

- Before going to sleep, elevate the upper body slightly with pillows, or raise the mattress under the head of the bed with a few bricks or wood blocks. Keeping the head higher than the feet may help prevent stomach acid from backing up into the esophagus.

If these methods don't bring relief, the next strategy is to use antacids such as Mylanta or Maalox, which neutralize acids, or acid blockers such as cimetidine (Tagamet) or ranitidine (Zantac), which act to block their production. The bedtime dose is especially important in controlling reflux. If symptoms of reflux or hiatal hernia persist, discuss them with your doctor, who may want to schedule a workup to rule out a narrowing of the esophagus, called a stricture or, in the rare case, a tumor of the esophagus.

Esophagitis—inflammation of the lower esophagus—and gastritis—its correlate in the stomach—often involve too much acidity. As with heartburn, they are usually associated with burning pain. Neither will show up on an X-ray, and only to some extent on an endoscopy (in which a flexible fiber optic tube is passed through the mouth into the esophagus and, if indicated, into the stomach). Both problems may respond partly to a drink of water and more completely to taking antacids and acid blockers described earlier. The symptoms overlap; indeed, the symptoms of gastritis can even overlap those of peptic ulcer disease. Both gastritis and esophagitis can usually be treated to resolution with a program of antacids and acid blockers over the course of several weeks.

Ulcers

The stomach completes the first phase, or preparatory work, of digestion begun when you chew and swallow food. A powerful muscle that resembles a deflated football, the stomach churns the food and mixes it with digestive juices or enzymes that are stimulated by powerful hormones and released from the stomach lining. In this scorchingly acid environment, solids and semisolids are turned into a smooth paste and moved on into the small intestine, the main site for digestion and absorption. Owing to the intensely acidic conditions needed for digestion, peptic ulcer disease can occur in the stomach and in the first section of the small intestine, or duodenum. Most ulcers occur in the duodenum and are, in general, more likely to be benign than those in the stomach. Just as esophagitis often responds well to simple treatments, so do ulcers, as we describe later. However, stomach ulcers especially need careful follow-up, including endoscopy, to be certain the ulcer heals.

Ulcer disease used to be thought of as primarily a "male" disease, but as more women enter the occupations that traditionally have kept men actively stressed—often while maintaining their roles as homemakers and mothers—there has been an increased incidence of peptic ulcer disease among them.

The hallmark of an ulcer is a persistent burning sensation in the pit of the stomach, usually more noticeable after meals and often during the night or in the morning. The ulcer develops in part of the stomach or duodenal wall, in craterlike fashion. This part of the wall is destroyed or eaten away by gastric acid, exposing nerves to the acid and causing pain. The ulcer may bleed. If it bleeds over a long period of time, the individual may become anemic (see page 104).

Only an upper GI (an X-ray of the esophagus and stomach using barium) or an endoscopy can really diagnose an ulcer, although several symptoms point toward the diagnosis, especially in the context of known risk factors. Poor health habits aggravate symptoms and may be contributing factors in causing ulcers. Factors such as stress, too much coffee, and smoking all have a high correlation with both the onset of the disease and its recurrence.

Often a person will have symptoms of gastritis or ulcer disease, and yet the tests will show negative. In this case, the diagnosis is usually excessive acidity—an important and very real entity, especially if stress is involved. This ulcerlike problem when no ulcer is involved will often respond to antacids and acid blockers like cimetidine (Tagamet). Sometimes, a glass of tap water helps, probably because it dilutes acidity.

Treating Ulcers

Diet is still a prime consideration when it comes to treating an ulcer, but now the approach is much simpler, much less restricting, and much easier than it was in the past. With the exception of those elements which increase acid secretion—cigarette smoking, alcohol, and caffeine—there are no longer any "forbidden foods."

For many years, ulcers were treated with a bland diet that included large amounts of milk and cream. Thirty years ago, some patients with ulcers were served cream that was 45 percent fat. Sufferers were directed to avoid fiber, acids, alcohol, caffeine, and spicy foods, and to take frequent sips of milk because milk was believed to coat the ulcers. Thus evolved what was referred to as a "sippy" diet.

As research continued and new drugs were developed, it became clear that the ulcer diet did not have to be this restricted—except perhaps in the very beginning. In fact, milk and other proteins that slow down acid production temporarily can often lead to an acid rebound; that is, while the milk is in the stomach little acid is released, but after it passes into the duodenum and jejunum, the stomach actually produces more acid than it did before the milk was introduced.

Today acid production is controlled by medication, either antacids or, more commonly, the acid blockers already noted in the treatment of hiatal hernia. The initial course of medication is usually at least six weeks. Although milk and dairy products are still important for general nutrition, most individuals with ulcers can enjoy more foods; in fact, they are actually encouraged to do so, since too strict a diet may lead to nutrient deficiency. Borderline ascorbic-acid deficiencies have developed when the diet tightly restricts fresh fruits and vegetables, as was the case with an elderly lady who came in with symptoms indicating the beginning of scurvy. She had stopped eating fresh fruits and vegetables when she'd had an ulcer—years ago. Though the ulcer had long since healed, she was still restricting the main sources of vitamin C in her diet. If a diet high in fiber causes a problem when there is an active ulcer, obviously high-fiber foods are to be avoided, but once the ulcer has healed, there is no reason not to go back to a high-fiber diet that includes plenty of fruits and vegetables—in fact, there are good reasons to do so.

Here are general guidelines for speeding the healing of peptic ulcers:

- Proceed without restrictions but with caution, especially when you suspect your favorite plate of enchiladas or bowl of chili or curried chicken is causing you stomach upset. Avoid specific foods that cause problems, but enjoy the ones that don't.
- When the preference is to start out on a bland diet, do not rely on milk alone but rather on a combination of easy-to-digest foods like rice, noodles, mashed potatoes, chicken (not fried, of course), boiled carrots, or applesauce. To these, add the glass of milk.
- Avoid alcohol, which may irritate an ulcer since it stimulates secretion of gastric acid.
- Avoid both regular and decaffeinated coffee (yes, decaffeinated; stomach irritants still remain from the roasting process).
- Proceed cautiously with soft drinks and soda, since they bother some people; also, if they irritate, avoid other acidic liquids such as vinegar and lemon, pineapple, orange, tomato, and cranberry juices. You may be able to tolerate them simply by adding them to your meal in a different sequence—for example, by eating your breakfast and then having your fruit or juice.
- To help reduce the pain of ulcers, eat small meals and eat often. An empty stomach still produces gastric acid, which makes for a highly acidic environment. Food and liquid lower the pH and buffer the stomach so that the juices do less damage.

The key in treating active peptic ulcer disease as well as acidity requires persistent, cooperative work with your physician, well after the ulcer has healed. If you have ever had an active peptic ulcer, you will always be at some risk for a recurrence. In some cases, chronic acid blocker use may be needed, but just as healthy eating decreases the risk of esophagitis and gastritis, so too it will help relieve stomach acidity and peptic ulcer disease.

THE LOWER DIGESTIVE TRACT

The GI tract includes the small intestine, connected to the stomach, and the large intestine. The lower five to seven feet of the digestive tract is the site of common, related problems of constipation, diarrhea, and diverticulosis. If these conditions sound like nuisance issues relegated to old age, revise your thinking. In our society they are so closely intertwined with diet, stress, and hasty eating habits that many people in their thirties, forties, and fifties suffer from them.

In the small intestine (divided into the duodenum, the jejunum, and the ileum), digestive juices produced by the pancreas, and some that are stored in the gallbladder, complete the digestive process, passing nutrients through the intestinal wall and into the bloodstream where, through a variety of mechanisms, they are metabolized and carried to the vital organs, muscles, and other body tissues. In the pleated folds of its interior wall and millions of tiny villi "fingers," the small intestine performs its task of chemical absorption through a surface area that would, if stretched out flat, cover two tennis courts.

A healthy colon is a working colon—that is, one that gets the kind of high-fiber materials it was designed to use in the job of processing the body's waste for removal. But these foods are sorely lacking in most Americans' diets, replaced instead with foods so refined (that is, highly processed, low-fiber, high-fat foods) that not much bulk is left when the food finally reaches the colon. Thus, the active, muscular bands in the colon wall barely get a workout.

The main functions of the large intestine, or colon, are not digestion or nutrition absorption as such, but rather the reabsorption of water and electrolytes (potassium and sodium, for example) in the liquid stool, and finally the evacuation of waste.

If you were lacking a large intestine, you could actually continue to feed the body by ingesting food in the usual way, but you couldn't do so without the small intestine, which is where most nutrient absorption takes place. An inflamed small intestine, in fact, can result in malabsorption, with resulting weight loss and diarrhea. This is a common site of Crohn's disease, one of the inflammatory bowel diseases.

As with any other muscle, the less the colon functions, the weaker it becomes. In time, weak spots develop in the walls of the inactive, underused colon. Consequently, when constipation causes pressure to build in the colon, sacs or pouches called diverticuli can form. The presence of these diverticuli indicate the condition called diverticulosis.

Diverticulosis and Constipation

In our society, *diverticular disease* frequently develops in people 50 years of age and over; in this age group its incidence exceeds 50 percent—all because of life-style and low-fiber diet. Symptoms are not always obvious, and most people do not know they have diverticular disease, feeling only a vague discomfort or mild, intermittent pain in the lower left quadrant of the abdomen. While these symptoms do not necessarily get worse, they can become chronic and progress to full-blown diverticulitis with its active inflammation, infection, and in some cases (though by no means the majority of them), perforation. Once diverticula form, nothing can reverse the process, although diet can halt further progress.

Women over 35 take note: give the underemployed colon more work to do and modify your diet by increasing fiber so as to increase the bulk of the stool, reduce constipation, and relieve pressure within the colon. The earlier you improve the fiber content of your diet, the better your chance of preventing diverticulosis.

Constipation has been described in some of the earliest medical writings, yet it continues to present a challenge. Many physicians and health professionals tend to regard it as a low-priority complaint, a minor management issue that is part and parcel of the sedentary life-style so many Americans embrace. Most patients who complain about constipation have a poor knowledge of what their bowel function should be. While a bowel movement every other day is normal for some adults, having one daily or even twice daily is the ideal. In a survey of the general population, at least 10 percent of people of all ages indicated they actually *prefer* to be constipated; the remaining 90 percent simply ignore the dietary aspects of the problem and instead find their solution in widely advertised, so-called safe and gentle laxatives.

Actually, there is no one thing that works for constipation—no single laxative, food, or fluid. "Curing" constipation involves a combined effort to address motility and bowel function, both vital to the well-being of a healthy colon. Followed on a daily basis, our program has succeeded for people who have had problems with constipation for ten or twenty years. It works not only to cure constipation and hemorrhoids, but also to eliminate the cycle of alternating constipation and diarrhea that can be accompanied by cramps.

Preventing Constipation

CUT OUT LAXATIVES. That is, eliminate any existing dependency on laxatives, even those that claim to be "gentle."

Specific bulk-forming agents such as Metamucil or Konsyl are much preferred over regular laxatives, especially those such as Ex-Lax or Correc-tol. In the rare instances when a person occasionally needs a true laxative (after consultation with a physician), the old standby milk of magnesia probably is the safest.

INCREASE FLUIDS TO INCREASE BOWEL MOTILITY. Before launching a high-fiber diet, you should understand that fiber is not the be-all and end-all of good bowel function. You could eat oat bran muffins at every meal, but unless you take in adequate fluids, the transit time of the fiber through the system will be too slow to keep the contents of the bowel moving on a regular schedule. Ample fluids will keep the peristalsis going. This may seem obvious, but many women forget to drink all day long, and only have a cup of coffee in the morning, maybe two, then a diet drink at lunch and then nothing until they get home in the evening. You need water to prevent constipation. Apple juice, which is in itself a mild cathar-tic, is good, too. The fluid requirements for each person vary depending on total body size. A petite woman needs five to six 8-ounce glasses of fluids a day; a larger woman requires eight 8-ounce glasses. Coffee, tea, and other drinks count in total fluid intake, as do foods themselves, but drinking ample water is encouraged. Keep a carafe of water near your work area and make it a habit to drink water during the day.

A daily cup of coffee or tea has proved helpful in working against constipation. In some cases of very resistant constipation, a cup of herbal tea (senna) seems to have a mild cathartic effect—but don't drink more than one cup a day.

RELAX. While diet is the central issue in greater than 90 percent of all cases of constipation, it is not the only issue. As pointed out earlier, a hurry-up life-style with poor eating habits can affect digestion. It can also affect regularity. If you habitually postpone or suppress the urge—or, con-versely, you try to force a bowel movement—you will do little more than encourage constipation and hemorrhoids.

INCREASE FIBER TO INCREASE BOWEL FUNCTION. Apples, pears, green beans, and broccoli—fiber is supplied by many foods, not just wheat and oats, that should be part of your diet.

Fruit provides ample fiber, as do vegetables. Some vegetables, including broccoli, green beans, and cauliflower, tend to encourage intestinal gas when eaten raw; cook them if they affect you this way. Contrary to what you might hear, cooking vegetables does not destroy their soluble or insol-uble fiber content, no matter how long you cook them. Studies have shown as much as a 93 percent recovery of insoluble vegetable fiber passed in feces. Overcooking does, however, destroy many vitamins and makes most fresh vegetables less palatable.

At least one portion of fresh fruits or vegetables should be part of each meal, a recommendation that is further elaborated in the tips that follow. Wheat and oat bran are beneficial additions to a daily diet, not only for elimination but also to help reduce blood cholesterol. We think fresh fruit with an oat-bran muffin or bran cereal is an ideal way to start each morning. Although we universally advise having breakfast, when you get your bran is not critical. You could have a bran muffin or even cereal at noon, or as a midafternoon or late-evening snack. Here are other easy ways to increase fiber in your diet.

Kitchen-Wise Hints for Increasing Fiber in Your Diet

Every 35-plus woman (and her family) can benefit from increasing the amount of fiber in her diet, but there's no need to get overzealous about it. The current evidence indicates that daily consumption of 20 to 35 grams of dietary fiber from a variety of food sources is best. *Too much fiber actually may cause nutritional harm;* amounts of fiber exceeding 50 to 60 grams per day actually interfere with the body's ability to absorb certain vitamins and minerals, including zinc, iron, calcium, and magnesium.

1. Choose from a variety of high-fiber foods. (A list of them appears on pages 313–316). While both soluble and insoluble fiber are found in similar foods, they exert different physiological effects. Generally, water-soluble fibers (pectins and gums) slow carbohydrate absorption, a process which is especially important for diabetics because it allows for a slower insulin response. Soluble fibers also combine with bile acids, helping to reabsorb cholesterol into the stool for elimination. Insoluble fibers (lignin, cellulose, and hemicellulose) help prevent constipation by increasing fecal bulk.

2. Increase dietary fiber gradually, in tandem with adequate fluid intake. By adjusting your body slowly to increases in the consumption of whole-grain breads and cereals, fruits, and vegetables, and by increasing your intake of fluids, you will help avoid the possible side effects of a high-fiber diet, such as flatulence and intestinal distention.

3. Think of ways to turn low-fiber foods into high-fiber foods. Food—not dietary-fiber supplements—provides the best means of increasing daily consumption of both soluble and insoluble fiber. Whenever a recipe calls for bread crumbs, substitute bran or part bran. This works especially well with meatloaf—rolled oats are good, too—or as casserole toppings. Make noodle or spaghetti dishes with whole-wheat pasta. With a little imagination you can find many ways to keep a high-fiber diet from becoming dull.

4. Include at least one serving of bran or whole grains in every meal. Sources include whole-grain cereals, breads, muffins, or crackers; use brown rice and whole-wheat pasta.
5. Have at least two, preferably four, servings of either raw or cooked vegetables a day, and three servings of fresh fruit every day.
6. Try to have at least one large serving of cooked vegetables a day; you can usually eat more of a cooked vegetable than a raw one. If you make a spinach salad, for example, you may eat eight to ten leaves of raw spinach, but if you cook the spinach, you'll probably eat a good deal more.
7. Use the following guidelines to switch to cereal for breakfast. Not only will you cut down on fat and sugar by choosing cereal over other breakfast entries but you will also start your day with a high-fiber food.

Choosing a High-Fiber Breakfast Cereal

Americans consume more than 20 billion bowls of cereal annually. This certainly explains why cereal companies are willing to spend millions of dollars to advertise their products, each supposedly containing the most vitamins, protein, fiber, and good taste per spoonful.

If the bombardment of television commercials and print ads has you confused as to which cereal is best, you are not alone. But solving your dilemma is simpler than you think. Just skip the ad copy and read the nutrition information on the side of the box.

- Check for realistic serving sizes. Nutrients aside, the calorie count for a ½ cup serving is meaningless if you put a cup of the cereal in the bowl.
- Pick a high-fiber cereal that contains at least 5 grams of dietary fiber per serving. Increase fiber in hot cereal by adding 2 tablespoons of oat or wheat bran.
- Look for a cereal with less than 5 grams of sucrose, dextrose, and related sugars per serving (5 grams of sugar is 1 level teaspoon). Breakfast cereals are the only food products sold in stores today that provide detailed information about sugar content. Cereal boxes generally carry a chart on the side panel titled "Carbohydrate Information." Here, the amount of complex carbohydrates (starches) versus the amount of sucrose and other sugars is listed.
- Select a cereal with less than 200 milligrams of sodium per serving. Remember that if you use the usual ½ cup of milk on your cereal, it contains about 60 milligrams of sodium, and this must be added to the sodium in the cereal. The only cereals that contain no sodium are ones that contain no sugar: Nabisco's Shredded Wheat (unfrosted), Quaker Puffed Rice and Puffed Wheat, and Puffed Kashi,

made by the Kashi Company of La Jolla, California. The cereals with the most sodium per ounce are Kellogg's Product 19, General Mills' Country Corn Flakes, and Total Corn Flakes.

- Find a cereal that contains no more than 1 to 2 grams of fat in each serving. Granola cereals are especially deceptive. One serving (calculated on the box as a meager ¼ cup) can contain from 7 to 8 grams of fat. If you pour out what you are used to serving yourself of other cereals—close to a full bowl—you'll get at least double or triple the amount of fat and calories listed on the label. Check the type of fat on the label, too. At least some of the fat in cereals is from the tropical oils—coconut, palm, or palm kernel. All are highly saturated. With increased public pressure to eliminate these, however, a number of companies are switching to unsaturated fats. Look for the naturally occurring polyunsaturated fats contained in grains or nuts. If oil is added, make sure it is cottonseed, safflower, or another polyunsaturated oil.

Hemorrhoids

Often thought of as a simple if embarrassing nuisance, hemorrhoids can be truly painful if not debilitating. They are rectal veins that, under pressure, pop out from beneath the skin layer of the anus. In 35-plus women, they can occur with chronic constipation or during pregnancy, especially during the "pushing" stages of labor and delivery. They can also result from lifting heavy objects if straining is part of the lift. The management of hemorrhoids is symptomatic, but the "cure" begins with attention to proper bowel movements. If stools are hard or difficult to pass, the risk of getting hemorrhoids increases.

Most people don't realize that taking laxatives as a routine cure-all for constipation can actually *contribute* to hemorrhoids by producing loose bowel movements containing fluids normally absorbed higher in the colon which can irritate and chafe the anal canal.

For topical use, over-the-counter unguents like Preparation H may be helpful in dealing with hemorrhoid symptoms, but when all is said and done, nature provides the best cure. Our program for eliminating constipation is equally successful in curing or preventing hemorrhoids.

To alleviate discomfort when hemorrhoids are present, if possible take frequent sitz baths—that is, sit in warm water several times a day to reduce inflammation. Also, be careful and thorough with rectal hygiene. For rectal cleaning after bowel movements, avoid dry toilet tissue and use Tucks (medicated pads treated with witch hazel), Baby Fresh wipes, or similar premoistened towelettes.

If conservative treatment fails, you may want to consider surgical treatment. For external hemorrhoids, the simplest procedure is to tie them off, sometimes called a rubber-band or banding treatment, so that the hemorrhoids wither and drop off. Sometimes high-tech laser treatments are used, but these offer no dramatic advantage over banding in most cases. Internal hemorrhoids, if large and prone to bleeding, may be excised surgically by a traditional hemorrhoidectomy.

With any of these removal techniques, recurrence is a likely possibility if excellent bowel habits aren't adopted to prevent it. As with other problems in the digestive tract, the key is to eliminate cause rather than simply treat the symptoms.

Other Intestinal Ills

Before embracing dietary fiber as the wonder treatment for all intestinal ills, bear in mind that there are conditions in which factors other than diet come into play, particularly when there is abdominal pain and symptoms overlap. For example, abdominal pain can be caused by anything from gas to peristalsis, from inflammation of the colon (colitis) to irritable bowel syndrome. In these cases, diagnosis is often tricky, and consultation with a gastroenterologist may be called for.

IRRITABLE BOWEL SYNDROME (IBS).   This rivals constipation as a colon-related concern for many 35-plus women, and it is twice as common in women as in men. Using the term *colitis* to describe an irritable bowel actually confuses matters. Colitis accurately describes a visibly inflamed colon, and that is not the case in most instances of IBS. In fact, even when pain and gas are present in IBS, especially in the lower abdomen, they may not always be related to bowel activity. And while symptoms overlap with other colon problems and causes are not universally known, stress and diet play such a significant part in an irritable-bowel condition that often a thorough history and physical exam can reveal as much as any single test. As for treatment, antispasm medicines such as Librax or Levsin, also used in esophageal spasm, are usually helpful in treating IBS. Dramatic "cures" have been effected without any medications or change in diet, however— simply by resolving areas of stress. For specifics on IBS, see page 181.

COLITIS.   This is true inflammation of the colon—involving either Crohn's disease (also known as Crohn's ileitis or regional enteritis) or ulcerative colitis, serious lifelong illnesses frequently associated with diarrhea, weight loss, abdominal pain, and frank blood and mucus in the stool. More than 2 million people in the United States suffer from one of these forms of inflammatory bowel disease. Crohn's disease tends to have its onset in adolescence and young adulthood, however, so it would be unusual (but by no means impossible) for it to strike *de novo* after age 35. Ulcerative colitis, on the other hand, can occur in younger people and indeed, even in children, but it reaches its peak incidence in the third and fourth decade.

Accurate diagnosis of these disorders is absolutely essential, and usually full colonoscopy as well as blood tests are needed. Treatment of colitis has at its cornerstone a good diet, but diet is usually not enough and other medications, including cortisone preparations, are usually needed. Management of both Crohn's disease and ulcerative colitis is chronic and often difficult, so it is best shared by your personal physician and a fully trained gastroenterologist.

GAS. As with abdominal pain, gas also provides clues to a variety of disorders—or sometimes to no real problems at all. At times people perceive a normal amount of gas in the intestines as abnormal; a doctor can provide clarification.

LACTASE INSUFFICIENCY. This condition is found in varying degrees in many adults. Lactase is the enzyme needed to digest milk sugar. Some insufficiencies may be so slight they are barely noticeable, while others may be so pronounced they cause a type of diarrhea. In the latter case, the calcium and other nutrients provided by milk can be obtained in lactose-free milk, usually sold in supermarkets. Alternatively, Lactaid tablets or Lactaid enzyme are available at health food stores, and can be added to milk.

When there is abdominal distress, particularly in the lower abdomen, that is connected with pain or bloating, discuss it with a physician rather than attempt a self-diagnosis.

FLATULENCE. Usually no cause for great concern, flatulence is often related to diet, particularly in the case of high-fat diets. But it is also a side effect of eating beans, cabbage, lentils, legumes, various fruits, and other high-fiber foods. Another common source of gas in the colon is incomplete digestion (absorption) of carbohydrates or starches. To decrease flatulence, *gradually* increase your intake of complex carbohydrates and fiber. Gas doesn't usually represent a serious underlying disorder, and with the help of a physician it can usually be relieved with a relatively easy treatment program.

SUDDEN OR UNEXPLAINED CHANGES IN BOWEL CONDITIONS. Particularly with constipation and in women beyond the age of 50, these should always be checked by a physician. A full colon examination may be needed to rule out any possibility of cancer. This should include a check of the lower colon (called sigmoidoscopy), as well as a barium enema and possibly even an endoscope exam of the entire colon—all in consultation with a gastroenterologist. For more on colon cancer, see Chapter 19.

Most colon problems, of course, are not cancer but rather disorders of function, usually related to improper diet and often aggravated by stress and a sedentary life-style. If proper choices were made with regard to good diet, regular exercise, and stress reduction where appropriate, these lower-bowel and colon problems would be much less common in 35-plus women than they seem to be now.

PROBLEMS WITH RELATED ORGANS

No review of the stomach and intestines is complete without a discussion of the liver, gallbladder, and pancreas. Although not part of the intestinal tract per se, these organs literally are connected to it.

The Liver

While the heart and the brain can be sources of high drama, there are virtually no suspenseful episodes on television or in the movies that show doctors and nurses scrambling about while the fate of a patient's liver hangs in the balance. Still, the liver is no less vital to survival than the heart or brain. Unlike kidney failure, where artificial cleansing (dialysis) is possible, there is no such thing as liver dialysis. Experimental procedures are going on with liver transplants, but these remain fairly uncommon and are primarily used to treat children with congenital liver problems. An end-stage liver will, in fact, lead ultimately to death.

Situated in the upper part of the abdomen, the liver is connected to the intestine by way of bile ducts. It serves many very important functions. The liver stores certain food products such as glycogen, which it converts into glucose (see the discussion of diabetes, Chapter 11), as well as vitamins such as A and D. It produces cholesterol and protein, specifically albumin, as well as some of the factors that help blood clot. It also breaks down toxic substances such as alcohol.

The way to keep the liver healthy is almost exclusively through nutrition—that is to say, by providing it with the proper nutritional building blocks as outlined in other chapters of this book. It is important to avoid insulting the liver with toxins, the most common of which is alcohol. Exposure to toxins can also occur in a factory environment, and even through medications. Treatment with niacin or lovastatin to lower cholesterol, for example, can sometimes lead to liver inflammation. Other vitamin and/or mineral overdoses also affect the liver (see charts beginning on page 284).

Hepatitis
One of the main threats to the liver is hepatitis. In the United States, the most common kind of hepatitis is hepatitis A, which is often a somewhat

mild and usually self-limited virus infection of the liver, with no specific treatment and usually a very good outcome. Hepatitis B, contracted (albeit rarely) through transfusion, needle pricks, or the exchange of body fluids, is serious and occasionally fatal. In some cases it leads to chronic liver infection, which in the long run can lead to a form of cirrhosis.

Worldwide, most cases of cirrhosis are not caused by alcohol, as they are in the United States, but rather by the hepatitis B infection. If you or a member of your family is infected with either form of hepatitis, there is a definite infectious risk to the household, and vaccinations for everyone are in order. Linked to drug use and sexually transmitted diseases, the incidence of hepatitis B is more common among the poor and in dense urban populations than in the middle class.

Cirrhosis of the Liver

The second liver problem—cirrhosis—is of wide concern among the general population, since it is caused by alcohol abuse, which is far more pervasive in this country than drug abuse. "Cirrhosis" means a scarring of the liver tissue, analogous somewhat to emphysema in the lungs and for the most part irreversible. While there are less common forms of cirrhosis, the cirrhosis caused by heavy drinking will not reverse, although there are often long periods of stability. Cirrhosis presents a minimal risk to women who take only an occasional drink, but heavy drinking over a number of years puts women as well as men into a high-risk category.

The Gallbladder

Nestled under the liver is the gallbladder, a somewhat minor character in the process of digestion but one that takes on more significance for some 35-plus women. Women over 40, especially if they are overweight, run a greater risk of gallbladder disease, commonly referred to as *gallstones* (quite literally, little pebbles or conglomerates that contain a bit of calcium or bilious material) than do men the same age. In total, 10 million Americans have gallstones, 20 percent of them women between 55 and 65 years old. About 250,000 to 300,000 Americans a year have their gallbladders removed.

Connected to the small intestine by way of the bile ducts, the gallbladder stores bile juices that help in the digestive process but the gallbladder itself is not essential to digestion. If gallstones require gallbladder removal, you can live a normal life, with a functioning digestive process, without it.

The main symptom of gallstones is a recurrent pain in the right upper part of the abdomen, or bloating or pain after eating, especially in response to fatty or fried foods or alcoholic beverages. Sometimes the pain simply comes and goes—the so-called spasm of the gallbladder *(biliary colic)*. But in some cases the pain continues, leading to *cholecystitis*, an active inflammation and infection of the gallbladder associated with an elevated white-blood-cell count and fever. Whether a patient has cholecystitis or biliary colic, both have a common cause: gallstone formation.

Diagnosis for gallstones is very straightforward, either by way of an X-ray called an oral gallbladder test or by ultrasound, which has a very high accuracy rate in picking up gallstones. If they are found, and if you are having a lot of discomforting symptoms, the usual treatment is surgical removal. Attempts to dissolve the stones with medication have not really fulfilled their promise and this treatment is used only with certain patients, after consultation with a gastroenterologist. Most general internists and family practitioners rarely use it. But when there is recurrent pain or infection and surgery is required, the good news is that the operation is relatively straightfoward, with small risk.

Diet seems to play only a small part in this disorder. Although one current theory holds that a high-fiber diet can help prevent gallbladder attacks, this has neither been proved nor disproved. The only time a woman need consider diet is when she is having an acute attack. Between diagnosis and treatment (which in most cases means surgery), a low-fat diet may be prescribed to help keep bile secretion to a minimum and thus avoid aggravating the area. After treatment, no specific diet is necessary. As long as the liver functions normally, adequate bile will be available for digestion. Once the stones have been dissolved or the gallbladder removed, the patient can go back to a normal diet.

The Pancreas

High up in the abdomen, behind the stomach, the pancreas is the third organ of this trio that connects to the digestive tract, supplying enzymes which flow into the duodenum of the small intestine. The pancreas also functions as an endocrine gland, secreting insulin into the blood to regulate the level of blood sugar in the body (see also Chapter 11).

As with the liver, the pancreas can become inflamed through alcohol abuse, with the resulting pancreatitis causing either an acute attack—with vomiting, fever, lowered blood pressure, faster heart rate, and clammy skin —or a chronic condition with impaired fat digestion and fatty stools. Problems with the pancreas can be extremely serious, so prevention—in the form of good diet and minimal use of alcohol—is a priority.

CHAPTER 11

Endocrine Glands

THE ENDOCRINE SYSTEM comprises the endocrine glands—chemical control centers stationed throughout the body that secrete the hormones needed to regulate many essential functions of life. These include food metabolism (thyroid glands), normal growth (the pituitary gland), kidney function (adrenal glands), and reproduction and sexual function (the pituitary gland, as well as male or female gonads).

The female sex hormone estrogen regulates the physiological events of menopause (covered in Chapter 15), but two other hormones are also of prime importance to 35-plus women: insulin produced by the pancreas to regulate blood-sugar levels during food metabolism, and thyroxine produced by the thyroid gland which regulates other metabolic processes. Functional disorders with thyroxine include an overactive or underactive thyroid; with insulin, they include diabetes mellitus, or "high blood sugar," which is on the rise in this country, and the much-misunderstood hypoglycemia, or "low blood sugar," which causes general fatigue and malaise. Contrary to popular belief, symptoms of hypoglycemia for the vast majority of women are not caused by a true hormonal disorder but are easily avoidable discomforts brought on by erratic eating habits, as you will discover later in this chapter.

Similarly, while insulin remains critical for many diabetics, diet is now recognized to be the cornerstone of treatment for all diabetics, and the complex carbohydrates that were once prohibited are now proving to be beneficial in assisting control—that is, in keeping blood-sugar levels close to those of nondiabetics.

This chapter introduces up-to-date prevention and treatment of the hormonal disorders that relate to food and energy metabolism. We present specific diets and dietary guidelines that have been successful for many of our patients in preventing hypoglycemia and controlling diabetes. We explain the increasing prevalence of "hidden sugars" in our foods—and why they may be linked to the increase of adult-onset diabetes—and describe the current medical approach to insulin use and treatments of thyroid disorders. All of this we consider vital information *every* 35-plus woman should have at her fingertips to ensure good health.

DIABETES MELLITUS

Diabetes mellitus involves abnormalities in the body's ability to produce and use insulin, the hormone which regulates the uptake of sugar (glucose) from the blood to body cells during the process of metabolism. The result is an abnormally high, or concentrated, level of sugar in the blood.

When this happens, the possibility of a potentially serious acid-base imbalance in the body arises, and the body begins to take protective measures, moving water out from its cells to try to dilute and remove the excess sugar. This causes the kidneys to work harder than usual and results in frequent urination (polyuria), frequent thirst (polydipsia), and increased appetite (polyphagia)—all common symptoms of diabetes. (The related changes in kidney function during this process provides the basis for the name diabetes mellitus, which literally means "sweet urine." It also explains why accurate diagnosis of diabetes can be made from a simple urine test showing an excess of sugar.) Other symptoms of diabetes include unexpected weight loss, fatigue and weakness, itching (including persistent vaginal itch), and blurred vision.

Diabetes mellitus occurs in varying degrees and includes a spectrum of relatively mild to severe symptoms, accounting for two different categories, or types, of diabetes.

JUVENILE DIABETES (TYPE I).   This is actually a misnomer because it can occur at any age, although it most frequently occurs in childhood or early adolescence. This is the most severe form, accounting for about 10 percent of all cases. In type I diabetes the pancreas fails to produce enough insulin, and without regular replacement of insulin by injection, the patient swiftly becomes ill, hyperventilates, and without treatment lapses into a diabetic coma. In the past, type I diabetics eventually died, but the discovery of insulin allows most of them to live a much-expanded, although not always completely normal, life. Because they require regular doses of insulin, those who have true type I diabetes are referred to as insulin-dependent diabetics. Administration is always by injection, since insulin is a protein substance and would be destroyed by digestive juices if taken orally.

ADULT-ONSET DIABETES (TYPE II).   This is the milder version of diabetes mellitus and accounts for about 75 to 80 percent of all diabetic patients. In adult-onset diabetes, there is a gradual failure of the pancreas to produce insulin, coupled, it seems, with an increasing cell resistance to the insulin itself. The body's fat cells can eventually show such a resistance, which is why type II diabetes seems a more common risk among people who are obese.

Symptoms of adult-onset diabetes are similar to those of type I, although they are usually milder and come on gradually. Sometimes general fatigue is the only symptom, although frequent urination and thirst are the most common signs. Treatment or control may include insulin, but this is not always the case; many type II diabetics manage very well with specific dietary control.

GESTATIONAL DIABETES.   Also related to elevated blood-sugar levels, this can occur during pregnancy and requires careful monitoring by a woman's obstetrician. Symptoms are usually undetected, which is one good reason why regular urine tests are so important in prenatal care. In the majority of women who experience gestational diabetes, the blood-sugar level returns to normal after delivery. However, since women who develop gestational diabetes are more susceptible to developing diabetes later on, this complication during pregnancy can be viewed as a valuable early warning sign. Prevention—in the form of good diet and a program of regular exercise—is a priority.

Whether a woman develops gestational diabetes or is diabetic before pregnancy, strict control is extremely important to protect mother and child, but in neither case should oral hypoglycemic medications be taken (see Pregnancy and Diabetes, below).

Complications of Diabetes

The problems with both type I and type II diabetes do not just involve high blood sugar. Diabetes can lead to serious complications including nerve damage, especially in the feet and lower legs; cardiovascular diseases; impairment of kidney function and even kidney failure; and impaired vision including irreversible retinal problems involving narrowing, blockage, and often hemorrhage of retinal vessels. In some cases, nerve damage can be reversed with improved control, but not always. Signs of diabetes, therefore, must not be ignored. However mild the symptoms might be, if you suspect diabetes, get an immediate medical diagnosis. Moreover, the diabetic who takes a devil-may-care attitude about diet and proper control can have terrible problems down the road. Diabetes is a disease whose progress can be controlled. The earlier such control is begun, with a program that includes ophthalmologic and podiatric care as well as monitoring of blood-sugar levels, the better the chances of preventing these complications.

Pregnancy and Diabetes

While there is some debate over how strict control should be for nonpregnant women, there is solid agreement that the pregnant diabetic requires special attention. Studies have shown increased maternal *and* fetal mortality for diabetics, but authorities think that strict management could reduce much of this.

In the pregnant diabetic (either diabetic before pregnancy or diabetic related to pregnancy), there is no place for oral medication. Most patients will require split dose insulin (at least two shots per day), and home glucose monitoring is strongly advised. Excellent (or "tight") control would be a fasting blood sugar of less than 90 and a random postprandial—meaning after a meal—blood sugar of less than 140. Of course, such a program carries with it the risk of insulin-induced low blood sugar (hypoglycemia), which in and of itself can be dangerous to mother and child. Clearly, then, the management of the pregnant diabetic will require close cooperation between the obstetrician and the internist, and may require the expertise of the endocrinologist.

Diabetes in 35-Plus Women: Who Is Most Susceptible?

Women generally seem to be at greater risk than men in developing the more common type II adult-onset diabetes. Some think this may involve certain events that occur during pregnancy, but such specific causes are as yet undocumented. However, risk factors that make some women more susceptible to diabetes than others have been documented. These include genetic predisposition, obesity, and poor diet. Any woman who is 25 percent over her ideal body weight will incur at least some risk of diabetes, but more cases involve women who are significantly obese—50 percent over ideal body weight.

A simple urine test or series of blood tests is used to diagnose diabetes, since higher levels than what is called normal fasting blood sugar ("fasting" meaning that twelve hours have elapsed without food) are easily detected. A normal fasting blood sugar is usually less than 110 milligrams, and a positive diagnosis of diabetes can generally be made if at least two fasting blood sugars over 140 milligrams are documented. A very elevated nonfasting, or "random," blood sugar of more than 300 milligrams also probably diagnoses diabetes, although this test should be followed up with a fasting blood sugar test.

Controlling Sugar Consumption—A Number-One Priority for All 35-Plus Women

Of course the "sugar" referred to in diabetes is monosaccharide glucose, not disaccharide sucrose—the table sugar used in foods. Still, there appears to be an indirect but significant connection between dietary sugar and type II diabetes as well as a connection to hypoglycemia.

Diabetes and the Chromium Connection

Government research suggests that people who eat a diet high in total sugar may also be depleting themselves of chromium, a mineral involved in the body's proper use of insulin. Such a deficiency may turn out to be a factor in the development of adult-onset diabetes.

One sugar that is particularly suspect in connection with this theory is HFCS—high fructose corn syrup—now contained in many foods in the American diet. Researchers have found that the people who lost the most chromium were those who ate foods high in HFCS right after eating insulin-raising sugars such as sucrose—for example, they drank soda pop containing HFCS after eating a candy bar containing sucrose.

The Hidden Presence of HFCS

U.S. Department of Agriculture figures show that sugar consumption in America rose 11 percent between the years 1975 and 1987—from 118 pounds to 131 pounds of sugar per person per year. This means that the average American is eating almost a cup of sugar every day.

You might say, "Well, that doesn't apply to me, I hardly buy a pound a year." But that's not taking the hidden sugars in processed foods into account, particularly the HFCS found in abundance in such common foods as:

cranberry sauce	mayonnaise
cranberry juice	sherbet
fruit nectars	spaghetti sauce
ice cream	sweet pickles
jam and jellies	syrup
ketchup	wine
fruited yogurt	wine coolers

The result of a process that converts the glucose in corn syrup to fructose, HFCS is the food industry's cost-effective alternative to the more expensive cane and beet sugars. Major soft-drink bottlers use HFCS as a 100 percent replacement for sugar, accounting for about 65 percent of all the HFCS currently produced.

In 1975, the average American ate 5 pounds of high fructose corn syrup all year, a mere ½ of 1 percent of all caloric sweeteners. By 1987, each person consumed 47 *pounds* of the stuff, accounting for 35 percent of their total sugar intake.

Manufacturers of products like baked goods still use refined sugar (sucrose) because it provides bulk, browns well and prevents moisture loss. But slowly the figures are changing; today, 7 percent of the HFCS produced is used in baked goods. In addition, HFCS can also be found in health food stores packaged as an alternative liquid sweetener—so read the labels.

In light of the findings about chromium deficiency in the presence of high amounts of dietary sugar, USDA scientists express concern about the increasing amount of HFCS in our diet. The result over time, they say, could well be a significant chromium deficiency, a deficiency which may trigger the onset of diabetes. Large amounts of dietary fructose can also raise blood triglyceride levels, increasing the risk of heart disease.

Although the chromium connection is not yet absolutely documented, we recommend that all women, whether presently diabetic or not, limit their use of products high in fructose and avoid such products as soft drinks and fruit drinks containing HFCS.

Food Labels

Food labels provide the key to spotting the hidden sugars, but sometimes even these can be confusing. FDA regulations presently stipulate that ingredients be listed in descending order (by weight) on a food label, so that the closer to the beginning of the list that sugar appears, the more sugar-laden the food is. On soft-drink labels, for example, HFCS is listed second only to carbonated water. But if the food contains a variety of sweeteners such as dextrose, HFCS, and corn syrup, their individual weights may be less than other ingredients and thus they may appear farther down the ingredients list. When this is the case, don't be fooled. In total, these sugars may actually represent the bulk of the product's weight and contribute to most of its calories. So if combinations of corn syrup, HFCS, dextrose, or sucrose appear on a product label, beware.

Treatment of Diabetes

Diagnosis of diabetes, either type I or type II, is the first step in treatment. This may seem obvious, but it has been estimated that half of the Americans who have diabetes don't even know it.

Once the diagnosis of diabetes has been established, the course of action you and your physician choose will depend on which type of diabetes is involved. If type I, insulin will be required; if type II, insulin or oral medication will be one option and dietary control alone (initially including weight loss if that's a problem) will be another. Or your doctor may prescribe a combination of the two. With the majority of type II diabetics we encounter in our practice, we work together to attempt effective control through diet alone. We do everything possible within conservative guidelines to avoid the use of insulin, which can cause excessive accumulation of fat and weight gain and put the type II diabetic into a vicious cycle of weight gain, high blood sugar, and increasingly higher doses of insulin.

Of approximately 6 million diagnosed diabetics on record in this country, over 2 million type II diabetics are leading full and productive lives by controlling their diabetes without medication. They are doing so through diet, which is the cornerstone for all diabetic treatment. For the insulin-dependent diabetic, diet carries with it the hope of delayed complications; for the non-insulin–dependent diabetic, it offers the possibility of eliminating or avoiding insulin or oral medication.

Teamwork is essential. If you are diagnosed as a diabetic of either type and your physician's dietary approach consists of a brief pep talk and a printed diet list, you should not hesitate to request a referral to an internist or endocrinologist, as well as a nutritionist or registered dietitian. It is a rare physician who can handle all aspects of diabetic education and care alone. In our group practice, we have an excellent diabetes program run by well-trained and very caring nurse practitioners, so that the physician need not try to handle chronic management alone.

Whether oral medications are involved or not, dietary management should not be undertaken without medical supervision. In other words, if you are diabetic, it is *imperative* that you discuss the diets and dietary concepts provided here with your physician and dietitian first, before implementing them. A small number of individuals may experience an increase in serum triglycerides when implementing a diet high in complex carbohydrates, which is why we recommend triglyceride levels also be monitored when on such a diet.

Dietary Guidelines for Treating Diabetes

The three main building blocks in our dietary approach to treating diabetes involve complex carbohydrates, reduced fat, and high fiber. This combination gives most non-insulin–dependent diabetics good control. In addition, many patients once considered to be insulin-dependent have achieved good enough control with the diet to lower and in some cases do away with insulin injections.

Complex Carbohydrates—Old Myths Pass
It used to be argued that since diabetes mellitus is a disease of disordered carbohydrate metabolism, diabetics should restrict their carbohydrate intake to lighten the load on the body's metabolic machinery. This approach was widely accepted, despite lack of scientific evidence to support the practice. Over the past two decades, it has been recognized that not only is dietary carbohydrate restriction, at least of *complex* carbohydrates,

unnecessary in managing type I diabetes but increased intake of such carbohydrates may actually be beneficial.

There are two reasons for this reversal. First, most complex carbohydrates produce a less pronounced, more gradual rise in blood sugar than do simple carbohydrates such as those in fruits and fruit juices, sucrose, fructose, dextrose, honey, molasses, and any foods containing concentrated amounts of these sugars. Second, complex carbohydrates apparently enhance the ability of the body cell receptors (as in muscle tissue) to use insulin efficiently.

The Glycemic Index

Not all carbohydrate foods cause identical blood sugar and insulin responses. They have different weights and molecular forms, and thus are absorbed in different ways into the body. Some foods containing complex carbohydrates, like white bread and white potatoes, behave metabolically like sugar. The relative measure of how quickly a carbohydrate food causes increased blood sugar is called the glycemic index. It compares foods to some established standard, usually either glucose itself or a food like white bread. Foods that cause a rapid rise in blood sugar have a high glycemic index.

Many factors influence the glycemic response to foods. Carbohydrates that can enter the blood quickly, such as fluids that contain sucrose or fructose, give the blood a temporarily higher concentration of blood sugar than those that are digested and absorbed more slowly, such as lentils or cooked dried beans. Because beans are high in water-soluble fiber, they influence gastric emptying time; in fact, as one of the richest sources of soluble fiber, they have the lowest glycemic index of any other group of complex carbohydrates—that is, they are least likely to cause a rapid, high rise in blood sugar.

Even with simpler sugars there are variations. For example, if you were to sip apple juice over several hours, it would produce a much smaller increase in blood glucose than if you drank it down in a couple of minutes. In other carbohydrate foods the rate can be affected by protein or fat content, preparation (cooked or raw), texture, and consistency (coarse or fine). Even form can affect digestion time: bread, for example, can be digested more rapidly than pasta; fruit juice more rapidly than whole fruit.

While the specific usefulness of the glycemic index is still a subject of controversy, it does provide a useful guideline for making choices about foods that can improve your diet, particularly when controlling diabetes is your prime objective.

Complex Carbohydrates Come Out on Top

Junk foods, heavily laden with hidden sugars, are carbohydrates of the lowest order. They supply the body with nothing much more than empty calories and the simple sugars diabetics must avoid. In most cases, they predictably have a very high glycemic index. As we have stressed, the high-fiber, complex carbohydrates found in whole-grain breads and cereals and in enriched or wheat pasta are now widely recommended as healthful for everyone, including patients with diabetes, heart disease, or diverticulosis. Complex carbohydrates, whose value in glucose and lipid control has been demonstrated, can go far in controlling these conditions. This dietary approach has led both the American Diabetes Association and the British Diabetic Association to recommend a diet composed of 50 to 60 percent complex carbohydrates, an increase over the 40 percent usually recommended in the average diet.

The increase in complex carbohydrates should be made up at the expense of dietary fat—for good reason. Reducing the intake of saturated fat is healthful for everyone, but especially for diabetics who are already predisposed to atherosclerosis. In our practice, we have seen that in more than 50 percent of adult-onset (type II) diabetes, the patient who is overweight can totally eliminate or avoid insulin or oral medication if she achieves lower body weight, especially if she is significantly obese. Even in the rare cases where optimum body weight is already achieved and a type II non-insulin–dependent diabetic still requires tablet form hypoglycemic medication, an appropriate diet of reduced fats, high fiber and complex carbohydrates is still extremely important.

High Fiber

We stress the importance of dietary fiber throughout this book, but it is doubly important for diabetics. Because digestion and absorption take place over a longer period of time when fiber is present, soluble fiber is helpful in minimizing the rise in blood sugar after eating, thereby decreasing the demand on available insulin. Soluble fiber also appears to improve receptor sensitivity to insulin, so that it is used more effectively. Thus in diabetics, diets high in soluble fiber are associated with less sugar in the urine, lower fasting blood sugar, and lower insulin requirements. We have seen all of these results with both non-insulin–dependent and insulin-dependent diabetics when they switch to a high soluble-fiber diet.

Jean Spodnik's Diets for Diabetics

For most 35-plus women who are not on oral medication or insulin for their diabetes, I use the 35-plus diet to reduce weight as soon as possible and to lower blood sugar.

One patient comes quickly to mind as representing a typical situation with non-insulin–dependent diabetics. She had an inherited tendency to type II diabetes, had lost weight very nicely on the 35-plus diet, and had got along for five years on the diet alone, without the need for any medication.

One day her blood sugar was found to be quite elevated, and it appeared that she might need insulin, which she did not wish to take. By switching her to a semivegetarian version of the diet, with just 5 ounces of lean meat per day and the rest of her protein coming from complementary sources (see page 304), we brought her blood-sugar levels down to a normal range again, and she's done beautifully since.

If you find yourself in such a situation, you may find success with the following diet. But *please be sure to check with your doctor first.*

Diet for Non-Insulin–Dependent Diabetics

	FRUIT	VEGETABLES	FAT	STARCH	PROTEIN	MILK
Breakfast	1	0	1	2 (use soluble fiber)*	1	1
Lunch	0	as desired	1	2 (whole grain)†	2 (supplied by 1 c. cooked legumes)	0
Dinner	1	as desired	2	2	4 (Lean Protein)	0
Snack	0	0	0	1 (whole grain)	0	1 or ¾ c. plain yogurt

* See soluble fiber list; use as many as possible for all meals and snacks.
† An old-fashioned corn muffin made without sugar may be used here, or a piece of whole grain or pumpernickel bread. If you go out for lunch, get your bean soup at a vegetarian restaurant, as nonvegetarian restaurants are likely to make their soup with some meat.

For women who are true insulin-dependent diabetics, the following meal patterns work very well. Again, please be sure to check with your doctor before beginning the diet.

Diet for Insulin-Dependent Diabetics

SAMPLE MEAL PATTERNS	1,000 KCAL	1,200 KCAL	1,500 KCAL	1,800 KCAL
	(Serving based on exchange list)			
Breakfast				
Fruit	1	1	1	1
Starch	1	1	1	2
Lean Protein	1	1	1	1
Unsaturated Fat	1	1	1	2
Low-fat Milk	½	1	1	1

Diet for Insulin-Dependent Diabetics *(continued)*

SAMPLE MEAL PATTERNS	1,000 KCAL	1,200 KCAL	1,500 KCAL	1,800 KCAL
	(Serving based on exchange list)			
Lunch				
Vegetables	. . . .	as desired	. . . .	
Lean Protein	2	2	2	3
Starch	2	2	3	3
Fruit*	1	1	1	1
Unsaturated Fat	1	1	1	2
Dinner				
Vegetables	. . . .	as desired	. . . .	
Lean Protein	3	3	3	3
Starch	2	3	4	4
Fruit	1	1	1	1
Unsaturated Fat	1	2	2	3
Evening Snack				
Starch	1	1	1	1
Low-fat Milk or Plain Low-fat Yogurt	½	½	1	1
Lean Protein	0	0	0	1

* May keep for afternoon snack

David Cogan's Recommendations for Medical Treatment of Diabetes

Although tremendous success can be achieved with good diet control, many patients with diabetes will still need medication: insulin for all true type I diabetics and pills or insulin supplements for type II non-insulin–dependent diabetics.

Control of diabetes is the subject of many long articles and academic debates, but it is clear that the tendency in the diabetic world is toward stricter control. The reasons for this are twofold: to enhance a daily sense of well-being and to prevent or slow down future diabetic complications. Although not totally conclusive, studies do suggest that tight—as opposed to simply adequate—control helps in both of these. (Tight control is a fasting blood sugar of 110 or less and a random (post-prandial) blood sugar of less than 140.) You and your physician can evaluate the blood-sugar element of your control by doing blood-sugar checks—fasting or random—and using the newer test for long-term control (hemoglobin A lc). For those patients on insulin, I strongly advise home blood-sugar monitoring with the new glucometers, a procedure taught and encouraged by our diabetic educators.

Insulin

Insulin, derived either from animal or synthetic proteins, has two uses. One is the continuation of use begun early on in women with type I, or juvenile diabetes. The other is initiation of use in some 35-plus women with adult-onset diabetes when a high degree of control is sought and oral medication is deemed particularly risky for long-term use.

The types of insulin commonly used can be classified by duration as short acting (regular) and intermediate acting (NPH). Many patients can be controlled reasonably but not perfectly on one shot a day of an NPH-type insulin, with or without a small amount of regular insulin mixed in. For excellent control, split-dose insulin (before breakfast and before supper) is often used; in these cases, home glucose monitoring is especially advised.

There are a variety of sources for insulins, and the new synthetic forms have gained favor over the traditional beef and pork types. But decisions involving dosages and types of insulin require close cooperative work between the patient and the clinical team. Once again it must be stressed that even for insulin-dependent diabetics, medication should only be part of a total treatment program. When it was discovered in 1921, insulin was hailed as the "cure" for diabetes mellitus. With insulin, diabetics would be guaranteed a normal life span; many even predicted it would eliminate the need to follow a strict diet. Time has proved, however, that while insulin has a valuable place in treatment, diet remains the true cornerstone of the management of diabetes.

Oral Medications

Oral medications—hypoglycemics—are used to lower blood sugar. While they do often prove effective, they remain controversial, specifically because of concerns over long-term safety and ultimate benefit. A study of oral hypoglycemics done nearly twenty years ago showed users to be at greater risk of death from heart disease, but showed no *overall* increased death rate. This study has been criticized as involving too few patients over too short a testing period to be completely reliable. It's a reason for caution, but not prohibition.

The main problem is that it is all too tempting for patient and physician alike to opt for oral medications rather than a program of strict diet, exercise, and/or insulin. It can be a lazy response to a situation that requires strong individual responsibility and lifelong discipline to ensure optimum long-term health.

While I prescribe oral medications for some patients, I use insulin more readily now than in the earlier years of my practice. But with either medication, I stress that the diet and exercise components are as important as they would be if no medication were being used.

Should a 35-plus woman become diabetic, it is unlikely she will be diagnosed as truly insulin-dependent and more likely that the problem can be improved or resolved through diet and exercise. In this context, then, the use of medication should be discussed with your doctor. If it is advised, use the lowest dose possible (consistent with good control goals) and work intensively with your physician–dietitian–diabetic educator team.

Exercise and Control of Diabetes

Exercise has positive short- and long-term effects on blood sugar. By improving the body's ability to use insulin, exercise helps lower blood sugar after meals, a time when the levels normally rise. When established in consultation with your doctor, a program of regular aerobic exercise—such as running, walking, swimming, or using stationary equipment—performed three or four times a week and lasting 20 to 30 minutes each time will have the overall effect of lowering blood sugar. Exercise increases the sensitivity of insulin receptors, and helps normalize the body's glycogen (sugar) storage in muscle tissue.

In some cases, it may be necessary to bring down high blood-sugar levels before beginning an exercise program—another reason why medical consultation is necessary before you begin exercise. Also, extra calories will be needed to "cover" vigorous new exercise—as much as 20 to 30 grams of extra complex carbohydrates per hour of exercise. This means two more servings from the starch exchange—one small bagel, for example—if you exercise an hour a day; one serving if you exercise half an hour.

HYPOGLYCEMIA

Suffering from depression, lethargy, or fatigue, many women are quick to diagnose themselves as having hypoglycemia (low blood sugar). But when the tests are performed, hypoglycemia rarely turns out to be the diagnosis. Symptoms almost always point to erratic eating habits coupled with a diet high in empty carbohydrates—the classic case is the person who gets up for work, drinks a cup of coffee, skips breakfast, grabs a midmorning doughnut or pastry, downs it with more coffee, and by then is feeling terrible. The caffeine lowers her blood sugar, the sugary doughnut or pastry on an empty stomach makes it suddenly rise, and then, exacerbated by more coffee, blood sugar takes a precipitous fall—leaving her feeling truly wiped out. In cases like this, symptoms usually come on quickly and can be readily avoided by eating properly—that is, by eating a bit of breakfast that includes protein and/or a complex carbohydrate, and steering clear of sweet snacks which, because they're so quickly metabolized, cause the sudden peak and equally sudden drop in blood sugar levels.

True hypoglycemia can be divided into two main types: fasting hypoglycemia and postprandial, or reactive, hypoglycemia.

FASTING HYPOGLYCEMIA. This can result from hormonal disorders, liver disease, kidney failure, and even tumors, but in a well-nourished person it is most likely from some aspect of diabetes. It can be a result either of too much insulin in self-administered doses, as a reaction to oral hypoglycemics, or in rare cases, from an insulin-producing tumor, called an insulinoma. Symptoms include nervousness, a fast heartbeat, sweating followed by dizziness or weakness, and at the extreme end, low blood pressure or shock.

REACTIVE HYPOGLYCEMIA. This is by far the more common type of hypoglycemia, although it is neither all that common nor is it a chronic phenomenon, as some women believe. However, it does occur more in women than in men because women normally run a lower blood sugar, even in a fasting state. Of those women who seem most susceptible, at least in our practice, the most prevalent type is the older woman who is either obese or slightly obese and has mild adult-onset diabetes, or, on the other hand, an older woman who is quite thin. Symptoms of reactive, or postprandial, hypoglycemia can include fatigue, excessive drowsiness, or malaise and sometimes jittery nerves—all far less acute or dramatic than the symptoms seen with fasting hypoglycemia and involving an insulin reaction.

The postprandial symptoms usually, but not necessarily, occur two to three hours after eating, and often after eating a meal that's high in simple sugars. Symptoms are usually short-lived, lasting an hour or two and, unlike symptoms of fasting hypoglycemia, go away by themselves, without treatment. Once again, they are very rarely noted less than an hour after eating, since blood sugar has not had a chance to fall in that time. Symptoms improve when food is ingested.

Taking a careful history usually leads to a diagnosis of true hypoglycemia, but if the diagnosis is not clear, consultation with an endocrinologist is in order. If symptoms of reactive hypoglycemia are evident, they can be a sign of early diabetes, which is why it is wise to determine the diagnosis with blood tests and sometimes even oral glucose-tolerance tests.

Jean Spodnik's Dietary Considerations
for Treating Hypoglycemia

The following suggestions really work for my patients who are susceptible to hypoglycemia, including those whose blood sugar is normal but who bring on bouts of low blood sugar with poor dietary habits. For true hypoglycemics needing greater control see the diets on pages 148–149.

1. *Eat at regular intervals, at least once every three hours during the day, and don't skip meals.* Typically, this means regular meals and "grazing" snacks—at least five or six times a day and chosen carefully for nutritional

content. Obviously, you want to pay close attention to what you snack on, monitoring your total daily calories.

We have described erratic eating habits. Often the woman who complains of hypoglycemia will have let up to sixteen hours elapse since her last meal; no food between dinner the night before and ten or eleven o'clock the next morning. If you can't schedule a good breakfast for yourself, as many women cannot, have something on a morning break that will hold you over until lunchtime—but not the proverbial danish, full of sugar, and coffee, full of caffeine. This kind of quick fix can wreak havoc with your blood-sugar levels. A better choice is a toasted bagel with light cream cheese ("light" because the low fat version contains more protein than regular cream cheese), or maybe a cube of cheese with a toasted bagel; a piece of whole-wheat toast will do, but steer clear of the jam.

2. *Be wary of caffeine and alcohol consumption, both of which bring on hypoglycemic episodes.* At most, one cup of coffee a day consumed with milk and in the presence of a meal is the limit for anyone who suffers from hypoglycemia. Caffeine causes blood sugar to drop, as does alcohol.

3. *Combine protein and complex carbohydrates in each meal.* For years, hypoglycemia was treated exclusively with frequent high-protein meals. Now complex carbohydrates—fresh fruits, vegetables, whole grains, and starchy vegetables—have been integrated into the diet. For ideas in combining both, refer to the meal plans below.

4. *Get your weight down to its normal range.* Weight loss in obese women will change their body chemistry to eliminate reactive hypoglycemia. Use the 35-Plus Diet for Hypoglycemia (page 150) along with the exchange lists in Chapter 22.

5. *Avoid sugar.* True hypoglycemics should avoid eating any sugar at all. Of course you can have complex carbohydrates—fresh fruits, vegetables, whole grains, and starchy vegetables—but avoid sweet desserts. If you harbor a hard-to-control sweet tooth, have a small portion of dessert after a well-rounded meal—never by itself.

THYROID PROBLEMS

The thyroid is the master gland of metabolism, so that when there is an imbalance of any kind, it surely will affect the body. Mrs. Dawson represents the kind of common thyroid disorder that can occur in 35-plus women. Thirty-eight years old, mother of three, and full-time homemaker, she described herself as "so nervous lately": she slept poorly, yelled at the children "more than usual," and felt anxious all the time. She also described how she perspired with minimal exertion, felt occasional heart flut-

Diet for Hypoglycemia *

	FRUIT	VEGETABLES	COMPLEX CHO	LEAN LOW FAT PROTEIN	UNSATURATED FATS	LOW-FAT MILK
Breakfast	1		2	1	1	½ c.
Midmorning snack	none	cooked–½ c. raw–1 c.	½ to 1	1–2	none	none
Lunch	1	2 servings	2	2–3	1	none
Midafternoon snack	1	none	½ to 1	1–2	none	½ c.
Dinner	1	3 servings	2–3	4–6	2	none
Evening snack	none	1 if desired	½ to 1	1–2	none	½ c.

* Avoid caffeine and use decaffeinated beverages. Also, alcoholic beverages should never be used without food, and even then minimally. If you wish to have anything sweet you may have a small amount, occasionally, as a dessert with your largest meal (never alone).

Hypoglycemia Sample Menu

Breakfast	½ grapefruit or ½ cup orange juice 1 c. cooked oat bran or 1 c. cold whole-grain cereal ¼ c. egg substitute cooked in 1 tsp. polyunsaturated margarine ½ cup low-fat milk Decaffeinated beverage
Snack	Celery & carrot sticks 3 whole wheat crackers 1–2 slices cheese, less than 5 gms. of fat/ounce
Lunch	2–3 oz. lean turkey 2 slices whole-grain bread 2 tsp. diet dressing Raw or cooked vegetables 1 apple Decaffeinated beverage
Snack	2 melba toasts (rye or whole wheat) 1 tbsp. peanut butter ½ c. low-fat milk 1 peach or another fruit
Dinner	Baked fish with lemon margarine, or lean meat Baked potato, large Cooked broccoli Tossed salad/diet dressing Canned pineapple slice (drained) Decaffeinated beverage 4 oz. glass, white semi-dry wine (if desired)
Snack	Half a sandwich (1 slice lean ham or turkey ham 1 slice rye bread) Lettuce and tomato, sour pickle, if desired ½ c. low-fat milk

35-Plus (Weight Loss) Diet for Hypoglycemia

	FRUIT	VEGETABLES	COMPLEX CHO	LEAN PROTEIN	LOW-FAT MILK
Breakfast	0	1	1	1	½ c.
Midmorning snack	1*	1	0*	1	0
Lunch	0	2	1	2	0
Afternoon snack	0*	1	1*	1	0
Dinner†	0	3	1	4	0
Evening snack	1*	1	0*	1	½ c.

* At snack time, you may substitute a serving of complex carbohydrate (such as whole wheat crackers) for the fruit, but have at least one, if not two, servings of fruit each day.
† Dinner may be accompanied by 4 ounces of dry wine, if tolerated and desired.

Sample Menu

Breakfast	1 c. V8 juice 1 c. cold whole-grain cereal or 1 slice whole-grain toast ¼ c. egg substitute or ⅓ cup low fat cottage cheese ½ c. low fat milk or ⅓ c. plain yogurt Decaffeinated beverage
Mid-morning Snack	1 piece of fruit in season or 2 whole-wheat crackers ⅓ c. low fat cottage cheese or 1 oz. lean meat Vegetables as desired
Lunch	2 oz. lean meat or ½ c. water-pack tuna 1 small pita pocket or 2 slices reduced-calorie bread No-fat dressing if needed Raw or cooked vegetables (2 servings) Decaffeinated beverage
Afternoon Snack	2 rye crackers ¼ c. water-pack tuna Celery and carrot sticks
Dinner	4 oz. baked chicken (marinated) ½ c. brown rice cooked in broth Cooked green beans with carrots Large vegetable salad with no-fat dressing 4 oz. glass white wine if tolerated and desired Decaffeinated beverage
Evening Snack	1 fruit or 2 slices crispbread 1 oz. low fat cheese Vegetables as desired ½ c. low fat milk or ⅓ cup plain low fat yogurt

ters, and despite a strong appetite, had lost 10 pounds over the course of a few weeks. On examination, her resting heartbeat was 120, her ankle reflexes were very active, her skin was warm, and her palms were sweaty. While awaiting results of a blood test and thyroid scan for further evaluation, Mrs. Dawson was given a beta blocker for partial relief—at least until the diagnosis of Graves' disease, a common form of hyperthyroidism, was made and specific treatment was begun.

HYPERTHYROIDISM.   This is an overactive thyroid, meaning there is too much thyroid hormone in the system. Situated around the larynx, the thyroid gland is readily seen or felt if enlarged. It produces thyroid hormone, a major factor in body metabolism, or energy consumption. If too much thyroid is produced, the body's machinery is speeded up to a rate that, if sustained, will wear it out. Full-blown hyperthyroidism—called thyrotoxicosis—can actually lead to death.

Mrs. Dawson's symptoms were strong indications that she was suffering from hyperthyroidism; the question was, what type? Her thyroid tests—especially the T4 and the nuclear thyroid scan—were consistent with Graves' disease; the fact that other specific tests for thyroiditis (inflamed thyroid), another cause of an overactive thyroid, were negative helped confirm it. Lastly, the nuclear scan ruled out nodular goiter, another cause of hyperthyroidism.

The treatment for Graves' disease needs to be individualized and discussed carefully with the patient's physician. The preferred therapy for most women is radioactive iodide, which is easy to administer and well tolerated. The disadvantage of this treatment, however, is a predictable rate of hypothyroidism, so that most patients end up on maintenance synthetic thyroid (L-thyroxine). Nonetheless, this seems a better option for most than either the oral thyroid-suppressing medications or thyroid surgery. In this situation, get a second opinion or consultation from an endocrinologist.

HYPOTHYROIDISM.   This is a deficiency of thyroid activity. Sometimes, women who are overweight and chronically tired believe they have an underactive thyroid. Since this disease may or may not produce an easily recognized change in thyroid size, blood tests are usually diagnostic. If the diagnosis is confirmed, treatment with synthetic thyroid hormone (L-thyroxine) will correct the situation but in most cases it must be continued indefinitely.

GOITER.   An enlarged thyroid, or goiter, must be investigated even if you feel well, so as to rule out the possibility of a tumor. Diagnosis is made through a thyroid scan and sometimes a biopsy.

The vast majority of 35-plus women will not experience these or other less common thyroid problems. But if you notice changes in your body's metabolism, whether it seems too fast or too slow, consult your doctor. A review of your history, an examination, and specific tests will usually determine the source of the problem.

As a final note, be wary of any recommendation to take thyroid pills to "speed up" your metabolism. These are offered by some questionable diet centers and should be avoided at all costs, since no good—and potential harm—can come from their use.

CHAPTER 12

Bones, Joints, and Muscles

MANY WOMEN WHO ARE "into fitness" have discovered for themselves why keeping bones strong and muscles and joints flexible is one of
the best things you can do for your 35-plus body.

Others, those 35-plus women leading sedentary lives, have discovered
something quite different: along with an accumulated bulge or two and
perhaps a few gray hairs, there is probably no area of the body that reveals
the hard facts of aging more than do the muscles, bones, and joints. Common midlife stories from couch potatoes attest to the little pranks the body
plays to put that message across. There are the "near miss" events—a
twisted ankle rather than a broken one; a pulled muscle in the back rather
than a spine in traction. There are common complaints of aches and pains
where none existed before. The body's get-up-and-go may not have "got-up
and went," but in sedentary 35-plus women it may be slipping away.

If all this sounds familiar, take heart. Health choices made in the thirties and forties about the condition of your bones, joints, and muscles can
determine their performance well into your seventies. Starting right now,
you have ample time to implement a plan of action for reversing the small
signs of aging that may have already begun and dealing with more serious
problems, such as osteoarthritis and osteoporosis.

In this chapter, you will find guidelines every 35-plus woman can follow
to prevent small aches and pains, as well as the more problematic signs of
aging that can crop up in midlife joints and bones—osteoarthritis, the risk
of osteoporosis, and back problems lead the list.

Fitness and muscle strength are essential to musculoskeletal health,
and here a regular exercise program is indispensable. In this chapter we'll

review the musculoskeletal system and concentrate on bone and joint health, but this is only half the story. Chapter 24, Changing a Sedentary Life-style, is the all-important second half.

THE BONES

In the old days, hands could tell a doctor much about a person's life-style and the influence it might have on areas of health and disease. Those whose hands showed the marks of physical labor usually had a very different body from those who didn't engage in physical activity. Human bones also leave behind an impression of how a person lived. Archaeologists have found signs not only of illness and disease but also of life-style and level of activity in the remains of ancient, primitive people.

Bone is living tissue. Gradually, it changes and even can be altered by constant stress and wear—in the osteoarthritis that appears in weight-bearing joints, for example. Bones also adapt to a lack of physical activity and exercise by losing calcium and growing weak. When doctors report that they see more bone injuries in people whose most strenuous activity is brushing their hair than in people who participate in riskier activity, what they mean is that inactivity weakens the bones and makes them more prone to injury. In time, inactivity can increase the risk of hip fractures, back injuries, and problems with the extremities.

Of course, inactivity is not the only factor that influences bone health and well-being. The shape, length, and bulk of the bones are part of the genetic blueprint that dictates basic body type and even the kind of physical activity a person is best suited (or not suited) to do.

Fortunately, whatever their shape, bones are only part of the miracle of movement, and a program of strengthening the muscles can help protect vulnerable spots in the bones as well. And the fact that bone mass forms and reforms gives us a chance to actively take part in shaping its health.

Bone Basics

When we say bone is tissue, we are speaking of collagen, a protein that forms a matrix to hold calcium, the mineral that provides bone density. Physical activity increases the production of collagen and, consequently, mineral content. Bones become stronger with exercise. "Super seniors"— 75-year-olds who play a regular game of tennis or run a mile a day—are living proof that calcium mass can be maintained at a good level throughout an active life.

In fact, calcium does many things for the body besides keeping the bones strong. It appears as a kind of "glue" in every cell in the body, causing muscles to work and nerves to function. It performs a protective function as well, acting as an essential element in the clotting action that prevents excessive blood loss from minor injuries.

Bones are the storage centers for calcium, containing 98 percent of the body's total supply. Hormones regulate the storage and release of calcium from our bones—what gets left behind after those needs are met is what determines bone strength. Thus it is a 35-plus woman's stores of calcium that are of primary concern, particularly in the years before menopause. After menopause, lack of estrogen significantly reduces the body's ability to absorb dietary calcium and incorporate it into the bones. But, before *and* after menopause, we can make more calcium available through diet so that the body need not deplete bone stores.

Osteoporosis

Many women worry that in their senior years they will become stooped little old ladies with dowager's humps who risk hip fractures or broken ankles every time they negotiate a street corner. This condition is the hallmark of osteoporosis, the thinning of the bones from loss of calcium that leaves them brittle and prone to injury. But even though reduced estrogen levels after menopause prevent the bones from absorbing calcium at the same rate as before, acute osteoporosis is hardly inevitable.

True osteoporosis is most apt to occur in a particular group of women —small-framed Caucasians, who are even more at risk if they are physically inactive smokers—though it is by no means limited to this group.

Osteoporosis is a degenerative condition that begins long before it becomes evident, and it should be of concern to all 35-plus women. You can do a lot to prevent its occurrence by paying attention to nutrition *now*. Keeping a good supply of calcium in your diet is where a successful strategy for preventing osteoporosis naturally begins.

The 35-Plus Plan for Preventing Osteoporosis

1. *Tailor your diet to provide extra calcium.* Studies have shown that the majority of women obtain only 500 to 700 milligrams of calcium a day from the food they eat. What women in midlife really need to maintain good bone strength is *double* these amounts—1,000 to 1,500 milligrams of calcium a day.

Some of the best sources of calcium are the following foods: milk and milk products, some fish and certain vegetables. Calcium content in low-fat milk is slightly better than in either whole or skim, with 1 cup of 1 percent fat milk containing 310 milligrams of calcium; 1 cup of skim milk 300; and 1 cup of whole milk 290. Yogurt, part-skim ricotta cheese, canned mackerel and sardines, collard greens, turnip greens, and bok choy are all excellent sources of calcium (see pages 317–318 for a detailed list of foods containing calcium).

2. *Rule out or compensate for possible lactose intolerance.* Clearly the easiest and best sources of calcium are dairy products—unless you have an intolerance for lactose. As discussed in Chapter 10, this digestive problem occurs when there is insufficient production of lactase, the enzyme that helps digest milk sugar, or lactose. Such an intolerance can produce a good deal of digestive distress, including bloating and flatulence, when dairy products are consumed.

If you suspect symptoms of lactose intolerance (a condition which can develop gradually in adults), discuss it with your doctor and perhaps switch over to milk products that have been pretreated with the lactose enzyme. Alternatively, you can buy the enzyme itself in health food stores and add it to regular milk.

3. *To help adjust to lowered calcium absorption in the perimenopausal years, take calcium supplements.* Choose them wisely, however, and do not depend on them entirely for supplying your body's needs.

According to the May 1988 issue of *Consumer Reports,* the best and least expensive calcium supplement is Tums, the antacid tablets, which contain 200 milligrams of elemental calcium in the form of calcium carbonate (which contains more calcium by weight than any other compound). Very recent research, however, indicates that calcium citrate may be more effective in aiding bone mineralization than other forms of calcium.

Tums and two alternative supplements—Oscal and Caltrate—are easily dissolvable in the stomach. There are others, however, that go straight through the digestive tract without being absorbed. These pills also contain calcium carbonate, but it is too highly concentrated to be of use; when large amounts of calcium carbonate are compressed into small pills, it is difficult for stomach acids to dissolve them sufficiently to be absorbed by the blood.

To gauge absorbability, Ralph Shangrow, Ph.D., of the University of Maryland School of Pharmacy, devised the following simple test: Place one of your calcium-supplement tablets in a few ounces of room temperature vinegar and stir vigorously for five minutes; after thirty minutes, the tablet should be dissolved. If it's not, choose another brand.

4. *Enhance absorption of your calcium supplement by taking it at mealtimes, and with six to eight ounces of fluid.* The presence of food in the stomach maximizes acid secretion and thereby helps dissolve the supplement, as does the presence of a liquid.

5. *Keep your vitamin D consumption up.* Vitamin D is found in dairy products and fish oils; it is also manufactured by the body in the presence of sunlight. If lactose intolerance limits your intake of milk products, you can get the extra vitamin D in a multiple-vitamin tablet, taken daily at

mealtime. Absolutely do not take vitamin D "straight," since it can be toxic if taken in excessive amounts; as little as five to twenty times the recommended daily allowance of 400 IU is harmful.

6. *Make sure your diet contains plenty of complex carbohydrates.* Studies have shown that a well-balanced diet rich in complex carbohydrates can help prevent osteoporosis. Diets that go to extremes—for example, weight reduction diets that are disproportionately high in protein—actually have been shown to increase the risk of osteoporosis. The trace element *boron* seems to help prevent osteoporosis. While there is no known dietary requirement for it, researchers have found that a diet rich in fresh fruits and vegetables (which contain boron) helps minimize bone demineralization.

7. *If you smoke, stop.* Nicotine lowers calcium absorption.

8. *If you have no regular exercise program, start one.* Even if your calcium level is normal, it appears that bone mass is lost in the absence of exercise, so you increase the likelihood of osteoporosis simply by being inactive. (See Chapter 24 on midlife fitness for more on the role of exercise and bone health.)

Medications for Osteoporosis
As the median age of the general population increases, so too does the interest in finding new ways to deal with osteoporosis. In this context, *estrogen replacement therapy* is a hot topic right now because it has been shown that it not only helps bones retain calcium, but in some cases appears to help restore bone mass. But it can have certain side effects, including the possible reappearance of menstrual flow after menopause. More serious are concerns that have arisen recently over the general use of estrogen and its possible link to breast cancer in some women. This has caused controversy over its use in birth control pills, in treating symptoms of menopause, and in treating osteoporosis. At this time, estrogen therapy for preventing osteoporosis is not a common preventive strategy, although when combined with progesterone (as it is in most birth control pills today), the side effects and risks seem to be much lower.

The whole issue of taking estrogen seems to come down to personal choice. Whether the issue is birth control pills or estrogen therapy for osteoporosis, a woman must first weigh her own situation against the possible risks and then choose what's best for her. If you are a small-boned Caucasian woman and other women in your family have been afflicted with osteoporosis, this may outweigh any other factors. As for taking estrogen during menopause, advantages and disadvantages (see Chapter 17) must be viewed in light of your individual situation.

Older methods of *sodium fluoride* treatment in severe cases of osteoporosis remain undesirable in most cases, since they were shown to have several drawbacks, including fairly significant risk of intestinal side effects and toxicity. But treatment with the new delayed-release form of sodium fluoride shows promise for advanced spinal osteoporosis. Recently, researchers at the University of Texas Southwestern Medical Center in Dallas reported that in clinical trials over a five-year period, they had success with a new treatment involving sodium fluoride in a timed-release form. Coupled with a calcium supplement, this treatment appears to inhibit the occurrence of tiny fractures that collapse spinal bone and cause the spinal curvature known as "dowager's hump," at the same time that it restores lost bone mass in the spine at a rate of up to 6 percent a year. While subsequent controlled studies will be needed to validate these findings, and while this treatment can't straighten a dowager's hump once it is formed, this front-page news was particularly welcomed by the 5 million Americans affected by spinal osteoporosis, and by the 500,000 who have suffered spinal fractures. The hitch is that the treatment does not appear to improve overall bone mass, and there were indications that the new treatment might actually damage other afflicted areas such as the hip, where the bone is very different from bone in the spine. Researchers reporting positive findings in the treatment of spinal problems cautioned against any other application. Nevertheless, this development may point the way to new fluoride treatments that could have broader use in treating osteoporosis.

THE JOINTS

Back, hips, knees, ankles, wrists, and shoulders—the major joints are the body's architectural wonders, providing flexibility and support, motion and stability. To meet these contradictory objectives, each joint is a complicated amalgam of muscles, tendons, ligaments and bone that are called on to perform carefully defined tasks within a specialized range of motion. Let's take a closer look at each of these elements.

Cartilage and Joint Fluid

The cartilage at the end of each joint bone enables the bones to move smoothly, ideally in a comfortable, competent range of motion. Joint fluid "greases" the joints, flowing in and out of membranes around the joint as the cartilage compresses and releases during physical movement. Additional cushioning of the joint is also provided by the fluid-filled sacs called bursae, which lie just outside each joint.

Physical activity encourages the production of these fluids. In a sedentary life-style, the body produces less joint fluid, so that in time cartilage can deteriorate, resulting in the wear-and-tear condition known as osteoarthritis.

Since cartilage has a modest blood supply, injuries that involve a tear don't heal as readily as they do in other body tissues, so that removing torn cartilage by surgery sometimes is the only option. Protecting your cartilage means keeping active—safely active, with sports that minimize joint stress, and exercise that helps strengthen surrounding muscles so they give support.

Tendons and Ligaments

Tendons and ligaments bind the intricate, interrelated musculoskeletal system together. Attaching the muscles to the bones, tendons provide tensile strength along with elasticity, thus influencing the range of motion, or flexibility. When muscles and joints tighten up—which can happen even in a positive program of fitness—flexibility exercises in the form of slow, easy stretches are critical. Both tendons and muscles benefit when stretching is an integrated part of regular fitness.

Ligaments stabilize the bones, connecting them across the joints. Muscle strength, tendon flexibility and warm-ups before exercise help prevent ligament sprains and injuries.

The Major Joints

The elbows and knees are obvious hinge joints, but the gently curving back is a hinge joint as well, consisting of twenty-five vertebrae attached by ligaments and separated by cartilaginous disks. With each of its parts so closely interrelated, the back truly is only as good as its weakest link. And at 35-plus, it deserves kid-glove treatment for the rest of your life—in a program of prevention that includes both strengthening and stretching exercises. Poor posture, tight muscles, and general overwork result in more injuries to the back than to any other joint in the body. Strengthening the muscles in the abdomen is critical to protect the back, since the abdominal muscles are part of the back's support team.

The knee joint is a complex hinge, providing full flexion, extension, and limited rotation in certain positions. Protection from injury involves strengthening the quadriceps muscle in the thigh, which give the knee stability.

The hips and shoulders are ball-and-socket joints, providing full range of motion. The hip is the strongest joint in the body, consisting of a socket in the pelvis and the ball end of the femur. The hip is subject to a good deal of wear and tear, particularly when a person is overweight, with overuse of the surrounding bursae and muscles. Since the hip is often the first joint to succumb to degenerative joint disease (osteoarthritis), a specific midlife program combining flexibility (stretches) with strengthening exercises can go far in preventing hip problems later.

Types of Arthritis

Arthritis—inflammation of the joints—is grouped into categories depending on how and what part of the joint is affected. It can result from a metabolic disorder, trauma, viral and bacterial infection, or other diseases, and it can affect joint membranes or cartilage.

RHEUMATOID ARTHRITIS.   This chronic, often deforming arthritis has its peak incidence between ages 35 and 45. It affects more women than men, at a ratio of about 3 to 1. Representing a spectrum of forms and intensities, it afflicts more than a million American women.

The management of rheumatoid arthritis should involve an internist with special expertise, a rheumatologist, or both. Treatment can range from simple anti-inflammatory medications to gold, antimalarials (Plaquenil), steroids, and even chemotherapy drugs such as methotrexate.

SYSTEMIC LUPUS ERYTHEMATOSUS.   This form of lupus is another serious arthritic illness involving joints and other connective tissue. Kidney involvement is common, as well. It predominately affects women and often is treated with steroids (cortisone). Its management should be directed by a rheumatologist.

OSTEOARTHRITIS.   By far the most common type of arthritis to affect women in their middle years is osteoarthritis, or degenerative joint disease. It is an uncomfortable, often progressive condition in which the cartilage at the joints begins to wear away. Osteoarthritis can begin as early as the thirties, depending on the life-style of the individual and the kind of joint stress involved. Because it helps keep joints lubricated, activity—that is, use of the joints—helps defer osteoarthritis. But genetic makeup plays a significant role; overuse, age, and physical abuse are not solely responsible. This can be seen in comparisons between symmetrical weight-bearing joints, such as the hip, when one hip is fine and the other shows signs of cartilage deterioration.

Early symptoms of osteoarthritis include stiffness, particularly in the hips or knee joints, but also possible in the nonweight-bearing joints of elbows, wrists, and hands. In the early stages, changes may not show up in an X-ray, which is the common way to confirm the diagnosis. Sometimes there is stiffness and pain, with a slight swelling or tenderness that dissipates during the day as the joints are exercised.

Medications for Osteoarthritis
Inflammatory substances have been found in the joint fluid of patients who suffer from osteoarthritis, so it is clear that the inflammatory component can be modified by anti-inflammatory medication. In its early stages,

the best treatment of this form of arthritis seems to be control of discomfort and pain with anti-inflammation medications. Leading the list is plain or buffered aspirin, or coated aspirin, such as Ecotrin.

Many women find that two aspirins taken when pain and stiffness are most noticeable in the morning is all they need, without further dosages the rest of the day. If aspirin products don't work, however, there is a large category of noncortisone, anti-inflammation agents to choose from. For many years, indomethacin (Indocin) and ibuprofen (Motrin) were the two medications that dominated this group, but now there are other choices; discuss them with your doctor.

It is important to remember, however, that there are different classes of anti-inflammatory medications. Indomethacin and ibuprofen, for example, are each in different chemical subclasses, so if one doesn't work, try another. Working with your physician, try as many as three different anti-inflammatory medications—each from a different chemical subclass—before you give up hope with this route.

Neither aspirin nor the newer anti-inflammatories can cure osteoarthritis, but they can usually control it. In addition, they have the big advantage over many other pain medications in not being habit forming, and thus can be used for years if necessary, barring such side effects as stomach upset and stomach or intestinal tract bleeding. In any case, most of these agents do not have to be used continuously, although effectiveness should be tested over the course of at least three to four weeks. While they can be used year-round, this is not always necessary. One good strategy is to take medications only when flare-ups occur and then to gradually taper off as the arthritis subsides. It is always better to ease off over a period of days or weeks rather than to go from full-strength medication to none overnight.

Cortisone (steroids) is somewhat controversial. Compared to other medications used in treating osteoarthritis, it is only sparingly used, if at all, by physicians and rheumatologists, and then in pill form. When inflammation is severe, steroids can be injected into the joint space, but this route requires the utmost skill in the hands of an experienced physician.

Alternative Treatments for Osteoarthritis

Medications are not always the first step in controlling osteoarthritis. Physical activity is vital to maintaining good joint function, and this includes joint function in the presence of osteoarthritis. When you feel pain, it is very tempting to lay low and pull back from regular exercise. Paradoxically, exercise may be just what your body needs most. Exercise that moves through a range of motion helps keep joints from stiffening up and losing function. Even when there is discomfort, try to do the stretches and physical movement (within reason) that are imperative to halt further deterioration.

Walking at a brisk pace for an extended period—of, say, 15 to 20 minutes—each day is an ideal way to keep joints limber and burn calories at the same time. In itself, being overweight can exacerbate arthritis pain. One 35-plus woman found the arthritis in her right hip to be all the incentive she needed to keep her weight down. One pound over 135, and her pain invariably began to increase. Swimming a few times a week at the local Y helped her control her weight and exercise her joints; she feels she's better off now than ever before.

In fact, swimming, preferably in a heated pool, is an ideal exercise for those with osteoarthritis in weight-bearing joints. Year round, warm-water exercises in a pool have been shown to significantly decrease pain and mobility problems in those who suffer from this condition. Moist heat from a hot bath or shower, preferably with a series of careful range-of-motion exercises for the upper body, can also help. Some people with joint inflammations prefer cold-pack applications, but for the vast majority heat gives the best relief.

Attitude certainly plays a significant role in managing arthritis. Women who succeed best in keeping pain at bay do what they can with exercise and medication, but they also diminish their pain by keeping busy and being distracted from it. Even in cases where deterioration of the joint has progressed so far that surgery or stronger medications are appropriate, by opting to fight the pain and keep physically and mentally active, 35-plus women have managed very well; they have postponed radical and not always successful options such as joint-replacement surgery.

Nutritional Reflections on Arthritis

Bookstores abound with titles that promise to "cure" arthritis—any arthritis —with special diets and nutritional strategies. Clearly, in view of the diversity of arthritic diseases, no one treatment could ever cure all forms of arthritis. Moreover, only controlled studies can verify claims that a given diet really works, yet it's hard to find any arthritis "cures" documented by any such controlled studies. Coupled with the fact that many forms of arthritis sporadically flare up and die down, so that discomfort might have subsided anyway, the success rate of any given arthritis diet has to be viewed with a skeptical eye. We don't intend to throw a wet blanket on the hopes of those arthritis sufferers who long for a dietary cure; but we do stress caution and wise choices in what you choose to eat.

It has been clearly demonstrated, for instance, that joint inflammation can be a manifestation of a food allergy, which explains why some people experience marked improvements when they eliminate certain foods from their diets. Such allergies can result from a range of foods including soy sauce, coffee, eggs, milk and milk products, potatoes, apples, lettuce, oranges, different types of alcoholic beverages, beef, and pork. In light of this, the "no nightshades diet," for example, which eliminates potatoes, toma-toes, peppers, and other vegetables in the nightshade family, can help peo-ple allergic to these foods. Testimonals do indeed apply—provided the beneficial results can be confirmed by an allergist.

Other Aches and Pains

Often overlapping osteoarthritis in their symptoms are the related "-itis" conditions, although these are more likely to be acute and nonrecurring, if treated promptly, rather than chronic.

BURSITIS. This occurs when the small fluid-filled sacs that lie just outside the joint spaces become inflamed. Especially troublesome are the bursal spaces of the knee, elbow, and hip, but bursitis can occur in the shoulders as well. Usually diagnosed by physical examination—that is, in-spection and palpation by a doctor—bursitis is treated in a similar manner as osteoarthritis. Cortisone injections are fairly easy and often effective, and not nearly so risky as for osteoarthritis.

TENDONITIS. This is an inflammation of the tendon, the connec-tive tissue or gristle that connects muscle to bone. Rest proves to be the prime course of effective treatment, along with aspirin and other anti-inflammation medications such as ibuprofen (Motrin) or indomethacin (In-docin). Often the intermittent use of cold packs helps.

COSTOCHONDRITIS. This is an inflammation of the rib-sternum joints, evident when there is marked pain when pressure is applied to the breastbone. Usually there is very good response to the same medications as used to treat tendonitis, but when this condition becomes chronic, treat-ment requires persistent and careful monitoring by your physician.

FIBROMYALGIA. This is marked by diffuse aches and pains, and ten-derness to touch and pressure in a range of muscles and joints. It is a condition of non-articular rheumatism, associated with stress, fatigue, and sleep disturbances. Fibromyalgia has been more widely recognized only in recent years, so some doctors may dismiss complaints that indicate this condition. This approach is unacceptable. Along with stress reduction, sufferers respond positively to moist heat or cold packs, gentle massage and stretching, walking, swimming, and periods of rest, as well as to anti-inflammation agents. As with a migraine, sometimes a low dose (25 mg) of a trycyclic antidepressant such as amitriptyline (Elavil) can help.

THE MUSCLES

We have two kinds of muscles: voluntary and involuntary. The involuntary muscles are the ones we don't think about, involved in digestion, respiration, and circulation, as well as in contracting the heart and controlling the pupil dilation of the eye. The voluntary muscles—those we choose to move —operate and protect the joints.

Muscle Activity

There are over 600 muscles of voluntary movement in the body—quick-acting muscles that are mostly arranged in two-muscle, push-pull teams, providing flexion and extension. These muscles complement each other, as demonstrated whenever you push (extension) a vacuum across a rug (for example) and pull (flexion) it back. If you put your left hand on the front of the right upper arm, make a fist with your right hand, and curl it up toward your shoulder, you can feel the biceps under your hand. That's a pull muscle. You can also feel its push partner when you press your right hand against a table. As you push, feel the muscle in the back of the right arm; your triceps are working against the resistance of the table. Muscles in the upper chest and in the shoulders, the inner thighs and the outer thighs, the abdomen and the lower back are all opposing muscle teams that need to be kept in good shape to perform well and protect one another.

Muscle fibers get their store of energy from the carbohydrate glycogen, which is produced by the liver. Using the muscles in physical activity encourages the production of glycogen, increasing muscle stamina and endurance. Muscle fatigue is a direct result of glycogen depletion.

While most ordinary tasks require work from both muscle partners, they don't necessarily require equal work from both. When one set of muscles is used more than its opposing set, it becomes stronger than the other—an imbalance that can cause discomfort and injury. The common discomfort known as shin splints, which occurs in the shins at the front of the lower leg, is an example of such an imbalance. When the calf muscle is overworked and becomes tight (after jogging, for example, when there's been no warm-up or cool-down stretching), it pulls on the weaker, opposing partner—the tibialis anterior—so forcefully that in extreme cases the muscle can tear or the shin bone can even be damaged.

Backaches

Although some backaches can be traced to osteoporosis or arthritis, the main cause in 35-plus women is a strain or inflammation of the muscles and ligaments of the back, especially the lower back. Sometimes, there is a specific strain or injury episode—or a flare-up "out of the blue." Provided the pain does not radiate to the legs and hinder movement or cause numbness (in which case, medical consultation is necessary to rule out a disk problem), the treatment of backache is symptomatic:

1. Brief periods of rest on a firm surface, although studies have shown that improvements are rare beyond the first two or three days.
2. Periodic applications of moist heat.
3. Anti-inflammation agents, including aspirin, often combined with muscle relaxants.
4. Initial avoidance of strenuous activity, including exercise, particularly when it involves the back.
5. Gentle exercises for the back as soon as pain permits.

When backache pain continues beyond three or four days, treatment strategies seem to dwindle. If you're faced with chronic back pain, it is worthwhile to consult a doctor, and perhaps through your doctor, seek nonmedical treatment referrals. Acupressure, acupuncture, and mechanotherapy may be considered unorthodox in this country, but they have worked extremely well in certain cases of chronic backache. More important than treating symptoms, of course, is preventing backache in the first place, which is where our program for fitness comes in.

Back problems also occur when there is an imbalance in the strength of the supporting muscles. Carrying heavy objects or leaning over to pick things up without bending the knees to put the greater burden on the legs (the quadriceps muscles) are examples of the everyday overuse of the back that causes the muscles to become so tight they lose their flexibility. Stretching these muscles and taking pressure off the lower back can prevent back injuries, as can strengthening the abdominal muscles, the back's opposing muscle partner. After a balancing-out program, in which the weaker muscle partners do their share of work, they will also look better—firmer, toned up, free of flab.

Foot Pain

Foot pain can be caused by inflammation of the muscles, but there are other considerations as well—some of them superficial ailments such as corns and calluses (see Chapter 6), others more serious, such as the joint deformities known as bunions. A bunion is a deformity and enlargement of the joint at the base of the big toe, coupled with a sideways deviation of the big toe itself. Although tight shoes don't cause them, they can exacerbate swelling and cause pain. The long-term treatment of bunions includes good shoes and molds (arch supports) that reduce stress on the area. Sometimes surgery is warranted, the latter by a qualified podiatrist or orthopedist, in which case molds must be used even after surgery for a good long-term result.

Circulation, arch structure and evidence of inflammation in the tissues surrounding the heel and foot bones (see Chapter 24) may be dealt with by your primary physician, but depending on the extent of the problem, referral to a podiatrist or orthopedist may be warranted.

Comfortable shoes that fit well and lend support are essential in preventing both foot pain and low back pain. High heels, because they pitch the body out of alignment, can contribute to back pain. Fortunately, running shoes (and their cousins), which are specifically constructed to provide comfort and support, are a perfectly fashionable part of today's casual attire, but it's dress shoes that cause problems. Men rarely experience the problems with their feet that women do, and it's not simply because they don't wear high heels; it's that their shoes are not usually as closely fitted as women's dress shoes are. If you can afford to spend a bit of money on any one part of your wardrobe, make it this one. This is especially true if you spend five days a week in an office where very casual shoes are out of place. Whatever the style, outside of the extremes, good quality, properly fitted shoes will give you a lot of comfortable mileage and look good through many wearings. Choose lower rather than higher heels, and alternate pairs from day to day. Absolutely avoid high heels on days you'll be spending much time on your feet.

SUMMING UP

In addition to increasing your intake of calcium to meet your body's increased needs for this mineral, the choice to keep bones, muscles and joints healthy involves a well-rounded program of regular exercise. If you're not already exercising regularly, now is the time to change your sedentary lifestyle, and the midlife fitness plan mapped out in Chapter 24 will get you started.

CHAPTER 13

The Brain and Central Nervous System

SITUATED HIGH ABOVE THE intricate network of glands, muscles, organs, and bones that constitute the human body, the human brain acts as computer system, memory bank, video terminal, copier, and communications center all rolled into one—sorting, collating, surveying, orchestrating, dictating, processing, and regulating physical and mental activity as well as giving rise to the feelings and creativity that make us different from other creatures on earth.

Through sophisticated technology, new discoveries about the function of the brain are rapidly coming to light. These include most notably the role of the chemical neurotransmitters—tryptophan, serotonin, glutamate, and others—and their complex effects on such areas as digestion, mood, and mental health. By focusing on how the brain uses and stores neurotransmitters, as well as how they may cause things to go wrong, this new frontier in neurobiology points the way to promising medical treatments and nutritional therapies unheard of in the past. But they are treatments many of us are destined to benefit from, possibly as soon as five years from now.

THE MENTAL POWERS OF THE MIDLIFE BRAIN

The body may crumble, but the brain continues to serve us well—some might say, even better—as we move through midlife.

Many middle-aged women begin to worry about memory loss and what they fear as signs of oncoming senility or Alzheimer's disease, a progressive dementia that becomes more common, although not epidemic, over age 70. Mild forgetfulness is not Alzheimer's, and anxiety only worsens simple forgetfulness. If there is a question of dementia, psychological testing can often separate *organic dementia* such as Alzheimer's (which involves deterioration of brain cells) from *psychological problems* such as depression and anxiety (which can also diminish intellectual function).

As the median age of our population increases, we have a broader base on which to study aging. In reality, a normal aging brain is very much like a young brain. While the brain cells do not regenerate at the same rate as do other cells in the body, neither do they wither and die, at least under normal circumstances.

Challenging a long-held theory that brain neurons decrease in number with age, in 1988 neuropathologist Robert D. Terry and his colleagues at the University of California concluded from their study that normal elderly people are largely intact intellectually, with the same number of brain cells they were born with. Terry found that some brain cells may simply shrink, as muscle mass does with age, rather than die. There's a parallel to be drawn here, based on such research, that carries increasing weight: just as physical exercise helps maintain muscle and keep the body fit, so mental exercise helps maintain brain cells and keep mental ability strong.

Another study, conducted by the National Institute on Aging in Baltimore, concludes that not only do brain cells normally stay intact as we age, it seems that our powers of concentration improve—our minds tend to wander less. Two self-exams were given to adult men and women aged 24 to 71, and when the exam was given again six to eight years later, the participants reported a steady *decline* in mental "wandering" over that period. This is in line with what many 35-plus women report: that they seem to be able to channel and exploit information as never before, using experience and accumulated knowledge as a resource for new creativity.

This phenomenon is documented by women in our lifetime whose greatest accomplishments have come with age. Georgia O'Keeffe, the configurations of her body and face reflecting the spirit of her beloved southwestern landscape, found new artistic confidence in her forties and fifties and went on to create some of her best paintings well into her nineties—at which point she began making pottery as well. She once confessed of her work, "It's as if my mind created shapes that I don't know about."

The crime novelist P. D. James, after years of supporting her children and a husband who was wounded in World War II, began writing fiction when she was 40 and went on to write the bestseller *Innocent Blood* when she was 60. Several books later, and just turning 70, she has set a standard against which crime novels are judged.

Of course personal achievements are not always so public, and most women don't become celebrities by the time they reach 50. However, the fact that their mental victories are private makes them no less rewarding.

At 35-plus, you have the chance to shift your attention from the superficial concerns of youth. You can risk expressing what you believe in, discovering what you really like, and, perhaps, who you have become. Barring specific organic disease, if you've got mental curiosity, an open mind, and the desire to explore new areas of knowledge, and if you actively seek change, there's no reason why the power of your brain won't continue to expand well into old age.

KEEPING THE BRAIN HEALTHY

The brain is dependent on the same good diet and protective care required by the rest of your body. Although sleep needs vary among individuals, adequate sleep is critical to mental function, particularly creative thinking.

This was demonstrated in a study conducted last year by Dr. James A. Horne, a psychophysiologist at Loughborough University in Leicestershire, England, and an expert on sleep. Expanding on the theory that sleep "repairs the cerebral cortex from the wear and tear of consciousness," he put twenty-four healthy college students through an array of tests to measure their performance at divergent thinking—the basis of creativity—when deprived of sleep. There were no right answers in the test; rather, measurements were taken based on the number of interpretations and creative responses given, thinking time, fluency, flexibility, and originality of thought, as well as the ability to elaborate on thoughts. After the first night of no sleep, the students showed a marked decline in creative thinking but relatively no decrease in practiced, or programmed, responses to known challenges such as making things with their hands, taking multiple-choice tests, and coping with well-defined emergencies for which they had been trained. After two nights of no sleep, the programmed tasks required more concentration but could still be done; the more spontaneous, creative thinking was seriously impaired. Lack of motivation was ruled out as a factor; even when they were offered money, the sleep-deprived subjects did poorly when called on to use insight and imagination.

While these findings have their most important implications for long-distance airline pilots, hospital interns, students, and others who are called upon to respond creatively—often in emergencies—after little or no sleep, they point out that a crucial brain function—creative thinking—needs as much good care and "nourishment" (in this case, adequate sleep) as does the rest of the body.

The brain is also affected by more serious abuses than sleep deprivation. The alcohol and drug use, smoking, obesity, lack of exercise, and poor diet that are factors in other health problems can also contribute to mental deterioration, weakening the arteries of the brain and leading to blood clots and strokes. In a stroke, subsequent damage largely depends on the age of the patient and the location of the stroke—whether the damage occurs in the "old," or lower, brain (the brain stem responsible for maintaining bodily functions), or in the "new," or higher, brain (the cortex responsible for higher cerebral activity). In either instance, there can be dire consequences affecting motor coordination and involuntary bodily functions as well as language ability, memory, and emotional response.

With therapy, some physical and mental recovery is often possible after a stroke, but even then such an episode can seriously and adversely affect the quality of the rest of your life. This is why minimizing the risk of a stroke—cutting out the abuses mentioned—is a top priority in the middle years.

As for recovery, new discoveries about the neurotransmitters—in this case, glutamate—may actually help prevent certain brain damage that results from strokes.

Glutamate, Oxygen Depletion, and the Brain

Researchers are now beginning to consider the possibility that glutamate— the common amino acid and neurotransmitter contained in all cells—may actually work to destroy cells, at least in cases where brain tissue is deprived of oxygen. If proved, this theory could lead to powerful new drugs for preventing the damage that occurs when oxygen is cut off from the brain, as in heart attacks or strokes, head injuries, seizures, and various neurological diseases such as epilepsy.

Glutamate, as in the substance monosodium glutamate (MSG), is an excitatory amino acid that under normal circumstances is stored securely inside cells, including the cells of the brain. But when the brain's oxygen supply is cut off (as can happen when a blood clot causes arterial blockage), and some of the cells storing glutamate begin to shut down, the glutamate "comes pouring, oozing and flooding out of the cells," according to Dr. Dennis Choi, an assistant professor in neurobiology at Stanford University and an expert on the subject. As reported in the *New York Times*, Dr. Choi says that this release of glutamate kills the master brain cells, or neurons, in a chain reaction that quickly destroys brain tissue. Ultimately, drugs that block glutamate receptors may halt this destructive process.

Difficult as it is to accept that a common substance in the body becomes toxic when cells are deprived of oxygen, the glutamate theory is rapidly gaining ground. There is convincing evidence, however, that other neurotransmitters such as dopamine, which is also released in abnormal amounts when oxygen to the brain is cut off, may figure in cell death as well. While the glutamate theory is the most complicated, neuroscientist Dr. Fred Gage at the University of California in San Diego predicts that, while physicians or neuroscientists may not be familiar with these concepts now, they will be soon, and experiments with glutamate blockers are already under way.

Mood, Food, and Metabolism

Since many of the brain chemicals, or neurotransmitters, responsible for normal brain activity are derived from certain food nutrients, there have been studies that explore how the food we ingest specifically affects normal brain function. One such metabolic study focuses on the food nutrient tryptophan, an amino acid which the body needs to manufacture the brain chemical serotonin. Good levels of serotonin in the brain produce feelings of well-being. When the amount of serotonin in the brain falls below normal, feelings of depression or problems with sleep patterns can result.

Tryptophan is supplied to the brain directly from the protein we eat—from dairy products, for example, or from meat. It can also be supplied by ingestion of the amino acid itself, especially if taken together with an insulin-releasing carbohydrate like crackers, fruit, toast, or muffins. After being digested and absorbed, the tryptophan attaches itself to the blood protein albumin, circulates in the blood, and gets to the brain. However, getting to the brain from the bloodstream can become a real transportation problem.

Protein foods contain many amino acids, large and small, that the brain needs for different purposes, all competing for transport through the cellular membrane called the blood-brain barrier. Other amino acids are more plentiful, larger, or more aggressive than tryptophan, so that when there is a "commuter crunch" on the transport system and there are not enough spaces for all the amino acids, the tryptophan is often the one that gets left behind, so that there is no elevation in mood following the high-protein meal. "Commuter assistance" comes in the form of carbohydrates which, when consumed with the protein, enhance the entry of tryptophan into the brain by releasing insulin. The insulin lowers the level of other competing amino acids in the blood, allowing the tryptophan unimpeded entry into the brain.

Studies on the brains of rats document that after they consume a high-protein meal, very little tryptophan gets into the brain; but after they eat a meal that includes carbohydrates, there is a definite rise in the brain's tryptophan level. In the human brain, mood elevation or relaxation will not occur until the carbohydrate in concentrated form is absorbed and serotonin is produced. At bedtime, serotonin can bring on drowsiness. If your grandmother brought you a warm glass of milk and cookies before bedtime, she was right in thinking the combination would help you get to sleep.

Dr. Adam Drewnowski at the University of Michigan disagrees with certain aspects of the carbohydrate theory. He says these changes in mood and attitude involve the interaction of carbohydrates, fats, and endogenous peptides—molecules that appear to act as neurotransmitters at central nerve ganglia throughout the body and whose functions are only now beginning to come to light. In the brain they may modulate pain; in the gut they appear to inhibit gastrointestinal motility and secretion. In any case, no less than fifteen of them have been discovered to have dual distribution in the brain and in the GI tract, indicating a relationship that is far more complex than initially supposed. Dr. Drewnowski's theory is that when stimulated in the presence of fats and sweets, these peptides may produce mood elevation and help regulate or control satiety levels in the brain during the process of digestion. His studies on obese women demonstrated a preference for sweetened, high-fat foods over an equally sweet solution of sugar and fat-free milk. In other words, it was not just sugar these women craved; it was also richness. This theory does not dispute tryptophan as the nutrient precursor of serotonin, but proposes other elements besides serotonin—in this case endogenous peptides—that trigger similar effects in the brain.

Another interesting aspect of this craving for fats involves the seasonal affective disorder, or SAD, which is characterized by symptoms of depression almost exclusively during the fall and winter months—symptoms usually abated by rich foods, most often desserts. Although the causes of this disorder are not yet completely understood, signs to date point to a possible food-nutrient deficiency linked to one of the brain's many neurotransmitters—once again, serotonin and/or endogenous peptides. Dr. Richard Wurtman, a psychiatrist at MIT and a leader in serotonin research, lays it all on the carbohydrate theory, while Dr. Drewnowski points to fats, carbohydrates—and the endogenous peptides. (Treatment of SAD currently includes exposure to sunlight and the use of special full-spectrum indoor lighting that simulates sunlight.)

While numerous studies are being done on cravings for fat, obesity itself is also being scrutinized as a kind of disorder—at least when there might be a deficiency of the protein adipsin. For more details, see page 23.

Depression, Mental Illness, and the Neurotransmitters

Treatment of depression and some forms of mental illness involve antidepressant and antipsychotic drugs which regulate the amount and release of neurotransmitters. In these cases, precursors come not from foods but rather from the medications that contain them in pure form, such as antidepressant drugs containing the nutrient choline, the food precursor of the neurotransmitter acetylcholine. Like serotonin, acetylcholine has been implicated in various neuropsychiatric disorders. Other drugs contain tyrosine, the food precursor of the neurotransmitter dopamine, which is involved in stimulating still another neurotransmitter, norepinephrine, deficient in people who suffer from depression.

Further studies of neurotransmitters may well lead to development of new medications for preventing and treating a wide range of psychological problems related to stress, depression, sleep disorders, schizophrenia, and perhaps ultimately, even some of the effects of PMS.

In the meantime, tricyclic antidepressants are one category of drugs that effectively treat depression and have a clear connection to the brain's synthesis of neurotransmitters. Based on the idea that depression is caused by or associated with decreases in neurotransmitters such as serotonin and norepinephrine, the tricyclic medicines presumably work by increasing these substances in the central nervous system.

Amitriptyline (Elavil) is a very common tricyclic in clinical practice. The dosage range is usually 25 milligrams up to 150 milligrams, usually taken at bedtime, once a day. In most instances initial dosage is 25 milligrams, working up to at least 75 milligrams a day for a therapeutic effect. Although improvement may be noted in a week, full benefit may take one to two months at a given dose. The most common side effects are dry mouth and constipation (anticholinergic effect) and drowsiness (antihistamine effect).

Doxepin (Sinequan) is another commonly used tricyclic, with a dosage range similar to Elavil but usually with fewer anticholinergic effects. Some patients who won't tolerate Elavil will tolerate Sinequan. Also, though efficacy should be similar, in clinical practice it is always reasonable to try a second antidepressant if one doesn't work. In this situation, a drug such as *desipramine* (Norpramine) or *nortriptyline* (Pamelor) might be used. With these latter two antidepressants, in many cases patients experience less sedation and fewer anticholinergic effects than with the others.

Apart from the almost certain metabolic connections between pure forms of drugs and nutritional deficiencies in the brain, there is no clear-cut proof that minor amounts of vitamins, for example, make a difference. Only in full-blown cases of mental dysfunction can we pinpoint vitamin deficiencies that can affect the mind—a lack of niacin in dementia or thiamine in Wernicke's disease, for example; otherwise vitamin therapies are of little value.

HEADACHES

Although headaches can occur off and on all through life, during the years around menopause their incidence can increase, bringing new health concerns. This is something we have clinically observed, although it does not seem to be purely physical in cause. Rather, it seems that as some people advance in years, they become more prone to stress at the same time that they become less active, thus reducing their opportunity to relieve stress, which is a prime factor in most headaches.

It is important to keep the nature of 35-plus headaches in perspective. Free yourself from imagining you have an inoperable brain tumor or an oncoming stroke. While headaches are a nuisance, and in some cases temporarily debilitating, over 90 percent of all headaches are muscular. Brain tumors are *very* rare.

Tension Headaches

"Tension," or muscular, headaches are the most common. They are usually characterized by a general tightness that often begins in the back of the head or neck and spreads around to the front in a circular band of pain. Such headaches produce a dull aching or throbbing sensation in the muscle tissue, and the sufferer usually becomes more aware of it as the day wears on. With a careful review of the day's events, such headaches can usually be traced to a specific incident that has produced stress or tension.

Of course any headache or pattern of headaches that lasts more than a couple of weeks, is new to the person, or is more severe than usual should be evaluated in concert with a physician. Those are the red flags that warrant a screening of ears, eyes, sinuses, neck, and blood pressure. Also, any new headache of unusual intensity warrants a physician's evaluation.

Usually, treating a tension headache with aspirin or acetaminophen (Tylenol) is sufficient to bring relief, but if your life situation is chaotic and your normal patterns are askew, relief will be fleeting, and the headaches will recur. In such cases, treatment begins by moving beyond the symptoms to the real source of the headache, beginning with an assessment of your total life situation, pinpointing stresses in work and family life, and seeking opportunities for exercise and relaxation, proper nutrition, and rest. Many women who complain of headaches skip meals—especially breakfast, drink coffee all day, and allow little or no time for sleep. They are oblivious to how these habits can fuel a cycle of pounding headaches. In such cases medication is useless, whereas alternative approaches such as relaxation exercises (perhaps with audiotapes), biofeedback, and yoga techniques practiced consistently can be of real value.

Prescribed medication for treatment of stress or muscular headaches requires cautious decision making and careful monitoring. Pain medications such as Fiorinal and Darvocet-N 100 and minor tranquilizers like Valium, Librium, and the like are potentially habit forming. In a trial period, some headache sufferers benefit from small bedtime doses—as small as 25 milligrams—of tricyclic antidepressants such as amitriptyline (Elavil), doses considered quite low for treatment of depression.

Vascular Headaches

A category that includes migraines, these headaches are usually more severe or intense than muscular headaches. In some women, *migraine headaches* can occur three or four times a month, often preceded by nausea and accompanied by any number of characteristic symptoms including pain on one side of the head, a sensation of flashing lights affecting the eye on the same side as the pain, and varying degrees of incapacitation. Hormonal variations, particularly estrogen in premenopausal women, may also be a factor, which adds to the perception that they are more common in women than in men, although this is not the case. In contrast to muscular headaches, vascular headaches seem to decline with age, so that in clinical practice we don't seem to see nearly as many older men and women having these headaches as we do younger patients.

Studies have shown that the occurrence of migraines may be directly related to certain foods, and thus can be managed without any medication at all (see pages 176–177). Newest findings on the causes of migraines point to abnormalities in the brain functions of the neurotransmitter serotonin, discussed earlier in this chapter; these suspicions arose when it was found that the same drugs that work to prevent or relieve migraines also affect serotonin levels in the brain.

For the acute migraine headache, ergotamine drugs such as Cafergot, which act directly on the blood vessels causing the pain, can abort the headache if used quickly—that is, at immediate first onset and again, if needed, 30 minutes later. When nausea prevents the taking of ergotamines, they can be given under the tongue in pill form, or by injection.

For prevention of migraines, beta blockers such as propranol (Inderal) have proved their worth for large numbers of sufferers. These medications must be taken on a daily basis to be effective (a challenge for some), but in the low doses used for migraines they don't usually produce the side effects of drowsiness, fatigue, lethargy, and even (occasionally) depression that may occur in higher doses.

A less common but more excruciating form of vascular headache is the *cluster headache,* in which there probably is a release of vasoactive substances that cause constriction and dilation of the blood vessels that produce the headache as well as some other odd effects like nasal stuffiness or tearing. These are sometimes the worst headaches to treat in terms of intensity, since they often occur at night and produce a pain so strong that some women claim that had they had a gun, they would have shot themselves. Fortunately, these headaches are relatively uncommon.

Treatment for cluster headaches is more difficult than for migraines, but doctors frequently use cortisone (steroids) in brief, tapering courses of one to two weeks. The drug Sansert works well for brief periods, but it has very serious potential side effects. Its use requires close supervision by the prescribing doctor.

Managing Migraines and Other Headaches—A Dietary Approach

While the exact causes of most migraines and cluster headaches remain unclear, studies link these and other headaches to certain dietary components, including food additives, some naturally occurring substances in food, and alcohol. As we get more information we may get better clues to what triggers many migraine headaches; in the meantime, what we do know suggests following headache-prevention strategies.

1. *Avoid food additives.* Watch for reactions to certain food additives, and avoid these substances if suspect. These include:

- *Monosodium glutamate (MSG).* A flavor-enhancer, this substance is found in over 2,500 food products. MSG is a stimulant to the central nervous system and has also been thought to trigger migraine headaches.
- *Nitrates (sodium nitrite).* Sodium nitrite is used as a coloring agent and preservative in smoked ham, bacon, hot dogs, pepperoni, sausages, and other processed meats. It dilates the blood vessels and can cause severe headaches in susceptible individuals.

2. *Avoid tyramine.* Watch for headaches that occur in the presence of certain foods high in tyramine, which can cause allergic reactions in some individuals. Tyramine is an amino acid that occurs naturally in certain foods. It causes the vessels in the brain to alternately constrict and dilate. Under ordinary circumstances, tyramine is broken down by metabolism, but in some individuals—those who suffer from migraines—there may be a metabolic deficit that prevents them from processing tyramine, causing it to build up in their blood and create a migraine attack. The higher the level of tyramine in a food, the greater the risk of experiencing a migraine. Foods with a concentrated or high level of tyramine include:

AGED CHEESES *	BEVERAGES	OTHER FOODS
American	Beer	Avocados
Blue	Chianti	Overripe bananas
Boursault	Coffee	Chicken livers
Brick	Colas	Chocolate
Brie	Cognac	Fava beans
Camembert	Scotch	Peanuts
Cheddar	Tea	Pickled herring
Emmentaler		Pepperoni
Gruyère		Sausage
Mozzarella		Soy sauce
Roquefort		

While headache evaluation may include a visit with an allergist who can do skin tests for certain foods, from which an elimination diet can be

* Some cheeses are blends that contain aged cheeses. People who are very sensitive should read labels carefully.

derived, aside from tyramine the correlation between headaches and food allergies is very rare—fortunately—since intolerance to many foods can result in a very restricted diet that's hard to follow.

3. *Avoid alcohol.* Consider alcoholic beverages suspect; proceed with caution. Apart from the tyramine issue, alcoholic beverages in general can provoke headaches. Alcohol not only dilates blood vessels but some by-products of the fermentation process, found in great amounts of cognac and Scotch whiskey, have been shown to provoke headaches. For many headache sufferers red wine is also a particular culprit.

4. *Limit or avoid caffeine.* Keep daily caffeine levels at 100 to 200 milligrams—that's one to two cups of coffee or tea in 5- to 6-ounce cups. If you are presently drinking more, cut down very slowly, since when excessive amounts of caffeine are stopped abruptly, severe headaches can result. Ideally, eliminate one serving at a time over a month or so, until you are in a safe daily range of 100 to 200 milligrams. (See pages 320–321 for guidelines in controlling caffeine intake.)

Also note that caffeine is an ingredient in over 1,000 nonprescription drugs and numerous prescription drugs. If present, it must be listed on the label.

5. *Limit your intake of chocolate.* Chocolate is doubly suspect when it comes to a possible link with headaches. Not only does it contain caffeine but it also has phenylethylamine, a naturally occurring substance that affects blood vessels in the same way that tyramine does.

6. *Don't skip meals.* Just as eating certain foods can trigger headaches, skipping meals can have the same effect. Prolonged fasting can make blood-sugar levels drop and bring on a headache. Often the problem is compounded by consuming large amounts of caffeine-laden foods or beverages, which lower the blood sugar even more. The result can be a terrible headache.

Headache Patterns

If you feel you get headaches more often than what you would consider normal, discuss them with your doctor—again, without jumping to conclusions and causing yourself undue alarm. Obviously, a headache that is not responding well to treatment requires further evaluation, but remember that brain tumors are very rare, and they are usually accompanied by other marked symptoms. Chances are you and your doctor will be able to formulate a management program long before a CAT scan is called for. As Woody Allen demonstrated in a memorable scene from his movie *Hannah and Her Sisters*, a CAT scan is a good test to rule out a brain tumor, but only a small minority of headache patients need to spend the money to free themselves from this largely unwarranted fear.

If you get headaches that cause concern, keep a written record of them, including the date and time of occurrence, the symptoms, the treatment, and general comments. This record-keeping can ultimately be very revealing. Some 35-plus women unduly chastise themselves for allowing what they presume is tension to cause a headache, when in fact their headaches have a biological base in the normal and predictable fluctuations of their blood supply and hormone levels. Premenstrual syndrome (see Chapter 15), certain birth-control pills, changes in early pregnancy, postpartum depression, and menopause—any of these can be real factors in the occurrence of headaches. Often a pattern emerges that tells you whether these correlations exist. Hard-to-pinpoint stresses may also be revealed, and you may discover that adjustments in life-style are all that is needed to eliminate the headaches.

DIZZINESS

Unless you are familiar with the range of possible causes, the feeling of dizziness can be more alarming than headaches. But, dizziness, the feeling of unsteadiness or lightheadedness without losing consciousness (fainting), is rarely a sign of anything dire. Often such a feeling is caused by a quick change of position, as when you move from lying down to standing up, for example, or by inadequate rest, poor nutrition, becoming overheated, or stress. Dizziness is not uncommon during early stages of pregnancy either, when rapid changes are occurring in a woman's circulation and increasing blood supply.

Whatever the possible causes, however, repeated episodes of dizziness should not be ignored. A medical evaluation can rule out anemia (low blood count), blood sugar or electrolyte imbalances, heart problems, or high blood pressure. Sometimes consultation with a neurologist is in order, but remember that dizziness caused by a tumor or blood vessel problem is very rare.

Acute rotating-type dizziness, where the room starts to spin, is often associated with nausea. This type of dizziness is usually diagnosed as an infection of the inner ear, or labyrinthitis; it is often viral in origin and responds to rest and fluids as well as antidizziness medications such as meclizine (Antivert).

On a final note, be aware that dizziness and headaches can also be the first signs of carbon monoxide inhalation, with symptoms that may even be confused with flu. Carbon monoxide is an odorless and colorless lethal gas generated by incomplete burning associated with certain fuel sources and situations: open flames heating a closed space; gas cooking stoves used for heating a room; room heaters and wood stoves with malfunctioning flues; fireplace smoke drifting into a room; machine exhaust without properly functioning catalytic converters. If you have the smallest suspicion that any of these situations exist, attend to it immediately.

DECLINING VISION

The eyes have been referred to as the windows to the brain. To keep them clear and healthy, have them checked every two years, both for vision (refractions) and for eye pressure (early detection of glaucoma). While there are always exceptions, most men and women benefit from using reading glasses by the time they reach 50. A gradual decline in vision is normal, and adjustments can be made easily—with glasses, that is.

Other routes to improving vision have proved somewhat dubious, if not dangerous, and we cannot recommend them. Evidence has recently come to light that the high-tech surgical procedure known as *radial keratotomy*, used to correct nearsightedness, is not as successful as touted, although 200,000 Americans have undergone such surgery. This is one example of the wide latitude given surgical procedures in this country. Had the treatment been a drug or implant, stringent FDA testing would have been required before such a procedure was allowed on the market, and it would have taken at least five years to confirm its safety and effectiveness.

Radial keratotomy involves making four to sixteen incisions radiating out from the cornea across the eye surface, ultimately to achieve the same objective as using corrective lenses—that is, to change the angle of light rays entering the eye so that objects won't appear blurry. As revealed in *Consumer Reports* (January 1988), the long-term results are still not fully known, since the cornea takes four to five years to fully heal; and serious complications can occur, including vision that fluctuates during the day, possible infection, and overcorrection—eyes that end up farsighted, which occurred in 16 percent of those who had the operation and took part in the study. These farsighted cases may not incur problems at first because, as Dr. Walter Stark, director of corneal services at Johns Hopkins School of Medicine, explained in the same issue of *Consumer Reports*, "you can see very well as a young person while you're farsighted, but by the time you get to age 40, you'll need reading glasses and by 50 you'll need other glasses to see at a distance. These people are happy until 40 and then they could be miserable."

Cataracts and degeneration of the macula, the "seeing" part of the eye, rarely if ever become problems in women under 70. Cataracts gradually cloud the lens of the eye; successful treatment is surgical removal of the lens and replacement with a synthetic lens. Glaucoma is a buildup of intra-ocular pressure (pressure inside the eyeball) caused by inadequate drainage.

Untreated, it leads to blindness. It is now well treated with eye drops, and in some cases with laser treatments, and as a result blindness from it has become rare. Unlike cataracts and degeneration of the macula, however, glaucoma is a concern for younger 35-plus women and your eye examinations should include a glaucoma check.

Diabetics face special problems involving the blood vessels of the retina, but fortunately laser technology is making rapid strides in this area and often these problems can be stabilized. Regular checkups by an ophthalmologist are an essential part of monitoring diabetes.

As with your skin, it makes good sense to protect your eyes against UV light when you are out in the sun, and you can do so by wearing sunglasses. Glasses offering the most protection are labeled "absorbs UV up to 400 nm." However, as almost any sunglasses will offer eye comfort and protection, you won't necessarily sacrifice quality by choosing an inexpensive pair —but be sure to check the lenses for distortion.

Good vision is an important part of overall prime health. Even when no problems are evident, an ounce of prevention by way of a periodic eye exam is worth a pound of cure.

PSYCHOSOMATIC MEDICINE:
THE MIND-BODY CONNECTION

A busy clinical practice quickly reveals that there are many paths to wellness, and that even in medicine, things are not always as they seem. Very often symptoms that would indicate a straightforward diagnosis need to be scrutinized more closely and viewed with an open mind to discover their true source, which may lie in a specific mind-body interaction. This leads into the area of psychosomatic medicine.

In a sense, everything in medicine has some mind-body interaction, even the illnesses or physical conditions that appear to be absolutely cut-and-dried. Diagnosis and treatment of strep throat, for example, involves significant mind-body interactions, including the very decision to seek care and to follow up on the advice and medications given. In coronary artery disease, coronary artery bypass grafting, which is a benchmark of technical prowess and medical progress, will avail little if the mind-body interaction is ignored.

Psychosomatic illness, as defined by the American Psychiatric Association, is a "psychophysiologic disorder of presumably psychogenic cause." In other words, physical symptoms that are caused or linked to emotional or psychological factors, such as stress or anxiety, anger or conflict. And it often involves an organ system that is under autonomic nervous-system control, such as respiration or digestion. For the person suffering from the very real symptoms that psychosomatic illness can cause, tracing the problem back to the mind is often a difficult and unacceptable route, which is why mutual trust between patient and physician is especially important in dealing with psychosomatic illness.

The following conditions and problems are some of the many that can have a specific mind-body connection and are commonly encountered among 35-plus women.

Irritable Bowel Syndrome (IBS)

The focus of IBS is either on the upper abdomen—the so-called nervous stomach—or the lower bowel. When it involves the upper abdomen, there often is a grinding feeling in the pit of the stomach. If it is centered in the lower bowel, there will be either diarrhea or constipation, or alternation of the two. Actually, IBS is a frequent cause of pain and variable bowel function, hence discomfort, and seems to affect many 35-plus women. It does not seem to be as common in elderly women as in those who are young or middle-aged, and it almost always seems to be a sign of stress—a factor that may well be apparent but that is not always dealt with effectively.

The medical approach to IBS—as with any other illness—begins with the doctor's taking a careful history and doing a physical exam. Usually the diagnosis can be fairly well established by history alone, while the physical exam, other than showing some generalized tenderness, often is not too revealing. X-rays or endoscopy sometimes are done to rule out specific physical causes, but treatment primarily involves attending to the psychological roots—in this case, stress reduction and perhaps, but not always, specific pharmacological treatment.

There is often excellent treatment for IBS among one of the antispasmodic medications, which slow down the smooth-muscle contractions of the stomach and intestines. Since at least a portion of the distress of IBS is caused by muscle contractions, antispasmodic medications can decrease the pain.

Sometimes, when the patient's history is very consistent with IBS, antispasmodics are used before any extensive testing is done. Then, if there isn't a good and prompt response, tests are appropriate and can include contrast studies, such as an upper GI, a barium enema, or endoscopy. If the patient is still unsatisfied after all these tests are run, she should consult a gastroenterologist.

Chest Pain

Another common psychosomatic problem of 35-plus women is chest pain of an unclear type, with or without chest-wall tenderness. This seems to be very common, probably because many people are worried about heart disease and have it in their minds that the main way people die in our society is either from heart disease or cancer. If someone is thinking along these lines, any pain in the chest can immediately elicit a fear of heart disease.

As with IBS, addressing this problem begins with the doctor's taking a careful history. In most cases, this is far more important in sorting out the underlying problem than the actual laying on of hands. There are various ways in which chest pain can be expressed, and various causes for it. There could be skeletal-muscular spasm, as in actual chest-wall pain, or smooth-muscular spasm, causing esophageal spasm and chest pain. Or there could be tenderness at the junctions of the ribs and the breastbone, leading to a type of arthritis called costochondritis (see Chapter 12).

The approach to each of these varies, and the therapy itself may serve to confirm the diagnosis. Indeed, a therapy that has failed can be used to diagnose the actual problem, as when a lack of response to an anti-inflammatory medication, such as Motrin, points away from the diagnosis of costochondritis; or a lack of response to one of the smooth-muscle relaxants means the problem isn't spasm. As always in psychosomatic illness, you need to identify the inciting stress, deal with that, and then use medication as needed.

Tension Headaches

One of the other major players on the psychosomatic stage is muscular or tension headaches, as discussed on page 174. Here again, attention needs to be given to identifying and reducing stress once the diagnosis has been made, and the approach should emphasize nonmedicinal treatments. Often these involve nothing more than a break from the stressful routine of the day, with time off for regular exercise. But biofeedback, yoga, and other forms of relaxation training are also effective in dealing with these headaches. Once life-style changes are initiated, supplementary medication can be used. In cases where pain is intense, even incapacitating, medication can begin at the same time; however taking this route requires careful monitoring, since many of the medications used for treating tension headaches can be habit forming. Your prime emphasis must always be on eliminating the stress that brings on the headache, which entails a straightforward communication between you and your doctor.

Chronic Fatigue Syndrome

Medicine has its trends, and just as hypoglycemia was for a while used to explain many of life's ills, now the media report on "chronic fatigue syndrome," a condition marked by chronic fatigue of several months' duration and an inability to manage the tasks of daily living, often associated with general muscle and joint achiness and poor sleep habits.

Previously thought to be associated with chronic Epstein-Barr virus—

the same virus that causes mononucleosis—chronic fatigue syndrome seems to overlap fibromyalgia (see Chapter 12) and chronic depression. In fact, a major university study found that the majority of people referred to their "chronic fatigue" clinic were in fact clinically depressed. This illustrates how important it is in the area of psychosomatic illness to do a careful evaluation before any firm diagnosis is attempted. Though organic illness must never be prematurely ruled out, the zeal to have a diagnosis can lead both patient and physician to mislabel hard-to-understand symptoms.

In the case of fatigue per se, a physical examination with tests is the first order of business to rule out problems such as anemia, underactive thyroid, or chronic infection. However, even after these tests have turned up nothing, it is often hard to believe there's no physical cause for the fatigue; it's also difficult to accept the fatigue as a sign of depression, which is frequently the case. Physicians often hesitate to introduce the idea that chronic fatigue might have a psychological base, but when this is your situation, you may well find significant benefit from antidepressant medications, started *before* you become psychologically incapacitated by the depression. Here the stoics among you should jettison the idea of toughing this out, and put a proper value on your time—how it's spent, and the quality of it. This is one area where antidepressants really do work, lifting the fatigue state and breaking through its persistent, disabling cycle.

Somatization and Hypochondria

Linking many of these psychosomatic conditions is the concept of somatization, defined by psychologist D. Z. Lipowski as a "tendency to experience and communicate psychological distress in the form of somatic symptoms that the patient misinterprets as signifying serious physical illness." A phobia of heart disease, cancer, or some similar life-threatening disease is often at the heart of the problem, and it becomes such an obsession that even physicians can't be of help. Patients who somaticize greatly will relentlessly seek medical diagnosis and treatment, and often become "doctor-shoppers" going from physician to physician. They continue this even after exhaustive tests have been done, sometimes letting themselves be put through the same tests (even painful ones) on a repeated basis because they are convinced that the previous physician has missed something dire. Ever alert to life-threatening symptoms, they become disproportionately alarmed by any symptoms.

Somewhere along the line, a physician may eventually be able to convince the somatizer that her problems do not have a physical basis. But it seems more common for these patients to resist such a diagnosis, remain disabled by nonexistent physical problems, and refuse to seek psychological treatment. Help for this sort of dilemma, for both patient and doctor, seems to be on the way, however.

In a new research study conducted by Dr. Arthur Barsky, a psychologist at the Harvard Medical School, the focus was on hypochondriacs, a group of people with a different somatoform disorder than somatizers. Hypochondriacs usually focus on one organ system as opposed to many—often as many as ten—that somatizers concentrate on. Dr. Barsky and his colleagues targeted hypochondriacs as supersensitive people who respond with unusual intensity to their body's normal aches and pains—so intensely, in fact, that the sensations become obsessions.

As reported in a recent issue of *Psychosomatic Medicine,* evidence backing Barsky's theory came from the study he and his colleagues did involving 115 patients who sought help for upper respiratory infections at the Massachusetts General Hospital clinic. Those who described symptoms far more severe than indicated during medical examination were also people who said they were very disturbed by loud noises, very uncomfortable in extreme heat or cold, and quick to sense hunger—in short, who were ultrasensitive to physical stimulation.

Pinpointing such patients provides a possible route to treatment—that is, a way to give these patients the means to manage their symptoms. Dr. Barsky has developed several strategies to accomplish this, including helping them change their intense perception of their symptoms by paying less attention to them; helping them change their opinion that normal aches and pains are alarming, and helping them concentrate on bodily sensations in a more positive way. When there is no medical basis for a diagnosis connecting symptoms to illness, coping strategies such as these will surely prove far more effective than trying to convince the patient that her symptoms don't exist, or that her perception of them is distorted.

In the meantime, such scenarios are commonly played out daily in medical offices all across the country, by people who find it more and more difficult to separate the symptoms of life-threatening diseases from those of nuisance ailments, and those that originate in the mind from those that start in the body. It has been estimated that since the 1930s the average number of visits Americans make to physicians has doubled, to five per year. Though seeking help for what seems to be a sign of illness is justified, statistics also indicate that as many as 60 percent of all patient visits have no serious medical basis. This is not to imply that these patients are all somatizers or hypochondriacs. But, according to Dr. Barsky, it does suggest the presence of "a cultural climate of alarm and hypochondria, undermining feelings of well-being. It is harder to feel confident about one's health when sensations . . . are portrayed as ominous, when every ache is thought to merit medical attention."

It is important to realize that the world of medicine does not always provide a cure, certainly not for every little ache and pain and especially when nothing is medically wrong. The thrust of psychosomatic medicine in general, and of all issues that deal specifically with a mind-body interaction, must be to establish trust in your physician. If you have symptoms that you or someone who cares about you thinks might be psychosomatic, it is important to review them with your physician. If the doctor you have chosen meets the criteria of compassion and competence discussed at the beginning of this book, she or he should be able to help you get to the source of the problem. The goal in this area is the same as in all the others —a strong mutual commitment to physical and mental health and a positive outlook on life, which is the ultimate choice.

CHAPTER 14

David Cogan on Alcohol and Chemical Dependency

THE GOAL OF GOOD HEALTH is more complicated with the brain than with any other part of the body. With the heart and lungs, for example, you enjoy a state of well-being and comfort by taking care of yourself, whereas with the brain, you can create such good feelings by abuse as well. The sensation of feeling good is so appealing that the brain is easily seduced by harmful, inherently repulsive substances—nicotine, drugs, and alcohol —that momentarily alter mood or alleviate anxiety, soothe the central nervous system, and yet act against the ultimate well-being of the entire body. Elsewhere in the body are reflexive mechanisms that work to protect against inherent dangers; any part of your body will recoil from the heat of a flame, for example, even before you mentally register the danger. Not so with the brain.

When nicotine, alcohol, or habit-forming drugs are first introduced, the body usually rebels. Lungs react to the first pack of cigarettes with sputtering coughs and the brain may second the motion with dizziness. Nonetheless, for the vast majority of people who begin smoking, the pleasurable, highly addictive effects of nicotine—the increased alertness and momentary high it affords—soon take over, ensuring a nicotine fix that can become a lifetime commitment. (Indeed, next to crack, nicotine may be the most addictive drug around.) In similar fashion, the stomach may rebel against liquor by involuntarily emptying its contents and the brain may punish further with a headache, but within a short time and with repeated use, the relaxing effect of alcohol is so rewarding as an escape from stress and inhibition that the user is willing to suffer the consequences.

Not everyone abuses these mind-altering substances, of course. But when there is a problem it exists because the choice of using nicotine, drugs, and alcohol bypasses the rational brain, leapfrogging over channels of sound judgment to reach for fleeting mind-body pleasures. If not carefully monitored, these substances can become a grave problem, extracting a high price of the user: true mental and physical deterioration, and in the case of alcoholism and drug abuse, irreparable damage to the human relationships that are valued most.

The issue of alcohol and drug dependency is deeply ingrained in our culture. It is an integral problem reflecting the turmoil of social change that has evolved as postwar baby boomers have grown up. These changes have been dramatic. Whether you turned on, tuned in, or dropped out, or had no interest in drugs, the high-flying 1960s seem a lifetime ago now. Lucy was in the sky with diamonds, but as Janis Joplin, Jimi Hendrix, and Jim Morrison tragically demonstrated, if you rode too high on drugs, you ran the risk of never coming back.

But even with its individual casualties, drug use in the 1960s and 1970s now seems almost innocent. Fueled by antiwar sentiments and the normal rebelliousness of youth, the vast majority of teens and young adults who wore tie-dyed clothes and smoked pot have moved on to raise their own children and succeed in professional careers. But the problem of drugs has only increased, cutting a wide swath through all ages, life-styles, and cultural influences. As a nation we are literally awash in illegal drugs, caught in a politically complicated drug war as unresolvable as any conflict waged in the dense jungles of Indochina.

The situation today is a far more deceptive one as well. The headlines may focus on illicit drugs like crack and heroin because they sell newspapers, but the "old news" legal substances of alcohol, prescription drugs, and nicotine account for the greatest number of blighted lives in our society. Moreover, while the media may focus on a resurgence of groups like AA or Al-Anon, these only serve those who *admit* they have a problem, a fraction of the men and women who continue hurting themselves and others close to them because of their substance abuse and dependency. This often overlooked abuse of alcohol and drugs has a big impact on the social and economic underpinnings of our culture and involves millions of Americans, directly and indirectly altering the lives of husbands, wives, children and coworkers—to say nothing of the people who are hooked.

These issues have a profound affect on women today. While the rates of alcoholism among men and women are probably about the same, the old double standard still applies in terms of social acceptability. Much of the general population still views it as macho for a man to get drunk in public, but sternly judges a woman who does so. In a busy medical practice that serves average men and women, I see far more hidden drinking among women than men, a situation that can make initiating treatment very difficult.

Prescription drugs are still perceived as more socially acceptable than alcohol; former first lady Betty Ford did this nation an enormous service with her openness and candor about her alcohol and legal drug dependence, as did Kitty Dukakis more recently. When it comes to alcohol abuse, such revelations are now beginning to be received in a supportive way, as witnessed by the good reviews and audience reception of journalist Nan Robertson's 1988 book, *Getting Better: Inside Alcoholics Anonymous*, an account of coming to grips with alcoholism. One hopes that social support will provide a new impetus for alcoholic women to seek help, to find strength in the positive reinforcement that coming clean can provide.

Are alcohol and chemical dependency diseases? An illness or disease is a group of symptoms and signs with a predictable rate of occurrence, a fairly predictable expression, and with treatment, a fairly predictable outcome. Without intervention and treatment, serious diseases have the potential to lead to death of the organism. Alcohol and chemical dependency are accurately covered by this interpretation—right down to the possibility of death—and thus can be defined and dealt with as diseases.

Fortunately, as with other diseases, using such a definition affords the chance for improvement—in this case, treatment based on abstinence that can lead to remission of signs or symptoms or, at least, their stabilization. How much of the disease actually "goes away" depends, of course, on whether there has been physical damage to the body. In this context, "cure" also requires an interpretation. Like insulin-dependent diabetics, a correctly diagnosed alcoholic or chemically dependent person is not cured. After diagnosis, it is not a question of good-bye and good luck. With treatment founded initially on abstinence and then proceeding to steps for recovery, the process can be controlled. Hence the terms *recovery* or *recovering* are also applicable—and actually more accurate.

DANGER SIGNS

Many committed career women suffer occasional but significant periods of high stress in their jobs and related anxiety about conflicts between career and family; they may turn to tranquilizers to get them through the hard times. Many women enjoy a drink before dinner, go to occasional cocktail parties, enjoy meeting friends at restaurants where good wine is a feature on the menu. In the great gray area between abstinence and abuse, what signals should users look for that indicate they're on slippery ground?

With alcohol, there are many small indications to be aware of. Do you often have more than two drinks a night? How much alcohol do you buy each week? Do you steer clear of social events where alcohol is not served? Do you begin to think about that first drink at three o'clock in the afternoon? Earlier? And—perhaps most telling—do you tend to hide your drinking? These are all warning signs: If you can back off and cut back now, you will be saving yourself some significant difficulties down the road. Aside from its direct impact on vital organs like the liver and brain, excessive alcohol has been linked to an increased incidence of breast cancer. It can wreck your complexion, lead to forms of malnutrition, and even encourage gingivitis, at the same time that it adds empty calories to your diet and flab to your waistline.

With drug dependencies, Valium, Librium and analgesics like codeine and Darvon are among the most abused prescription drugs, along with sleeping pills. If you are taking even 5 milligrams of Valium every day you may have withdrawal symptoms when you quit. This is a dependency. Sleeping pills more than once or twice a week, at most, should be avoided. Insomnia a few times a week is unpleasant, but it won't have any permanent effects, and chances are after one sleepless night you'll be able to drop off the next night. All sedative-hypnotics are potentially habit forming, but in no case do we recommend the use of barbiturates. Drugs in the benzodiazepine class may be used occasionally. (My preference is temazepam [Restoril], which is less likely to give you a "hangover" than flurazepam [Dalmane], which is a second choice.) Painkillers such as Talwin, Darvon, and codeine are all habit forming if taken for more than a couple of weeks, and alternatives (discussed later) should be sought.

A common characteristic of true dependence is increased tolerance, whether it be to alcohol, prescription medications, or illicit drugs, and a constant need for increased amounts. In all cases, a true sign of dependency is loss of control whenever the substance is used, so that there is no cut-off point, no stopping time.

It may seem that we're touting regular exercise as a cure-all for just about everything, but in truth few avenues of relief available to us are as effective in dealing with the tension, anxiety, depression, and pain that otherwise lead us to seek chemical balms. Regular exercise helps you relax: A good workout earlier in the day will help you sleep at night. Exercise relieves stress: It reduces muscle tension and gives you an outlet for working off the day's frustrations. Exercise produces feelings of well-being: A sustained workout lowers the level of triglycerides in the blood and produces endorphins, neurotransmitters (chemicals in the brain) that elevate mood and counteract feelings of anxiety and depression. Regular exercise makes the mind-body connection friendlier, and the man or woman who is happy in his or her body is also more attractive and open than the one who is not.

DETECTING DEPENDENCE

Excluding nicotine addiction, alcohol and prescription medications, espe-cially analgesics (pain pills) and sedatives, lead the list of legal dependen-cies. In a woman over age 35, abuse of either type may have gone on for many years: the problem at this point is recognizing the dependency. Often women with a dependency problem won't show up in their doctor's office until symptoms have become advanced. In the case of alcoholics, that may not be until there is cirrhosis of the liver or fluid in the abdomen, termed *ascites*. When sedatives or pain pills are involved, patients may not appear until they are seriously strung out or have become completely disoriented (which is not uncommon). At this end of the spectrum, of course, even abstinence can't reverse all the damage.

Whether the dependency is extreme or not, one reason why diagnosis is often delayed is that family members cover up—or, to use modern ter-minology, "enable"—the drinking. They love the person so they clean her up and tuck her into bed when she vomits on the carpet and goes to sleep on the floor, and then they call in sick for her the next morning. Denial is almost always a factor in alcohol or chemical dependency prior to diagnosis, even right up to the point of organ damage. Unless that denial is broken through, there can be no lasting progress, even if a patient is put in an alcohol-chem dependency unit for thirty days.

If there is a willingness to confront the problem of substance abuse, detecting it is really not too difficult. Positive proof lies in the evidence that the activities of daily life are in some way being impaired. Early on, a woman may successfully hide her use of alcohol or drugs, but eventually this will have an effect on herself, her family, and her work. Often the most dramatic (and sometimes most tragic) proof of substance abuse involves driving. For many people, the DWI (Driving While Intoxicated) charge is the first time their misuse of alcohol becomes apparent—to themselves and to others. Although such discovery and recognition varies with each per-son, rarely does an alcoholic or drug-dependent woman recognize she's on a crash course. More often, she's got to hit bottom first; and in our experi-ence, that usually involves poor function at work (the threat of job loss) or DWI.

TREATING THE PROBLEM

When a diagnosis of alcohol or chemical dependency is made, and when the problem is accepted by the individual, what is the treatment? In either case, treatment always begins with abstinence: ending the use of the sub-stance, whether it be alcohol, pain pills, sedatives, or illegal drugs such as cocaine or heroin. This is usually accomplished within a program of intense group support and self-education, which for most alcoholics in this country means Alcoholics Anonymous (AA).

Alcohol

AA flags its program with many mottoes and sayings. One of the most useful in the initial phase of treatment and recovery is "ninety in ninety"—that is, ninety meetings in ninety days. This often surprises alcoholics, who think, "My goodness, surely I don't really have to do that." But in fifty years of frontline work helping alcoholics stay on the wagon, the people of AA have discovered that even after successful detoxification, those who start to drift away from meetings early on eventually drift back to the substance. Consequently, "ninety in ninety" is but the first phase of a lifelong commitment to abstinence, a recovery process which will, in the overwhelming majority of cases, mean regular attendance at meetings. It is a rare patient who can "do it alone." It can happen, but my experience has shown this to be the rare exception rather than the rule.

One reason for this is that although an alcoholic may succeed at abstinence, and abstinence is better than nothing, it does not provide the full recovery that a true commitment to the entire process can bring about. That's why support groups can be so helpful, and why the message from health-care professionals, family, and friends must consistently be that willpower alone won't do it. Alcoholism and chemical dependency are chronic illnesses, and need continuing treatment and sustained support from family and friends to sustain recovery. A diabetic with extremely high blood sugar would never be told that she could use insulin for a few days until her sugar level was normal and then she'd be fine on her own. In treating alcoholism and drug problems, the best approach is teamwork, involving a strong outpatient emphasis that combines individual and group counseling, regular sobriety meetings, and strong encouragement to use AA and Al-Anon. When the health team is a large group, as is the case at Kaiser Permanente, it usually offers regular family meetings as well, for education, counseling, and sharing. People with alcohol dependencies do not exist in isolation. Although a woman is responsible for her own recovery, those close to her must also deal with the family and work issues that inevitably bear on the problem.

Assuming there is a diagnosis, treatment that begins with abstinence, and general agreement that treatment and recovery require continuing work—ninety in ninety—what else can be done? Certain women may require detoxification—that is, actual acute withdrawal from the abused substance in an in-patient facility. During this time there is intensive education, and the patient may receive short-term sedatives—for two to four days, if needed.

Emphasis must always be on the "real world," where the patient either will or will not remain in a recovery state. The woman who will not do outpatient group work or take responsibility for her own recovery usually also won't be saved by a multiweek program in a nice hospital in the country. Many people have the misconception that if an alcoholic can just "get away from the world" for a few weeks, her problem will be solved. Sadly, experience has shown this is not the case. The critical element is that she accept the diagnosis and begin to work on a continuing program.

Prescription Medications

Dependency on prescription medicines is a more widespread and insidious addiction than alcoholism because it is the most socially acceptable. And withdrawal is often a slower and more difficult process.

Sedatives and painkillers are the two most common prescription drugs that can lead to dependency, particularly among women. Among the sedatives, the minor tranquilizers, or anti-anxiety agents, such as diazepam (Valium) and chlordiazepoxide (Librium), have such wide use their brand names are considered household words. Among the painkillers, or analgesics, are propoxyphene (Darvon) and its compounds, codeine and its compounds, and meperidine (Demerol).

Despite all good intentions, dependency on prescription drugs sometimes emerges before either the physician or patient is aware of it, especially with the anti-anxiety agents. So many people today are chronically anxious. Those who don't suffer from that problem may find it hard to imagine taking anything when a rare bout of anxiety occurs, but the woman who is anxious about every business meeting or social encounter—and who initially turns to tranquilizers or sleep medications to tide her over tough, stressful periods—can very rapidly slip into dependency.

For anyone dependent on tranquilizers, sedatives, or analgesics, the ultimate goal is the same as for alcohol dependency: abstinence. Often this requires a gradual tapering off in tandem with intensive outpatient group work—similar to the approach taken with one of my patients who is down from 5 milligrams of Valium twice a day to 2 milligrams a day. Encouragement and counseling have not yet led to complete abstinence, but the goal remains and the work—in this case, persistence on my part as well as continuing responsibility on the part of the patient—continues.

With a woman dependent on sedatives and tranquilizers, the first priority is to introduce specific changes to help her cope with the anxiety or pain that initially led to the dependency. As we've noted, exercise is an especially therapeutic component of the recovery, as is diet, and the process can be noticeably hastened when attention is turned to these areas. There will always be some anxious people who will need pharmacological help to taper off a dependency; BuSpar is a new drug that can serve this purpose, assisting some chronically anxious patients without leading to dependency problems. However, the goal for society as a whole certainly should be to live without medication. Even those who consider themselves chronically anxious should seek to root out the causes of their anxiety, work to eliminate them, and move toward a drug-free life. Your doctor can help.

From Darvon to Demerol, the weaning process from painkillers has proved to be as difficult as from sedatives, especially when the drugs are taken to alleviate chronic pain.

"Pain centers," multidisciplinary clinics or hospital wards that stress counseling and educational and physical therapy, can truly help, provided there is a patient-physician partnership and a nonnarcotic pain-management plan.

In the treatment of pain, even more than that of anxiety, there are many helpful new alternatives to medication, including creative physical and occupational therapies, heat and ultrasound, home exercise programs for certain kinds of pain, and in the last few years, electrical stimulation— the so-called TENS (Transcutaneous Electrical Nerve Stimulation) units. These have helped many analgesically dependent patients decrease their pain and get off habit-forming medications. Even nontraditional healers— trained acupuncturists or therapists in biomechanics—can help get patients off of pain pills, so long as their therapies are conscientiously followed.

In dealing with chronic pain, good nutrition is tremendously helpful, especially a high-fiber diet to improve elimination and weight loss, where appropriate. Here again, regular exercise can't be overemphasized.

Many who suffer from chronic pain live in a very circumscribed world. They don't go out, don't exercise, take little interest in food, have a meager social life. Anything a physician, family member, or individual herself can do to help open up such a circumscribed world will probably in and of itself help decrease the pain she experiences. So the approach to chronic pain management, especially for those who have become dependent on pain medications, must encompass what the world outside of medication has to offer, not just substitute a new or different drug.

Illicit Drugs

Illicit drugs form an important category of chemical dependency and thus deserve some mention here, although they do not appear to have dramatic overt use among the middle class, especially not among those to whom this book is addressed.

Cocaine and the cocaine derivative crack are the most prevalent illicit drugs today; as with heroin, they create dependencies that are very hard to treat: chronic addictions that require nothing less than chronic treatment. Objectively speaking and as easy as it is to say, the treatment is, as with alcohol and prescription medicines, abstinence.

While not as widely used as in the past, marijuana remains a drug of choice for some members of the 35-plus generation who started using it in their youth. However, the situation has changed since those days, because research has shown that marijuana is by no means a bland drug. Chronic use may well lead to lung damage similar to that resulting from regular cigarette smoking. Certain studies have also tied marijuana to chronic impairment of the central nervous system, possible decrease in fertility, and even to genetic changes. Like all addictive drugs, if a person is dependent on marijuana, the only treatment is abstinence, ideally reinforced with a program of regular exercise and good nutrition.

When it comes to passing along drug dependencies—or getting hooked in the first place—many of us are better role models for our children than the parents of past generations ever were, particularly those parents today who have beaten their dependencies and can tell their children about it. The more the appeal of smoking regular cigarettes decreases, the less chance there is that a drug like marijuana will take hold with youth. One hopes that this pattern will continue, especially since it has also been shown in adolescent treatment centers that regular cigarette smoking really is a gateway to illicit drug use, especially use of pot.

So choice comes in again, and the ideal choice is to avoid all drugs. Taken literally, that would mean everything from any drinking at all, to using habit-forming medications at all, to using cigarettes at all. Total abstinence from all these substances may be unrealistic, but think hard about each of them: about the clear risks involved in their use, since each is toxic in varying degrees, and about the more insidious danger of addiction.

The choice of avoidance is probably one of the hardest to make in a society that glorifies anything that can lead to some sort of high. Giving something up can be hard to do, but in cases of alcohol, chemical, and drug dependencies and their significant health risks, giving up is really gaining: gaining good health, vibrant good looks, sharp mental powers, and a clear sense of who you are and where you are headed. All of life has risks, but risking the loss of your midlife assets can be counted among the greatest.

FOUR STEPS TO BREAKING DEPENDENCY

1. *Recognize it.* Look hard at its effect on the quality of daily life.
2. *Confront it.* Speak up about it to a doctor and/or clergy.
3. *Treat it.* Tap into medical resources and community health programs.
4. *Recover from it.* Actively embrace a life-style that includes time for fitness, good nutrition, and relaxation with family and friends.

PART FOUR

Midlife Reproduction and Sexuality

AS REVEALED IN THE chapters that follow, nowhere are changing health attitudes and discoveries more evident than in issues relating to female reproduction and sexuality. It may seem to us that each new revelation in this area only brings to light another health risk—from the specifics of breast cancer to the global threat of AIDS. But it only takes a glance at the past to see that in most areas of sexual and gynecological health, women today have truly been liberated from the worst complications of pregnancy, "female problems," and the premature aging associated with menopause.

As they generally do now, many women in the old days outlived men —that is, if they managed to make it to menopause. Pregnancy and delivery were high-risk propositions, and since the only sure way to avoid pregnancy was not to have sex, sexuality itself was fraught with danger. Mary Godwin, an early feminist, died of an infection after the birth of her daughter Mary Godwin Shelley—Mrs. Godwin spending days in delirious fever while the attending physician attempted to remove the remnants of a retained placenta. Two of Jane Austen's brothers went through several wives apiece before marrying women who survived the birth of their last children. While their emotional reaction to menopause was probably as mixed as ours is today, many women must have greeted it as a haven of safety. Issues of sexuality and childbearing began to be a relatively broad part of women's political thinking and writing only in the late nineteenth century, and it wasn't until the late twentieth that these issues took hold in the general population. If it seems that they have become overpoliticized or dominate too much of our thinking today, one can see the source, but in most cases we can only imagine the impact the ominous facts of life had on women of the past.

Liberated from unwanted or badly timed pregnancies by reliable birth control, from the monthly misery of periods by advances in treating PMS, and from many of the undesirable effects of menopause, women are faced with a lot of choices. The biological clock is still a reality women must come to terms with a lot sooner than men do, since one of the central questions of adulthood is whether or when to have children, and it's a question women must answer in their prime. By the time you've reached 35, the routine matters of coping with monthly periods and using birth control are probably so familiar that you rarely think about them. But approaching forty, you face new issues—waning fertility and choices about becoming pregnant; reassessment of birth control methods, particularly if you've been on the pill; dealing with subtle signs that you're now in your pre-menopausal years. Past forty the signs of menopause become less subtle, though they need not be calamitous—far from it. At 35-plus, you have more options and information available than ever before to help make the sexual passage through the middle years an enlightened one. In many ways, you're at the peak of your powers.

CHAPTER 15

PMS and Menstruation in the Middle Years

PMS

One sign that menopause may actually be on the horizon is the condition referred to as PMS, or premenstrual syndrome. It occurs in some women in the days just before the onset of their menstrual cycle, and it accounts for any combination of headaches, bloating, intense cravings for sweets and other foods, depression and general malaise. Genetic makeup plays a role in who gets PMS and who doesn't, but age also seems to be a factor. The perimenopausal years are generally considered to start at age 35, and many women between 30 and 40 report PMS symptoms when they never had them before, or else their familiar PMS symptoms become more intense during this time. While the causes of PMS are unclear, it appears to be a spectrum of illnesses and problems that in turn necessitates a spectrum of treatments and medications, many of which are still in the experimental stages.

Signs and symptoms of PMS in large numbers of women have been established in several studies, including those conducted by Dr. Jean Endicott, a professor of clinical pyschology at the New York State Psychiatric Institute at Columbia University. Based on detailed records of women's menstrual cycles, she and her colleagues found that about a quarter of all women report no PMS symptoms, approximately one-third have mild to moderate symptoms which do not disrupt daily life, another third have symptoms that exacerbate existing chronic conditions and thus cause temporary disruptions, and less than one-tenth of all women reported PMS symptoms severe enough to be incapacitating. In all cases of PMS, Dr.

Endicott confirms that it is critical for symptoms to be carefully sorted out to ensure proper treatment.

For years researchers and clinicians assumed that the cause of PMS was variations in estrogen-progesterone levels, but a new theory suggests that PMS is actually the result of sudden changes in levels of endorphins, the morphinelike chemicals made in the brain. As the Johnson study described below indicates, the fact that many women use exercise to combat PMS symptoms is one possibly vital clue that this is the case, since vigorous exercise has been shown to raise endorphins and produce the so-called runner's high, which many people experience after strenuous sports.

No more than a generation ago PMS theories were virtually nonexistent, and premenstrual "jitters" tended to be written off as an unfortunate emotional tendency somehow related to that "time of the month." Without an organized way of thinking about it, or medical confirmation to legitimize it, women who suffered from PMS were pretty much left to their own resources.

One 35-plus woman describes how she diagnosed herself when she uncovered a tell-tale pattern in her behavior—in her case, after she and her husband had begun to fight so intensely that their marriage was threatened. She began keeping a record of when the fights occurred, on the same calendar she used to mark her menstrual periods. After a few months she noticed that the bitter battles always preceded the onset of her period by two or three days, so that just as she was feeling apologetic, her period would begin.

Another 35-plus woman described her symptoms as a "wolfman metamorphosis." As the month progressed, she'd become wilder and woollier until she fell prey to a chocolate binge, which signaled the onset of her period and a return to normal. Still another woman was so overwhelmed by the anxiety caused by PMS that even when she knew its source, she felt she'd be better off spending those days in bed—if only she could.

Putting some perspective on the emotional side of a syndrome that used to be referred to as "female problems," Dr. Endicott noted that there was "nothing distinctive about the mood and behavior changes in women and men. The only difference is that in women these changes are cyclical."

Whatever the PMS symptoms, they do seem to disappear with the onset of your period, a fact that doesn't make them any less troublesome or less worthy of treatment. The good news is that PMS is taken much more seriously than in the past, with new medical and nutritional approaches evolving all the time to help control symptoms and enable women to formulate their own plans of action in dealing with them.

Current Medical Treatments for PMS

There are a number of standard options for treating PMS with medications.

If pain predominates, the use of nonsteroidal anti-inflammatory drugs such as Motrin or Ponstel is beneficial in many cases. When there is significant water retention, the cyclic use of diuretics, especially the week before menstruation begins, is a longstanding route that really can help. Vitamin B_6 (pyridoxine) may be helpful with mood swings, as are various hormonal treatments—usually progesterone-progestin medications used in a cyclic way each month. There is no definite way to know in advance who will respond to these treatments. The medication route generally represents a conventional approach to PMS, and new findings may in time supersede them.

The Johnson Study

In a fascinating study by Susan Johnson and colleagues, published in the *Journal of Reproductive Medicine* (April 1988), 730 nursing-school graduates (most of them married and well educated) were surveyed on their experiences with PMS. Although 87 percent reported at least some occurrence of PMS symptoms, for only 3.2 percent were they severe. How did these women manage to keep their symptoms under control? The answer has significance for all women who suffer from PMS. About 20 percent used vitamins, including B_6; about 25 percent changed their diet; and about 42 percent used exercise to relieve symptoms, thus supporting a 1971 study by Timonen in Finland which showed that women who exercised reported fewer PMS symptoms than those who were sedentary.

As for taking medications, the women in the Johnson study who did so often chose aspirin or nonsteroidal (noncortisone) anti-inflammatory drugs such as Motrin. Diuretics were the next most common category chosen, followed by hormonal preparations including progesterone and similar drugs, with less than 2 percent using these, although 17 percent had at some point had them prescribed. (In fact prescription drugs in general—including oral contraceptives, progesterone, bromocriptine, and lithium have had little, if any, overall effect on PMS.)

It is interesting to note here that a large group of medically educated women relied primarily on self-help measures for PMS control, and that only a very small number used hormonal treatments. This isn't to say that hormonal treatments are without value, but for many women the self-help approach centering on exercise or diet is a safe and effective primary choice. If such an approach doesn't work, then a gynecologist or internist with interest and experience in medication treatments can be consulted. In situations in which PMS symptoms and depression are intertwined, a trial of tricyclic antidepressants may be in order, provided such a route is taken with the advice of the primary physician and his or her consultants.

Other Approaches to PMS Treatment

While some promising research is under way in developing treatments for PMS, some of the nutritional therapies (vitamins and minerals) currently being used need clarification—and a few words of caution.

VITAMIN B_6. There is some controversy over the use of vitamin B_6 in treating PMS, although many experienced doctors seem to use it with good success. Some studies have shown B_6 treatment to be effective for many women in dealing with PMS-related anxiety and depression, but only in large doses—500 milligrams a day. These studies report no bad side effects at this level. Conflicting studies report possible side effects, including nerve damage, in doses of 200 milligrams or more. In treating PMS, individual doctors will use varying approaches, and those who use vitamin B_6 will base dosage on their own experience with regard to its safety and effectiveness. We believe that a therapy that calls for more than 100 milligrams of B_6 per day (41 times the RDA) should be carefully monitored by your doctor. You should not take large doses of B_6 without medical supervision.

VITAMIN E. Another vitamin sometimes recommended for PMS is vitamin E, in a daily dose of 400 IU. Supposedly this relieves both physical and psychological PMS symptoms, but these claims are unsubstantiated and this is a route we cannot advise. Not only does the dosage far exceed the RDA of 30 IU a day, but the possible side effects from such large quantities have not yet been determined.

TRYPTOPHAN. Supplementation with tryptophan has also been promoted as a cure-all for PMS. As explained on page 171, tryptophan is a precursor of the neurotransmitter serotonin, which sometimes helps with depression and sleep disturbances. There is currently no definite evidence to link it to any other possible symptoms of PMS, however, so we can't specifically endorse tryptophan to treat PMS, although we realize some readers might wish to try it.

MAGNESIUM. There have been claims that PMS is the result of magnesium deficiency, primarily by an advocate who heads a company that makes and sells magnesium supplements. We find little basis for the theory, which is based on a handful of animal studies and only a few poorly controlled human studies.

A study that plays devil's advocate to the general idea that vitamin or mineral supplements are effective in treating PMS was recently concluded in Australia. Participants included thirty-eight women who suffered from PMS and a control of twenty-three women who did not. In both groups, the blood levels of thiamine, vitamin B_6, vitamin A, vitamin E, magnesium, and zinc were measured just prior to menstruation, when the PMS sufferers exhibited symptoms. Blood levels of the six nutrients were no different in PMS sufferers than the blood levels in the nonsufferers. Whether or not the conclusion the researchers drew from this study—that there is no evidence PMS symptoms are caused by nutritional deficiencies—is considered definitive, the results do suggest that taking large amounts of any vitamin above the RDA—vitamin B_6 notwithstanding—is a speculative approach.

Finding safe ways to manage PMS through nutrition does not always lead to dead ends, as research with certain hormones is beginning to show. Many features of PMS, such as breast tenderness and swelling, are similar to effects produced by the injection of prolactin, the hormone that triggers the production of milk in a woman's mammary glands. Studies of this hormone and its connection to PMS have led researchers to theorize that some women who suffer from PMS may actually have an abnormal sensitivity to normal (as opposed to elevated) levels of prolactin. It seems that another hormone found in human milk can counteract the effect of prolactin. It is the prostaglandin derived from the essential fatty acid gammalinolenic. Interestingly, the only available therapeutic form comes from a plant—the seed oil of the evening primrose (Oenothera biennis). This oil is currently being researched in England as a possible treatment for PMS. When the results of more extensive studies on both sides of the Atlantic come to light, a derivative of evening primrose oil may well prove to be a safe and effective treatment for certain PMS sufferers.

One of the difficulties in dealing with PMS is the wide assortment of symptoms included under the term. Although some of these, like breast tenderness and general fluid retention, can be readily described in physiological terms, others, like mood swings and food cravings, are less easily pinned down, and the range and severity of symptoms can differ markedly from woman to woman. In some instances particular symptoms may be labeled as part of the premenstrual syndrome simply because they appear cyclically. In time more will be learned about specific causes and treatments for each of the symptoms categorized under PMS, but in the meantime you may discover that exercise, which has an impact on mood and on blood sugar levels, coupled with dietary changes that can reduce bloat and further manage blood sugar, may be all you need to relieve PMS symptoms—and these drug-free alternatives are available to you right now.

Jean Spodnik's PMS Diets: Two Safe Options to Relieve Symptoms

As a nutritionist and author, I was intrigued to hear that many women between the ages of 30 and 40 who had used my 35-Plus Diet reported that it seemed to relieve their PMS symptoms. I wished to observe this more carefully, so, in a small pilot study, I compiled data that included measurements of weight gain, breast tenderness and swelling, joint soreness, headache, abdominal cramping and bloat, nausea, and food cravings. My findings were based on records kept through six monthly periods by the participants in the study.

For their first two periods, I asked participants not to change their present diet, but to keep track of PMS symptoms so that severity on a scale of 1 (nonexistent) to 4 (most severe) could be established. For their next two periods, half the women in the study were put on a high-carbohydrate diet and the other half were put on a high-protein diet. For the final two periods, the women switched diets so that those who had been on the high-carbohydrate diet went on a high-protein diet, and vice versa.

While the number of women (15) completing the study was small, 218 measurements of the specified symptoms were obtained, with results clearly confirming a correlation between diet and PMS relief.

- Eighty percent of the women completing the test reported improvement in symptoms using one of the diets.
- Over half the women experienced a marked decrease in all symptoms on the high-protein diet. This result confirmed the many casual reports made by women who had used the 35-Plus Diet for weight loss. These women included both obese women who did not exercise, and women of normal weight who exercised 30 minutes daily. The latter reported that, because they had fewer of their usual symptoms, their mental attitude improved and they felt more inclined to keep up with exercise.
- Just under one third of the group in the study felt stress on the high-protein diet, but reported feeling well on the diet higher in complex carbohydrates. All but one of the women in this group were in their normal weight range, and all exercised daily. Although this form of the diet does not cope with fluid retention and bloating as well as the high protein diet does, it deals with cravings for carbohydrates in a healthy way, keeping blood sugar at a good level without adding unnecessary calories.

To reduce the incidence of transient hypoglycemia—low blood sugar, which has been documented to occur in women seven to ten days before the onset of their period—alcohol, sugar, and caffeine were restricted in both diets, although one cup of regular coffee (or tea) was allowed on the high protein diet, because the high protein diet tends to stabilize blood sugar levels in normal adults. Three meals and three snacks a day (to compensate for the increased appetite many women experience prior to their period) further ensured that blood sugar would never become low during this time. That both diets were low in fat and were either moderate or low in salt were two additional factors that seemed to contribute to the overall positive effects.

Although broader testing will enable us to better pinpoint the effects of the two diet variations, the diet higher in complex carbohydrates may be a better fit for relatively slender women whose PMS symptoms include food cravings, especially for sweets. The high protein version is more effective in relieving symptoms such as breast tenderness which are related to fluid retention. Since overweight women are more susceptible to fluid retention, they will probably find the high protein diet to be more effective, although women of normal weight were equally represented in the group that preferred this version. A side benefit of the high protein diet may be a pound or two of weight loss.

In the diets that follow, serving sizes and allowable foods are keyed to the 35-Plus Diet Exchange lists in Chapter 22. Vegetables in the diet refer to the "free" vegetable list, while complex carbohydrates appear under the starch list. Although all starches are technically complex carbohydrates as opposed to simple sugars, those carbohydrates closest to their natural state (starchy vegetables, brown rice, whole grain breads and pastas) will lead to more stable blood sugar levels than breads and crackers made with refined flours, which the body turns into glucose relatively quickly.

A PLAN OF ACTION FOR PMS

If you suffer or think you may be suffering from premenstrual syndrome, note on your calendar when symptoms occur and what they include. This is especially helpful for symptoms that aren't overtly connected (as cramps are, for example) to your period. If you can identify a monthly pattern that tends to center on the second or third week of your cycle, you'll know that symptoms like anxiety or food cravings are probably symptoms of PMS. But don't neglect to take other factors into consideration. If you have to make a monthly report to the boss or go over the family budget the third week of every month, you may be experiencing symptoms of stress that aren't organic in origin—or are only partly so. Stress factors such as these may be compounded by PMS.

Try management with exercise and diet. The good results of the Johnson study and of Jean's early research strongly suggest that exercise and/or diet may be all you need to manage moderate symptoms.

While an exercise program should be a regular part of your life, you can get good results from dietary changes without staying on a diet full time. If your periods and your PMS symptoms follow a very regular pattern, you should go on the diet two days before PMS symptoms normally occur, and stay on it through the first day of your period. If the onset of PMS

High-Protein PMS Diet (1,200 Calories)

	VEGETABLES	COMPLEX CARBOHYDRATES	PROTEIN	FRUIT	LOW-FAT MILK OR PLAIN YOGURT	UNSATURATED FATS
Breakfast	0	1	1	1	½ c.	1
Snack	as desired	0	1	0	0	0
Lunch	as desired	1	2	0	0	1
Snack	as desired	½*	1	0*	0	0
Dinner†	as desired	1	4	0	0	1
Snack	as desired	0*	1	1*	½ c.	0

Because the high protein diet is effective in reducing fluid retention, salt may be used *in moderation*, but you should avoid heavily salted foods. Caffeine should be limited to one cup of regular coffee or tea a day.

* With either of these snacks you may have either half a serving of complex carbohydrate, or one serving of fruit.
† Take one multivitamin with minerals with dinner.

Sample Menu
High-Protein PMS Diet

Breakfast	½ grapefruit
	1 c. Special K *or* 2 slices whole wheat reduced-calorie bread
	½ c. low-fat milk
	1 tsp. polyunsaturated margarine
	¼ c. egg substitute *or* ⅓ c. lowfat cottage cheese
	Coffee or tea (black, with artificial sweetener or part of milk serving)
Snack	1 oz. low-fat cheese
	raw vegetables
Lunch	Tuna salad (½ c. water pack tuna, 1 or 2 tbs. low-fat mayonnaise, chopped onion or celery)
	1 pita pocket
	Raw vegetables or small salad
Snack	1 apple
	1 oz. low-fat cheese
Dinner	4 oz. broiled sirloin steak *or* fish *or* skinless chicken
	1 small baked potato
	1 tsp. polyunsaturated margarine
	Steamed broccoli, carrots, cauliflower
	Spinach salad with diet ranch dressing
Snack	½ c. plain yogurt (with vanilla flavoring and sugar substitute, if desired)
	1 sliced peach

symptoms varies somewhat, try going on the diet ten days before your period is to begin, again staying on it through the first day of your period. Experiment to find out what timing is best for you. You may be able to get relief with the diet using it only one week out of the month.

If these measures aren't enough to relieve PMS symptoms, consult with your doctor about medications for PMS, but don't give up on the exercise and do monitor your diet to curb the food cravings—especially for sweets —that can increase bloat and wreak havoc with your blood sugar levels. As we've noted, in many women there is a tendency to hypoglycemia in the week before menstruation and it will be further exacerbated by alcohol and caffeine. These should be restricted during this week. Well-balanced lowfat meals, supplemented with small snacks of lowfat protein, fruit or complex carbohydrates can keep you on an even keel without adding pounds to your figure.

OTHER MENSTRUATION PROBLEMS

The menstrual cycle in 35-plus women usually averages twenty-eight to thirty days, with periods lasting three to five days. For many women, the

High–Complex Carbohydrate PMS Diet (1,300 to 1,400 Calories)

	VEGETABLES	COMPLEX CARBOHYDRATES	PROTEIN	FRUIT	LOW-FAT MILK OR PLAIN YOGURT	UNSATURATED FATS
Breakfast	0	2	1	1	½ c.	1
Snack	0	1	0	1	0	0
Lunch	as desired	2	2	1	0	1
Snack	as desired	1	0	1	0	0
Dinner*	as desired	2–3	3–4	1	0	2
Snack	0	1	0	1	½ c.	0

Salt should be restricted on the high–complex carbohydrate diet, to help reduce fluid retention and bloat. Avoid caffeine altogether.

* Take one multivitamin with minerals with dinner.

Sample Menu
High–Complex Carbohydrate PMS Diet

Breakfast	4 oz. orange juice
	½ c. cooked oat bran *or* ½ c. bran flakes
	½ c. low-fat milk
	1 slice whole wheat toast
	1 tsp. polyunsaturated margarine
	¼ c. egg substitute *or* 1 oz. lowfat cheese
	Decaffeinated coffee or tea (black, with artificial sweetener, or part of milk serving)
Snack	2 graham crackers
	2 tbls. raisins
Lunch	2 ozs. turkey (no skin)
	2 slices whole wheat bread
	Low-fat mayonnaise
	Lettuce and raw vegetables, or small salad
	1 apple
Snack	2 bread sticks
	½ c. orange juice
Dinner	4 oz. cooked chicken, fish, lean pork, or beef
	⅔ c. cooked brown rice *or* 1 c. whole wheat pasta, mixed with cooked onions, mushrooms, and green beans, tossed with 1 tbsp. grated cheese
	Garden salad with low-fat dressing
	Small bunch of grapes (12 to 15)
Snack	½ c. plain yogurt
	mixed with ½ c. crushed pineapple
	2 graham crackers

first signs of premenopausal change include changes in the menstrual cycle, with intervals between periods becoming longer or shorter than usual, or longer one month and shorter the next. The duration of periods can also vary, as can the heaviness of the menstrual flow and the intensity of PMS.

As at any other age, tampons can be used for normal menstruation, but they must be the smallest size necessary and frequently changed to avoid risk of infection. The problem of toxic shock syndrome, which surfaced several years ago, prompted a new awareness of tampon use. While the problem still occurs, it is not nearly as widespread as it was in the past. To avoid the risk altogether, many women prefer sanitary napkins, and there is now a wide variety of pads or sanitary napkins to meet individual needs.

If a woman is having a problem with menstrual cramps, nonsteroidal, anti-inflammatory agents such as Ponstel or ibuprofen (Motrin) can really help, and have the added benefit of not being habit forming. Many women who avoid medications in general are comfortable with these drugs.

Anemia might seem an odd thing to discuss in connection with normal gynecological issues, but as pointed out in Chapter 8, the most common cause of anemia in 35-plus women is iron deficiency owing to menstruation. Anemia, or low red-blood-cell count, is usually defined as a hemoglobin of less than 12 grams; for many 35-plus women, this is a normal consequence of heavy menstruation.

If you are experiencing unusual fatigue or pallor—or indeed, heavy menses in general—you should visit your doctor for a complete blood count, or CBC. If there is an iron deficiency, options include oral iron tablets, oral liquid iron, or even iron injections, as well as dietary changes. (For specifics, see Chapter 8).

VAGINAL AND URINARY TRACT INFECTIONS

Although these can occur at any age, nonsexually transmitted yeast infections and urinary tract infections commonly crop up in 35-plus women. Only occasionally do they pose serious health risks, but they usually do cause a high degree of discomfort. (For sexually transmitted diseases, see Chapter 18).

YEAST INFECTIONS. These infections, especially those caused by *Candida albicans*, are fairly common in women. Particularly susceptible are those who are on birth-control pills; who are immune suppressed, as when on large doses of steroids; who take broad-spectrum antibiotics, such as ampicillin; or who have diabetes and do not control it well.

Yeast infections are thus caused by an upset in the normal symbiotic balance among related organisms that inhabit the vagina. The imbalance results in an overgrowth of the *Candida* organisms that leads to infection. Symptoms include a white, cheesy vaginal discharge, itching, irritation, and a "yeasty" odor.

While not caused by sexual contact, once yeast infections set in, they can in fact be sexually transmitted to a partner, which is one reason they deserve prompt attention. Diagnosed by means of a direct microscope-slide examination (the "wet prep") in the office, treatment includes vaginal suppositories or creams. In the case of diabetics or women on steroids or antibiotics, control of the underlying situation, including a possible change in medication, should also be undertaken.

If you have recurring yeast infections and medication is not entirely effective, your diet may be partly to blame. If you are consuming a lot of sugar, your blood sugar levels will be elevated and this affects the growth of the yeast. Replace sugars with grains, fruits, and vegetables and your condition may well improve.

URINARY TRACT INFECTIONS. These are also very common in women. In clinical practice, the number of women we treat for urinary-tract infections exceeds the number of men by twenty to one.

Usually the problem involves a lower urinary-tract infection, sometimes called cystitis, or bladder infection. Acute onset is common, and symptoms include frequent urination accompanied by a burning sensation and possibly a fever. Diagnosis is made by laboratory examination of the urine to confirm the presence of white blood cells or bacteria. Often there will be an immediate positive reaction to a certain chemistry strip that indicates infection; in this case, the urine will still be sent out for lab culture, even if treatment is initiated before the culture comes back (in two or three days).

Treatment consists of antibiotics: most commonly, sulfamethoxazole with trimethoprim combinations such as Septra or Bactrim, sulfa drugs such as Gantrisin or Gantanol, or penicillin drugs of the ampicillin type. Years ago, it seemed all women with these infections were put on a traditional ten-day course of whatever antibiotic had been prescribed, but nowadays many receive shortened courses of antibiotics—often three to five days—especially if the symptoms are of cystitis only.

The general, nonspecific advice connected with treatment is to increase fluids: water to help dilute the urine or the time-honored cranberry juice to acidify the urine. If a urinary-tract infection recurs often, that is, three times in one or two years, tests are needed. Provided you are not pregnant, these usually include a kidney X-ray, called an IVP, as well as a visual look at the bladder in a process called cystoscopy, the latter done by a qualified urologist. This is to check for irritation or even a small tumor of the bladder.

To help prevent urinary-tract infections when they are recurrent, it is probably best to avoid tub baths, bath oils, and bath powders. In addition, patients are usually advised to get up and urinate after sexual intercourse, and to drink plenty of water each day so that urination is reasonably frequent. Occasionally, despite these measures, urinary tract infections continue to crop up. A recurring or persistent pattern warrants preventive treatment with a low-dose antibiotic. A common regimen is one-half of a Septra tablet each night, which often brings improvement. Urine cultures should also be taken so that if a patient does not respond to initial treatment, the bacteria can be checked to be certain they are sensitive to the antibiotic chosen.

Symptoms of a urinary infection can be generalized and more severe. In addition to frequent irritating urination there may also be backache, chills, fever, and malaise, indicating an upper urinary-tract infection. Sometimes called pyelonephritis, this is caused by bacteria—as with cystitis. It requires a longer course of antibiotics, and it may even require hospitalization so that these can be given intravenously.

ABNORMAL CONDITIONS OF THE UTERUS

There are two conditions that can develop at midlife (and sometimes before) which are not cancerous but which can seriously complicate pregnancy and cause difficult menstrual cycles.

FIBROID TUMORS. Fibroids, also called leiomyomas, are slow-growing, usually benign growths in the uterus, consisting of a mixture of smooth muscle cells and connective tissue. They are actually quite common, occurring in approximately one out of every four women of child-bearing age, especially when there is no pregnancy. As each month passes without implantation of a fertilized egg, the sloughing-off process of tissues lining the uterus become less efficient and thus fibroids can result.

Often, fibroids cause no symptoms and can be left alone, since they inevitably decrease after menopause. However, depending on their size and location, sometimes they can interfere with pregnancy by preventing the normal passage of an egg through the fallopian tubes, or they can impede a normal vaginal delivery. If fibroids are present when a woman conceives, their rate of growth can quickly increase, owing to the increase in hormones to the area, but they usually shrink again after delivery.

One advantage of cesarean delivery in this situation is that an obstetrician can observe the general condition of a woman's uterus; in some cases, he or she can remove significant fibroids on the spot. One woman describes how all along she'd thought the lump on the left side of her pregnant belly was the baby's foot, whereas it turned out to be a fibroid about the size of a lemon. Her obstetrician removed it during her cesarean delivery and then presented it, along with a healthy nine-pound baby girl, to her husband!

While the majority of fibroids present no problems, if they cause heavy, prolonged menstrual bleeding or if their size greatly increases uterine size (for example, to the size of a three-month pregnant uterus), hysterectomy may be considered. Generally, fewer hysterectomies are done for fibroids than in past years, and indications for surgery must be reviewed carefully with your gynecologist.

ENDOMETRIOSIS. This condition occurs when endometrial tissue (uterine lining) grows in places where it should not be, such as in or on an ovary, or elsewhere in the pelvic lower abdominal area. Although benign (noncancerous) endometriosis can cause pain and can be a cause for infertility, and is clearly an issue for 35-plus women, since the median age of diagnosis is 37. The diagnosis is visual, either by laparoscopy (insertion of a scope into the abdominal cavity to "take a look") or by laparotomy (limited exploratory surgery of the lower abdomen).

Treatment can be either surgical—varying from total hysterectomy with ovary removal to selective removal of the endometrial "implants"—or it can be medical—traditionally with the drug danazol (Danocrine), which decreases the output of the hormones from the pituitary gland that stimulate female hormone production. In either case, endometriosis requires the care of a well-trained and experienced gynecologist.

HYSTERECTOMY. The main reasons for elective (as opposed to emergency) hysterectomy, with or without ovary removal, are various forms of cervical or uterine cancer (these are covered in Chapter 19), and problems with excessive bleeding (with or without fibroids). Without doubt, a hysterectomy is a major operation, and the reasons for it must be clear. Though the situation is changing, there are still some doctors who may advise a hysterectomy when it is not essential, and even in cases where cancer is involved, we advise you to get a second opinion before proceeding with a hysterectomy. Should ovary removal be involved, it will bring on the condition known as surgical menopause, and in nearly all cases hormonal replacement is strongly advised, even if menopausal symptoms are mild. As noted in Chapter 17, surgical menopause clearly accelerates a woman's aging process, but this can be tempered by hormonal replacement.

CHAPTER 16

The 35-Plus Pregnancy: Nine Healthy Choices
Every Woman Should Make

BECAUSE THE KEY ISSUE for all pregnancies is making healthy choices, if you want to start a family at 35-plus you should begin making informed decisions as soon as possible: when to try to conceive, how to ensure the best prenatal care and birth experience, and even how you want to nourish your baby in the days following delivery—breast or bottle feeding.

1: TIMING

Whether premenopausal or otherwise, an erratic menstrual cycle affects the predictability of ovulation. This poses a special challenge to women trying to conceive in the years when their biological clocks are ticking away. The physiological challenges to conceiving, including on average a 50 percent decline in a woman's fertility after age 40, really do increase with age, as do certain known risks, the greatest of which is conceiving a Down's syndrome baby. Statistics show that the possibility for Down's syndrome leaps ahead in almost geometric proportion, from 1 in every 1,000 pregnancies in women of age 30, to 1 in every 350 in women of age 35, to 1 in every 100 in women age 40, and then to 1 in every 30 pregnancies at age 45.

Despite these risks, many 35-plus women are starting families later in life and are doing so with a happy outcome. The ultrasophisticated testing procedures now available, such as chorionic villi sampling (done when there have been previous miscarriages), amniocentesis, and ultrasound, make it possible to anticipate problems at an early stage, and are particularly helpful for women over 30. Up-to-date details on these tests are widely available, both in books that cover pregnancy as well as from your own obstetrician, so if testing is an area of concern, do some research. If you are anxious about a 35-plus pregnancy, what you discover can be very reassuring. But every couple should make their decision about when to start a family with the risks of postponed pregnancies in full view. Women on birth-control pills should note that at least three normal, nonpill menstrual cycles are advised prior to attempting conception. While the age factor is but one element in family planning, it is usually the most significant and timing should be a prime consideration. Having built-in time to conceive increases the chance of a healthy pregnancy and birth. Rabbits may conceive with every try, but not all ready-and-willing humans are so lucky.

Infertility is generally diagnosed and treated if a couple fails to conceive after one year of trying, but the 35-plus woman should probably be evaluated after six months. Since male infertility is easier to identify than female, an evaluation of the sperm count and motility should be the first diagnostic test. For women, a thorough exam should include a careful history and appropriate tests by a competent gynecologist. Assessment includes determining whether ovulation is occurring; evaluating the function of the endometrium and corpus luteum; and evaluating the cervix, uterus, and fallopian tubes to see if transport of the ova is blocked. If a woman is not ovulating but all other signs are normal, hormones may be prescribed to stimulate ovulation. In cases of blockage of the fallopian tubes or problems with fibroids or endometriosis, surgical correction may restore fertility; with endometriosis drug therapy may also be used. Beyond these, there are high-tech solutions such as *in vitro* fertilization, but you should know what you're getting into before venturing into this territory. The cost is high and the success rate low, and many infertility treatment centers give out confusing statistics in this regard. Resolve, a national support group for infertile couples, can help: it maintains a current bibliography of books and articles and publishes fact sheets on every aspect of infertility. You can get a list of Resolve's fifty local chapters and more information by writing to Resolve, 5 Water Street, Arlington, Massachusetts 02174.

2: CONFIRMING THE PREGNANCY

The accuracy of the pregnancy test (the HCG, or human chorionic gonadotropic test) increases with the length of time a menstrual period has been missed, so it is wise to wait at least two weeks past the estimated date of onset before having the test done. At-home tests are increasingly accurate and serve as a good screen, but your next step is to go in for a regular medical-office laboratory test—as soon as possible. This is especially important for the over-35 woman pregnant for the first time. With a positive test result, most obstetricians will advise an ultrasound or amniocentesis (or both) to assess any abnormal fetal development.

3: MINIMIZING KNOWN RISKS

Early confirmation of pregnancy enables a mother to prepare the best possible *in utero* conditions for her baby's fetal growth. Ideally, these preparations begin as soon as you start planning your pregnancy. Setting the stage for a healthy baby means there must be *no* smoking, since cigarette smoke has been strongly associated with birth defects, premature delivery, and low birth weights. In this regard, nature works in favor of the baby, causing many smokers to feel so nauseated by the smell of cigarettes during pregnancy that they gladly quit.

Although the pros and cons of alcohol consumption during pregnancy continue to be debated, it has been shown that in some women even small amounts of alcohol can adversely affect fetal development. This alone makes a strong case for abstinence, even from beer and wine, and certainly in the first three months.

It should go without saying that using illicit drugs including marijuana or cocaine is totally out of the question during pregnancy—and that includes even occasional use. But you must discuss all prescription or over-the-counter medications (including aspirin, laxatives, and simple cold remedies), with your physician before taking any of them. If you are diabetic, however, you must be closely monitored by your doctor and keep your blood sugar levels under strict control (see page 136).

4: CHOOSING GOOD NUTRITION

Because your unborn baby is totally dependent on you for its nourishment, a nutritious diet can be your most important contribution to its future well-being.

Monitoring your eating habits best begins when you first start thinking about getting pregnant. Many of the vitamins, minerals, and proteins that are transferred to the baby through your blood are provided by the reserve of nutrients accumulated well before pregnancy. If your diet during pregnancy can't supply the nutritional needs of the fetus, then these reserves will be called into play. Don't make the mistake of thinking that all the nutritional do's and don'ts we discuss below are strictly for the sake of your baby. This is a symbiotic relationship. For nine months your child is literally a part of you, and if he or she isn't getting enough nourishment, your body is going to suffer as well. Although the greater impact of poor nutrition is going to be on the fetus, you'll put extra strain on your heart and circulatory system, risk anemia, and deplete the calcium stores in your own bones if you try to get along on less than the two of you need.

Good diet is important, not just at the beginning but all through pregnancy, since the nutritional needs of both mother and baby are continually adjusted to meet new stages of gestational development. These adjustments are determined by several physiological events in the mother's body. Beginning in the third month, for example, your metabolic and blood circulation rates increase with the fetus's demand for more nutrients. The heart, kidneys, intestines, and other organs shift into high gear to make sure nutrients circulate freely to the baby.

There are specific ways a mother can adjust her diet to meet the changes taking place in her pregnant body. One of the first steps in approaching the question of diet is to develop a realistic "pregnant body image."

5: MONITORING YOUR WEIGHT

If you are in good health and in good shape when you conceive, it is perfectly normal to be concerned about the weight you gain as you watch your figure rounding out. You will naturally want to do everything you can to return to your prepregnant figure after the baby arrives. But if you think that because you are normally thin you should stay thin when you are pregnant, you are mistaken, just as it is a mistake to think you can use the next nine months to overindulge in calorie-laden treats because no one will know the difference.

Of course there is no way to have a baby and *not* gain weight. The purpose of the weight gain is to provide a nutritional boost that will nourish the growing fetus as well as provide adequate energy for you to meet the effort required in carrying a child. For an average healthy woman at term, weight gain should be about 25 pounds, depending on body size and type. A petite woman might gain 20 pounds; a large-framed woman could gain up to 30 or 35 pounds. Women who are underweight before pregnancy may need to gain more than the average, while women who are overweight may gain less (though in most cases pregnancy is *not* the time to go on a weight loss diet). It's especially important for both overweight and underweight women to evaluate their diets and make careful and nutritious food choices.

Here again usually nature helps out. If they get the right nourishment during pregnancy, very often women who are very thin will gain 30 to 35 pounds, while women who are somewhat overweight will not gain more than 20, and quite obese women have been known to gain only 15. These variations correlate with the prepregnant body stores mentioned earlier. An overweight woman comes to her pregnancy with more reserves of nutrients for the baby to live on, and thus will put on less weight than her under-weight counterpart.

Even with some understanding of the relation between weight gain and the nutritional needs of the fetus, weight-conscious women are often shocked to hear that a good part of what they gain is an accumulation of fat. But that's the way it is, and indeed was meant to be. While many women are better off only gaining between 2 and 4 pounds in their first trimester, at full term a pregnant woman should have accumulated about 3.5 kilograms (7 to 8 pounds) of extra fat. Ideally, these pounds are laid down in the second trimester (the middle three months of pregnancy), but usually where she least wants them—in the derriere, hips, and legs.

There are two good reasons for this: First, it helps with the ordeal of birth, probably the greatest physical endeavor a mother will ever take on. While it is obviously far less of a shock to give birth in a hospital or birthing room than in a field, your body doesn't know you are any different from your ancestors and it stores the greatest amount of energy possible. Second, the accumulation of fat provides the energy and fat stores that will be used in the first six months of breastfeeding.

Weight gain in the last trimester is primarily the baby's, giving it a layer of fat and a source of energy for its entry into the world.

Obviously, these changes are going to require changes in the way you eat. An active, nonpregnant 35-plus woman of small stature needs about 1,300 to 1,400 calories a day; one of average build anywhere from 1,600 to 2,400. Assuming she isn't chronically under- or overfeeding herself, the average woman needs to increase her daily intake by about 300 calories once she becomes pregnant. This is not a gross increase, but it is significant.

It should go without saying that where you get these calories matters a lot. A well-balanced prenatal diet consists of a wide variety of nutritionally dense foods.

Food that is nutritionally dense is usually more or less in its natural state when eaten—lean meats, fresh fruits and vegetables, for example. An orange provides vitamin C and potassium, among other nutrients; a piece of baked or broiled chicken provides protein, as well as niacin, iron, and thiamine. Food preparation makes all the difference. Broiled, a half-breast of chicken amounts to 165 nutritionally dense calories; deep-fried, it's over 300 calories, an increase in fat and empty calories that effectively cuts the nutrition-per-calorie figure in half. Dietary fiber is important, too, helping prevent the constipation and hemorrhoids many women suffer during pregnancy.

Jean Spodnik's Guidelines for Healthy Eating During Pregnancy

Your prenatal diet should include plenty of milk and dairy products, meats, complex carbohydrates (grains and vegetables), and fruit, plus a moderate amount of fat. Note that serving sizes are keyed to the exchange lists on Chapter 22, and that meat and starch exchanges, in particular, are in small units.

DAIRY PRODUCTS.   Four servings a day, as a source of calcium, phosphorus, riboflavin, and protein. Preferably two glasses of 1- or 2-percent low-fat milk and two other servings—low-fat yogurt or cheese, for example —of dairy products. I don't recommend skim milk because it does not contain any fat, and calcium is always absorbed a little better in the presence of fat.

MEAT PRODUCTS.   Six to eight servings (6 to 8 ounces) a day of lean meat, fish, or poultry. Or eat an alternative to meat, such as peanut butter or dried beans (see the exchange lists in Chapter 22).

The protein and nutrients from meat and dairy products are very important, especially in the last trimester. Ovolactovegetarians can meet these needs with cheese, milk, eggs, complementary proteins, and other foods. A daily prenatal vitamin-mineral supplement is important for all pregnant women, but especially so for those who eat little or no meat.

GRAINS AND STARCHY VEGETABLES.   Six to eight servings daily. Adequate amounts depend on the woman's size: if she's very thin and requires 2,200 to 2,500 calories a day, she should eat between eight and fifteen servings (please note serving sizes in the exchange lists, in Chapter 22). If she requires 2,000 calories a day, then six to eight servings is usually enough, although it can be as many as ten. Nutritionally dense foods— whole grains, whole-grain cereals or crackers, brown rice, baked potatoes —should be chosen over refined flours or sweets.

OTHER VEGETABLES.   Three to five servings of vegetables daily, some cooked and some raw, including dark green and leafy vegetables, and some that are deep yellow—tomatoes, carrots, sweet potatoes, and squash, for examples.

FRUIT.   Two to three servings a day, including ½ cup of juice. The diet should not be all juice, but should include plenty of fresh whole fruit, such as apples, oranges, and bananas, and other fruits in season.

FAT.   Indeed there should be some fat in the pregnant woman's diet, and dairy products will supply a bit of it. Other recommended sources include margarine, oils, and salad dressings made from unsaturated fats, rather than fried foods or snack foods high in saturated fat. Nuts are an acceptable source as long as snacking on them doesn't fill you up so much that other foods are ignored. Rich desserts should be kept to a minimum.

If you have a sweet tooth, satisfy it after the daily requirements have been met, preferably with a fruited yogurt or a small portion of ice cream, custard, or pudding, or a couple of cookies.

VITAMINS AND MINERALS.   It is difficult, if not impossible, to get all the iron you need from diet alone, so a prenatal vitamin-mineral supplement, taken as directed by your doctor, is advised.

FLUIDS.   Milk, fruit juice, and plain water are recommended. Alcohol is ill advised and caffeine only in moderation. The dangers of caffeine during pregnancy are not entirely known, but animal studies have linked it to bone malformation and cleft palates. A cup of morning tea or coffee, or a soft drink at lunch may be allowed, but use caution. As for artificial sweeteners, it is best to avoid diet drinks during pregnancy and also artificial sweeteners such as Nutrasweet, because of the chance that free phenylalanine in the blood can affect the fetus if he or she is prone to phenylketonuria (PKU). (Phenylketonuria is a genetic disease that, if not detected and treated, leads to developmental abnormalities, including mental retardation.)

6: KEEPING UP WITH REGULAR EXERCISE

In the past, any form of exercise during pregnancy was thought to be risky for both mother and baby. Today we know better. In an article published in *AFP*, the journal of the American Academy of Family Physicians (November 1988), Drs. Jan E. Paisley and Morris B. Mellion reported on the most up-to-date studies and recommendations for safe exercise during pregnancy. The benefits they list are many:

> Maintenance or improvement of maternal fitness
> Control of excess weight gain
> Improved mental outlook and self-image
> Increased sense of control
> Improved appearance and posture
> Increased energy
> Relief of tension
> Improved sleep
> Less backache
> Fewer problems with varicose veins
> Less water retention
> Possible decreased labor complications and shortened labor
> More rapid postpartum recovery

These are strong incentives for staying active while pregnant.

The type of exercise you choose depends on the physical shape you are in when your pregnancy test comes back positive. Many women athletes continue their training during pregnancy, and may even compete with no ill effects, as Mary Decker Slaney and others have shown. However, as the pregnancy progresses, even trained athletes are wise to reduce their levels of strenuous or vigorous exercise. Not only does the added weight put strain on the circulatory system but it can throw you off balance, and this indeed could result in injury. In consultation with your obstetrician you can gradually adjust an existing program down to meet your increasing size. Previously sedentary women should start slow and advance gradually. They should have no trouble with a walking program such as the one described in Chapter 24.

Many physicians feel that aerobic dance involves too much bouncing for the fetus, particularly in the second and third trimesters. But in a normal, uncomplicated pregnancy, exercise of the large muscle groups is beneficial. Many health clubs, YWCAs, and other organizations offer exercise classes designed specifically for pregnant women, who may be more cautious than they need be when it comes to exercise. A good instructor can provide reassurance in this regard with safe, enjoyable exercise routines.

The American College of Obstetricians and Gynecologists provides its own guidelines for exercise during pregnancy and postpartum. These are extremely useful in establishing a safe exercise program.

Pregnancy and Postpartum

1. Regular exercise (at least three times a week) is preferable to intermittent activity. Avoid competitive activities.
2. Don't do any vigorous exercising in hot, humid weather or during a period of illness with fever.
3. Avoid ballistic movements (jumping and other bouncy motion). Exercise should be done on a wooden floor or a tightly carpeted surface to reduce shock and provide sure footing.
4. Deep flexion or extension of joints should be avoided because of connective-tissue laxity. Joint instability is another reason to avoid activities that require jumping, jarring motions, or rapid changes in direction.
5. Always precede vigorous exercise with a five-minute period of muscle warm-up. This can be accomplished by slow walking or stationary cycling with low resistance.
6. After vigorous exercise, cool down with a period of gradually declining activity that includes gentle stationary stretching. Because

connective-tissue laxity increases the risk of joint injury, stretches should not be taken to the point of maximum resistance.

7. Measure your heart rate at times of peak activity (see Target Zones, Chapter 24), and don't exceed the target heart rates recommended by your doctor.

8. Take care to rise gradually after any exercise you do sitting or lying down, to avoid orthostatic hypotension (a drop in blood pressure to below normal). Some form of activity involving the legs should be continued for a brief period.

9. Liquids should be taken liberally before and after exercise to prevent dehydration. If necessary, interrupt your activity to replenish fluids.

10. If you have led a sedentary life-style you should begin with physical activity of very low intensity and advance activity levels gradually.

11. You must *stop* exercising and consult your doctor if any unusual symptoms appear. These include breathlessness, dizziness, chest pain or tightness, difficulty walking, decreased fetal activity, uterine contractions, vaginal bleeding, or leakage of amniotic fluid.

Pregnancy Only

1. Your heart rate should not exceed a maximum of 140 beats a minute.

2. Strenuous activities should not exceed fifteen minutes in duration.

3. Don't perform any exercise in a supine position (lying on your back) after the fourth month is completed.

4. Avoid exercises that employ the Valsalva maneuver—straining while holding your breath.

5. Caloric intake should be adequate to meet not only the extra needs of pregnancy but also of the exercise performed.

6. Maternal core temperature (true body temperature, usually measured with a rectal thermometer) should not exceed 38°C (100.4°F).

7: PREPARING FOR CHILDBIRTH

While regular visits to your doctor will ensure the healthiest pregnancy, prepared childbirth—the Lamaze method—can be one of your greatest allies during childbirth. We strongly advocate participation by both partners in Lamaze classes, which are readily available in most areas. Not only will the relaxation and breathing techniques serve a mother well all through labor but taking the classes together encourages camaraderie at a time when couples need it most. This is enormously valuable even if you end up having a cesarean birth.

Classes also cover current issues such as cesareans, as well as various options for pain medications administered during birth. Attitudes toward the latter are changing among women and health professionals alike, with many women opting for mild medications, timed to wear off before birth, that will not affect the baby's state of alertness as it comes into the world.

8: BREAST FEEDING

While we advocate breast feeding, the choice is strictly a personal one and you should not feel bad if you decide against it. Bottle-fed babies stand no less chance of being happy, healthy, or well-nurtured. The main advantages of breast feeding are that it helps encourage early bonding and the breast milk provides the newborn with a whole range of helpful antibodies in the early days after birth. In addition, breast feeding has been shown to be a positive factor in good breast health. Even if you are planning to go back to work, if you only breast feed on your maternity leave you will still reap the advantages. The colostrum will have been passed along to the baby, and it is this fluid that contains the antibodies which help build up the infant's immune system.

Women who breast feed need about 500 extra calories a day, obtained from the same good diet used during pregnancy but increased by one or two glasses of milk or servings of dairy foods to meet added calcium needs. Ordinary fluid intake should add up to about 2½ quarts a day, but a breast-feeding woman needs 3 quarts of fluid daily, 4 in hot weather.

Continuing with prenatal vitamins is also encouraged during breast feeding and for the first six weeks after delivery, even for women who bottle-feed, since this helps rebuild vitamin stores.

The initial few weeks after pregnancy is not the time to start a diet, but breast feeding itself can help you get back to your prepregnant shape quickly. Two factors work in your favor: breast feeding helps the uterus contract more quickly and it uses up some of the fat stores around your hips in the production of milk.

9: PLANNING AHEAD FOR THE POSTPARTUM WEEKS

Just as the experience of birth is never going to be quite what you expected, no matter how well you've planned, you can be sure that the notions you might have about being a parent will be very different from the reality.

In the postpartum weeks emotions usually run high—for some women, covering the full gamut from great euphoria and intense attachment to the child, to wishing someone else had to take care of it, to nostalgia and even longing for the quiet days before this small but demanding infant burst upon the scene. Having some negative feelings about the miraculous event is perfectly normal; the phenomenon of postpartum depression in the days and weeks after pregnancy is no myth. Hormone levels are in flux, and your body, in the aftermath of giving birth, is not the same body you knew before you were pregnant. With good eating habits and exercise, you'll get back into your favorite pair of jeans, but it may take a few months. Don't be too hard on yourself if this is the case.

Hormone levels stay up during breast feeding and may help postpone some of the emotional susceptability connected to postpartum depression. But if caring for a newborn has drained your energy and you're new at breast feeding to begin with, you may feel overwhelmed. If you decide to try it (and there are good reasons to do so), take the baby for all the feedings in the hospital, including those during the night, and ask the nurses for any tips they can give you about techniques that will make feeding easier.

Whether you breast feed or not, when you get home don't push yourself back to your normal level of activity right away. During your pregnancy, sort out who's going to do what in the weeks following birth. More than likely, your husband won't be able to do all the chores around the house, and you should line up some temporary help—if not a parent, possibly a close sibling or friend who is really willing to pitch in. If you can afford it, get paid help. Whether you're on maternity leave from work or plan to be a full-time mother, you'll be far better off if you do nothing for those first few weeks but lounge around caring for the baby, resting or sleeping on the baby's schedule, and savoring this time off from other mundane responsibilities to discover more about the tiny, special person you've brought into the world.

SOME RESOURCES

Many excellent books give couples safe, realistic, and encouraging guidelines for managing the pregnancy and birth experience. By all means invest in a few good reference books: Sheila Kitzinger's *The Complete Book of Pregnancy and Childbirth* (Alfred A. Knopf), or *Fritzi Kallop's Birth Book* (Vintage Books) are two good examples. To follow the miracle of fetal development, pick up Geraldine Flanagan's *The First Nine Months of Life* (Simon and Schuster) or the astonishing, full-color edition of *A Child Is Born* by Lennart Nilsson (Dell).

CHAPTER 17

Menopause

OF ALL THE gynecological issues that surface in the middle years, there is probably no more widely anticipated one than a woman's passage into menopause—an event that despite evidence to the contrary, still brings with it enormous emotional baggage that's been passed down for generations. But negative perceptions about menopause are currently undergoing an overhaul.

As reported in the December 1988 issue of *Psychology Today* magazine, in a survey of 2,300 healthy, middle-aged women conducted by psychologist Sonja McKinlay, president of the New England Research Institute in Watertown, Massachusetts, *only three women* expressed regret over their menopause four and a half years after it was over—the rest were vastly relieved to be free of concerns about pregnancy, contraception, and menstruation. Moreover, during their menopause, 85 percent of the women never experienced depression, 10 percent were occasionally depressed, and 5 percent were frequently depressed—these are statistics that parallel the general population of women, regardless of age.

In the book *Our Bodies, Ourselves*, women speak about menopause from personal experience, highlighting the diverse physical and emotional reactions that accompany this feminine *rite de passage*. One woman told of how her periods were "excessively lengthy and torrential" for two or three years, and then abruptly ceased; another noticed how the intervals between periods lengthened gradually. One woman described waking up in the middle of the night drenched with sweat and thinking something was very wrong with her body; another woman reported that while her "hot flashes" were uncomfortable, they were also manageable because she knew they were a normal part of menopause. Most women who had problems coping with their menopause conceded, in retrospect, a lack of knowledge about it; others confirmed that when you know what to expect, menopause is not always the calamity it's been made out to be. Supporting the Massachusetts study, women often reported *positive* changes when the "change of life" was over—better sex without the worry of pregnancy and nuisance of birth control and improved physical and mental well-being without cyclic changes or pain.

As menopause has become better understood, treatments have become more individualized than in the past and, for that reason, much improved.

Treatment depends on the clinical presentation of symptoms; as with PMS, these can vary. Some women have few if any definite problems with menopause—no hot flashes, no significant problems with vaginal dryness, thinning of the skin, or irritability and depression. Others are immediately hit with the full gamut of symptoms—drenching hot flashes, profound mood swings, irritability—that continue for years after menstruation has ceased. Still others stand on a middle ground, now and then noticing a few nuisance changes, but nothing intense or dramatic.

The *approach* to treating specific problems also varies, depending, first of all, on the attitudes held by your physician or gynecologist. Some gynecologists regard menopause as a purely normal phenomenon that requires minimal therapy. Others view it as a specific endocrine problem that should be treated aggressively with medication, in this case with the hormones estrogen and progesterone.

Both sides deserve consideration. While you do not necessarily lose thyroid or insulin as you age, all women do lose their estrogen during menopause. Clearly, over time this makes for major changes in your body. Because of genetic or physiological factors, certain women—those with a family history of heart disease, for example—actually may place themselves at a greater risk of serious illness without replacement hormones, while others who have a family history of breast or other cancers are better off with nonmedical alternatives. If you have had breast cancer yourself, estrogen replacement therapy must be ruled out.

In truth, estrogen replacement therapy (ERT) remains somewhat controversial, even with the lowered doses, in combination with progesterone, that are now generally prescribed. This is one issue that you must inform yourself about before you make a decision to go one way or another, and if your doctor's approach seems unsuitable to you, get a second opinion.

TYPICAL SYMPTOMS OF MENOPAUSE

Several areas of the body can be affected during and after menopause. The vagina and vulva may show increased dryness and irritation. The body's covering—skin and hair—can become thinner and drier. With the loss of estrogen protection, the risk of coronary artery disease increases, as does the risk of developing osteoporosis. There is also a whole range of neuropsychiatric changes that are prominent in some women and minimal in others.

As with any significant life change, sexual relationships can suffer, thrive, or weather the ups and downs that this change normally brings. While there may be genital changes (less vaginal secretion, for example), sexual desire does not necessarily diminish after menopause, although a woman's menopause can have an effect on her partner's libido. Any sexual dysfunction related to menopause should be treated, not only for your sake but for the sake of your relationship (see Chapter 18).

Symptoms of menopause can be acute if menopause is brought on surgically. In a natural menopause, changes occur gradually over the years, so there's a good chance the changes you experience won't be burdensome or dramatic. If the change is surgical—that is, due to surgical removal of the ovaries—then the change is abrupt. This sudden switch-off can rightly be viewed as a specific endocrine problem requiring specific medication. Studies in the field of menopause research bear out this differentiation.

With this brief overview, let's focus more closely on the most prominent symptoms of menopause.

HOT FLASHES

Nearly half of all menopausal women note hot flashes—a feeling of warmth, with or without actual sweats, that can occur day or night. These are real problems associated with changes in skin and body temperature and are related to the episodic release of hormones from the pituitary gland. They can usually be eliminated with estrogen replacement and are one of the main reasons for using estrogen in menopause.

BONE CHANGES AND OSTEOPOROSIS

As described in Chapter 12, osteoporosis is a decrease in bone mass that occurs at different rates in different women, depending on genes, diet, and level of fitness. While efforts made with diet and exercise can help most women prevent osteoporosis, nothing at the juncture of menopause will rebuild the skeleton, although there is some promising research on treating osteoporosis of the spine that may replace some bone mass there. It is not effective for—and may actually damage—the rest of the skeleton, however. The main causes of osteoporosis are indeed age related, but certain factors increase the risk in women who are smokers, who are anorectic, who have an excessively high protein diet, who consume excessive amounts of alcohol, or who are hypothyroid and are on synthetic thyroid replacement at too high a dose.

Medications

Whether the menopause is natural or surgical, estrogen will slow down bone loss, especially if it's taken early after the change of life. In this case, the minimum dosage that appears to be effective is .625 milligram of conjugated estrogen (Premarin) a day, taken for at least ten years following (or beginning just before) the last menses. Studies have not shown that higher estrogen dosages are better with regard to osteoporosis prevention and treatment. But consistent use of estrogen, in the dosage and time period noted, should decrease the risk of spinal and hip fractures. In addition, some studies have shown that estrogen and calcium taken together actually can add slightly to bone mass, although such an increase is seldom significant once the loss has begun.

Another medical treatment is use of the hormone calcitonin. This can be effective for osteoporosis, but because most women prefer to avoid frequent injections, and this is its route of administration, it is not very popular. Other ways to administer calcitonin are currently being researched.

For now, it seems that the most effective treatment for prevention of osteoporosis in high-risk groups is early and sustained use of estrogen on a daily basis. There may or may not be other factors in choosing this route, but there is no question of its beneficial effect on bone health. This is an option you must carefully review with your physician, bearing in mind that osteoporosis research is becoming more "pro-estrogen."

Alternatives

What about an alternative approach to preventing osteoporosis during and after menopause? Understandably, many women do not want to take estrogen. Women who have had breast cancer or breast fibrocystic changes usually should not even consider it. For these women the answer lies in not smoking, in avoiding the diet factors known to hasten osteoporosis (excessive alcohol, excessive protein, inadequate calcium), and in implementing a positive program of regular aerobic exercise. After all, for countless decades women managed well enough without synthetic estrogen. Now, however, you have a choice: make it an informed one.

CARDIOVASCULAR HEALTH

Research in the area of cardiovascular health is also clearly moving toward a "pro-estrogen" stance. The biggest reason for lower rates of coronary artery disease in women—and a major factor in their longer average life span—is the protective effect of estrogen on the heart and vascular system. Although the precise mechanisms are not fully known, the outcome is. Comparisons between surgical and natural menopause have shown a greater cardiac risk in the former group, with the risk factor of the latter group rising slowly to meet its male counterpart. Since a large number—40 percent—of all female deaths in this country each year are from cardiovascular problems, even improving the prospects of a segment of this group could lower the female death rate.

Medications

The consensus, therefore, is that in cases of surgical menopause—that is, bilateral ovary removal—the woman is advised to use estrogen (and progesterone, if her uterus is intact) on a regular basis, if there is no strong reason not to. The usage should last until the approximate time she would have experienced natural menopause and be of mid-strength, at least .625 milligram.

Although there is not yet a national consensus on estrogen use for cardiovascular protection for women with natural menopause, here again the medical community seems to be moving toward a "pro-estrogen" stance, although only a minority of these women currently use estrogen.

With any use of estrogen, you must pay careful attention to the health of your breasts. This includes monthly self-examinations, periodic exams by your doctor, and annual mammography.

Alternatives

Is there an alternative to estrogen? The nonmedication approach to heart protection after menopause follows the guidelines for osteoporosis, along with a low-cholesterol diet. For women with good "heart heredity," who are at low risk of heart disease, this approach is appropriate.

SEXUALITY AND CHANGE OF LIFE

As mentioned earlier, certain physical changes can occur in the genital area that are inevitably associated with menopause. These can lead to irritation in the vagina, dyspareunia (pain with sexual intercourse), or even vaginal bleeding.

Studies have shown that most couples experience a marked decrease in sexual intercourse at their change of life. Compared with an average of one to three times a week before menopause, sexual intercourse may drop to once or twice a month afterwards, though such a decline is not usually sudden. These studies dealt not only with the female partner but also with potential changes in the male partner, presuming he too is encountering age-related symptoms. Even when the latter is not the case, clearly there are higher rates of male impotence, either full or partial, in marriages where the woman has gone through menopause; this phenomenon is discussed further in connection with male health issues on pages 243–246.

The key to assessing sexuality, and the possibility of sexual dysfunction after menopause, is for both partners to discuss the matter, and for a physician to take careful sexual histories, in tandem with a detailed physical examination, of each partner.

Medications

If hormonal replacement is deemed necessary for the woman, the choice is between oral estrogen medication, one of the new estrogen patches, or possibly an estrogen cream, particularly when symptoms are limited mainly to vaginal dryness. If estrogens are not to be used, lubricants such as K-Y jelly may suffice. But the general approach toward improving the situation should be one of attitude and pacing, with partners proceeding more slowly and thoroughly through foreplay than in earlier years.

TAILORING ESTROGEN THERAPY TO THE INDIVIDUAL

In the final analysis, hormone replacement is something that needs careful consideration based on a clear rationale. In most cases these considerations are limited to the three major issues already mentioned: (1) prevention of osteoporosis, (2) cardiovascular protection, and (3) sexuality or sexual dysfunction—balanced against risk factors for cancer. Should estrogen prove to be an appropriate approach, then it becomes a matter of proper dosage.

If a woman no longer has her uterus, then only estrogen need be used. But if, as in the majority of cases, a woman has an intact uterus, the current recommendation is to use estrogen and progesterone combined.

Your doctor will explain that there are different ways to approach this. Based on the menstrual cycle, for example, you may be put on continuous estrogen on days 1 through 15, switching to a combination of estrogen and progesterone on days 16 through 25. Or, in a somewhat newer approach using lower dosages of each, a combination of estrogen and progesterone in one continuous treatment may be prescribed. The latter has the advantage of eventually stopping your periods altogether, while the common cyclical hormone use means your periods will resume after menopause.

The question that immediately comes up is, what kind of gynecological follow-up is necessary with estrogen therapy? It is extremely important that an experienced gynecologist closely monitor your gynecological health. Very definitely, you should have an annual pap and pelvic exam. Probably you should also have an endometrial biopsy to check the uterine lining; the experts in the field continue to be divided on how often, with some favoring an annual biopsy and others preferring one baseline biopsy and then re-biopsy only if there is a specific problem. We would also advise annual mammography after menopause, and indeed, this seems to be emerging as the national standard.

MAKING THE DECISION

How are you to judge what is best in your particular situation? This is a matter to discuss with your primary physician and gynecologist. Keep in mind that if your menopause is surgical, there is an accelerated risk of cardiovascular disease and osteoporosis without estrogen therapy. If the goal is to help prevent either cardiovascular disease or osteoporosis, estrogen should be used early on—that is, just as the menses are ending. One or two years later and the effect will be lessened. However, this is not the case if the goal is to eliminate hot flashes, which can occur off and on for one to three years after menopause. For this use, it makes no difference if there's a gap in time between menopause and the beginning of therapy.

How long should you use estrogen preventively for osteoporosis or heart disease? For most women, ten to fifteen years, with fifteen years apparently the upper limit. In cases of hot flashes and sexual dysfunction, use the estrogen as long as symptoms persist. In this country there's no uniformity in estrogen use. Many women with intact uteruses are on estrogen alone, an unwise practice because of an undue risk of endometrial carcinoma. Combined hormonal therapy in this case is something every woman must insist on.

SUMMARY GUIDELINES FOR COPING WITH MENOPAUSE

1. Check with your doctor when your periods show any sign of change, to be sure hormones are the cause.
2. Review all risk factors for osteoporosis and heart disease, and correct

as many as possible with a low-cholesterol diet, additional calcium, no smoking, regular exercise, and other good health choices.

3. If you are at significant risk for osteoporosis or coronary artery disease, consider estrogen-progesterone replacement early on—but not if you are in a high-risk category for cancer.

4. If you suffer significant hot flashes or hormone-related sexual dysfunction, consider estrogen-progesterone replacement, with close follow-up.

5. If estrogen-replacement therapy is chosen, close gynecological follow-up, as detailed, is essential.

CHAPTER 18

Female Sexuality Involving a Partner

BIRTH CONTROL

While contraception is a major sexual issue before menopause, it is rarely a new issue for 35-plus women. Sexual initiation usually occurs at a much earlier age and choices for birth control have already been made. Nevertheless, the average 35-year-old has another fifteen years to go before her menstrual cycle totally ceases, and after that she still needs to wait another year before giving up birth control.

With such a span of fertile years still ahead, the 35-plus woman should review the various birth-control methods. This is particularly true if you've been on the pill for many years.

The Pill

Other than abstinence or sterilization, the most effective method of birth control continues to be women's birth-control pills. Despite periodic articles in the media, the outlook for a male contraceptive pill seems dim. Contraceptive research in this area is very modestly funded, possibly because of an uncertain market and liability worries.

In nonsmoking women, the pill today is considered quite safe, especially with the newer, low-estrogen preparations. The doses prescribed are monitored much more closely than in the past, with the FDA's advisory committee recommending that all contraceptives with greater than 50 micrograms of estrogen be taken off the market. If you have been on oral contraception for years you should certainly check the dosage of the pill you're using. If it contains more than 50 micrograms of estrogen, review the situation with your prescribing physician to adjust down to a lower dosage.

As mentioned in Chapter 16, women wanting to conceive should go off the pill for at least three months—that is, they should plan at least three normal, nonpill menstrual cycles before they can expect to conceive. If they are not breast-feeding, most women can resume the pill after their postpartum checkup. Breast-feeding mothers should use another means of birth control until after the baby is weaned. Nursing itself is considered a form of contraception, but it is not at all reliable. If you don't want another baby right away, you must use another method, such as an effective barrier.

Barrier Methods

Diaphragms, condoms, and cervical caps are very safe, but not quite as effective as birth-control pills. Pills have an estimated 96 to 98 percent accuracy in preventing conception, while barrier methods are somewhere in the low 90 percent range.

Nonetheless, barrier methods can be a good choice for women who are smokers, who have a history of phlebitis, who suffer from cardiovascular disease, or who are generally worried about taking an extra hormone into their bodies. These methods represent the natural choice, so to speak, provided you can live with the slightly lower degree of effectiveness.

Of all barrier methods, the *diaphragm* remains the most popular in this country. It is highly effective if properly fitted by a physician (some physicians are more experienced than others in doing so). Also, it must be used with a spermicide and changed after each intercourse. A diaphragm can be safely left in as long as twenty-four hours. But if a woman loses as little as 10 pounds, she should have her diaphragm checked to see that it fits properly; some women using diaphragms have lost weight—and gained an unexpected baby.

There have been claims that spermicidal gels increase the risk of birth defects, but this has not been scientifically proved. Thus using them remains an option in helping decrease the chance of pregnancy. When the gels contain an antiviral agent, they decrease the risk of sexually transmitted disease as well.

Cervical caps, though not nearly as widely available as diaphragms in this country, have been around for about sixty years. Licensing is under way so that more cervical caps will be sold here, and we will surely see increased use—beginning with competent fittings—soon. One of the greatest advantages of the cervical cap is that it can safely stay in place for up to three days and is about 95 percent effective.

Condoms have become more popular in recent years, but there is still some male resistance to them. Used with foam or spermicidal jelly, condoms have an effectiveness rate comparable to a properly fitted diaphragm or cervical cap. Condoms have the added advantage of helping prevent the spread of sexually transmitted diseases, including AIDS. As we will stress later, any woman who has an active sex life with changing partners is strongly urged to carry condoms and to insist on their use.

Commonly used in the past, *intrauterine devices* (IUDs), including the popular Copper 7, had a very high success rate. They seemed safe and could stay put for several years, so they were popular for good reasons. At the time, women who were reluctant to take high-estrogen birth-control pills (the only such pills then available), and who liked the idea of uninterrupted sex, favored IUDs. But that was before problems with the Dalkon Shield, involving infection and infertility, which led to removal of all IUDs, including the Copper 7, from the market between 1985 and 1986.

While women were wise to be wary of IUDs, their risk of infection was often related to improper insertion. In well-trained hands, the Copper 7 IUDs were probably fairly safe. In 1988, a new copper IUD began to be marketed in some areas, but only several years' experience will tell if it passes the test, as both an effective contraceptive device and, more important, a safe one. In addition, a progesterone-releasing IUD called Progestasert, marketed by the pharmaceutical firm Alza, appears to be both safe and effective; but it is available only with a lengthy informed consent, and does not appear to be slated for wide general use.

The Rhythm Method

The rhythm method relies on the fact that there are relatively few days in each menstrual cycle when you're actually fertile—usually about two or three days after ovulation. The key to success is predicting ovulation. This means monitoring your basal body temperature, which increases slightly at ovulation, and careful record-keeping using a calendar. Even with scrupulous monitoring, it may be hard to predict ovulation with much precision and especially difficult if your periods are at all irregular. This method requires high motivation and self-control—which means limiting sex to non-fertile days, usually allowing a couple of days on either side as an extra precaution. Studies give the best estimate of effectiveness at 80 to 90 percent.

Sterilization

Sterilization as a contraceptive method certainly works. Both tubal ligation and vasectomy have a greater than 99 percent effectiveness if properly done, and they represent an ideal choice for many 35-plus women and their spouses. You must not go into this lightly, or think that either procedure is reversible.

Both vasectomies (for men) and tubal ligations (for women) are relatively simple procedures. A vasectomy can be done by a physician on an outpatient basis; it involves excising a segment of the vas deferens, the duct that transports sperm. While the procedure may be reversed with a degree of success up to a certain point, after several years reconnecting the vas deferens becomes more difficult and the resulting sperm count and motility may be low.

Tubal ligations involve tying off segments of a woman's fallopian tubes. It is now usually done by laparoscopy, which involves only a small incision near the navel and the insertion of a fiber-optic tube. The easiest time to perform a tubal ligation is immediately after giving birth—before the mother is discharged from the hospital—when the tubes are large and easy to see and manipulate.

In our experience, of all available means of contraception, the majority of sexually active 35-plus women and their partners choose either barrier methods or sterilization.

SEXUALLY TRANSMITTED DISEASES

Although the appearance of AIDS is the century's most harrowing phenomenon having to do with sex, many sexually active people perceive sexually transmitted diseases as something "out there"—an issue for members of other socioeconomic groups, for people with unconventional sexual proclivities, for anyone else but themselves. Short of absolute, long-standing mutual monogamy, however, no one—male *or* female—is home free. Moreover, as with other health choices such as smoking, 35-plus women are in a powerful position, by strong example and education, to influence younger women, especially young women in their teens who are bearing the brunt of sexually transmitted diseases and unwanted pregnancies. Few issues facing women in the late 1980s and early 1990s are more important than this.

For our ancestors, gonorrhea and syphilis were the major scourges; after these were conquered with antibiotics, it seemed that at least from the health point of view, sex could be enjoyed on a fairly casual basis, without risk of major infection. But then some years ago, along came the painful and recurrent disease of herpes which, although not usually fatal, brought with it other risks, such as risk of infection to infants born during active outbreaks. Now the focus has shifted from herpes to something far more ominous: the HIV infections, presumably caused by a retrovirus, that lead to acquired immune deficiency syndrome. The potential calamity of AIDS should not blind you to the risks posed by other sexually transmitted diseases, however, for they are hardly benign.

Gonorrhea

The bacterial illness often known as GC or clap, gonorrhea probably remains the most common sexually transmitted disease. It's at least ten times more common than syphilis, and it is relatively easily communicated by vaginal, rectal, or oral sex (not, however, by toilet seats). Because it is bacterial in origin, gonorrhea is successfully treated with antibiotics.

However susceptible to treatment the gonorrhea bacteria are, this cannot be thought of as a casual disease. Undiagnosed, it can lead to pelvic inflammatory disease in women, which, in addition to causing a great deal of general sickness, can often so scar the fallopian tubes that it results in sterility and even occasional mortality. Anyone who thinks gonorrhea is of minimal consequence needs to be set straight—especially male partners, who don't run the risk of sterility.

Men are not apt to miss the diagnosis; in at least 98 percent of all male cases there is a significant penile drip. In contrast, the symptoms are not so obvious in women. There may be nothing more than a mild discharge, or no visible signs of the disease at all. Many times (but not always) gonorrhea is picked up in a routine cervical culture, having been missed up to that point by both physician and patient.

If symptoms are present, they may include vaginal discharge, lower abdominal pain, or fever and lower abdominal pain. In addition, although it might seem totally unconnected, *any unexplained hot or swollen joint* could be a sign of gonococcal arthritis, not uncommon in 35-plus women who have unprotected sex (that is, without condoms) with multiple partners. While the cervical culture provides diagnosis, another clue for the doctor is evidence of inflamed or infected fallopian tubes, which would show up in the bimanual portion of the pelvic examination.

A doctor can make a proper diagnosis of gonorrhea in the office with a swab culture of the cervix, which is immediately plated on a special culture medium. If the culture proves positive, the disease is usually treated with penicillin, either by injection or taken orally; by tetracycline if the patient is penicillin allergic; or by one of the newer antibiotics—spectinomycin or ceftriaxone—which are particularly useful in treating the penicillin-resistant varieties prevalent in certain urban areas. Even before the culture is ready, the doctor can get an immediate indication of the diagnosis by examining the discharge from the cervix or penis on a specifically stained microscope slide. The culture then serves as confirmation.

Certainly if the gonorrhea culture is positive, treatment must be initiated and should be combined with treatment with tetracycline for the non-gonorrheal infections from *Chlamydia* bacteria, which are often passed along to a woman when she becomes infected with gonorrhea.

Treatment may begin with antibiotics, but the primary goal must be prevention. As described earlier, mutual monogamy—either lifelong or long-term serial monogamy—offers protection not only from gonorrhea but from most other venereal diseases; certainly it is your first line of defense.

If the male partner is new, or if he seems to be someone who "plays around," insist on condom use with a spermicidal jelly that has antiviral properties, such as the nonoxynol preparations. In truth, a male who won't use a condom shouldn't be a sexual partner; clearly he is not interested in what harm he may do to you. Furthermore, regardless of how intimate the relationship seems to be, the voice of reason in the cold light of day dictates that a woman never completely rely on what men say. In order to have sex, many of them will frankly lie about their sexual contacts and about possible risks, not simply in connection with gonorrhea but also with herpes or HIV. The one-night stand is a classic scenario—and one you are wise to avoid. In this context, no barrier is 100 percent effective, either as a contraceptive or as protection against infection.

If the partner is unknown, even if he is willing to use a condom, it is crucial to avoid rectal sex—period. Nor is oral contact any safer than vaginal. It is a delusion to think that if a woman performs oral sex, she is less likely to get sick than if she has vaginal sex. With regard to gonorrhea, oral infection is fairly common and has become an important issue in gynecological literature.

Syphilis

When sexually transmitted diseases were still known as venereal diseases, syphilis was the most dangerous, and the name is still well recognized by the general population. But it is much less common than gonorrhea or herpes. It tends to appear as an open sore, called a chancre, in the vulva or vaginal area, which goes away on its own. This is deceptive, since the syphilis has not left the body but rather has just "gone underground." At some point later, it will reappear in signs of what are called secondary syphilis, sometimes evident as a rash on the palms of the hands or soles of the feet.

An early diagnosis of syphilis is made by a scraping of the open sore or chancre, which is then examined under a special microscope. About six weeks later, a blood test (the VDRL) will turn positive; it cannot diagnose syphilis sooner. Late stage (tertiary) syphilis can result in serious neurological or heart abnormalities. Although it can be treated, total cure is uncertain at this stage.

The drug of choice for treatment is penicillin, but in a different dosage and somewhat different administration than for gonorrhea. As with other diseases that require antibiotics, there are alternatives if the patient is allergic; in this case, erythromycin is usually chosen.

The preventive tactics for syphilis are very much the same as for gonorrhea: know your partner and his health history, and practice safe sex.

Chlamydia Infection

A currently much-discussed disease is chlamydia, referred to earlier in connection with gonorrhea. It is so common a complicating factor in that disease that it is now standard practice to follow up gonorrhea treatment with a seven- to ten-day course of tetracycline for the chlamydia infection.

Any resistant urethral infection in a male or vaginal or urethral discharge in a female must be considered as a possible chlamydia infection. It is important to know that chlamydia will not show up in a routine culture for gonorrhea, so it must be tested separately with a special culture medium.

Herpes

Viral infections are an entirely different category of sexually transmitted diseases than those just discussed. One of the most prevalent is herpes. Herpes simplex is a chronic, nonfatal infection characterized by recurrent sores, usually in the genital area. The sores are painful, often forming little blisters that come and go with a variable frequency of weeks, months, or years. Infection is transmitted by an infected partner, usually—or so it is thought—when there are active sores and not from the ejaculate itself.

There is no cure for herpes, although there is antiviral therapy in the medication acyclovir (Zovirax), a pioneer drug that was synthesized in 1974 by Dr. Howard Schaeffer and studied carefully by the renowned Gertrude Elion of Burroughs Wellcome who, with partner George Hitchings, won a Nobel Prize in 1988 for medical research. Describing how she and her team pursued the properties of acyclovir, she says, "we worked out the whole metabolism" of the compound which, in a fascinating process, remains inert until it meets a herpes virus and then is converted by the virus into a substance that proves toxic to itself. According to Elion, this discovery "was a real breakthrough in antiviral research. That such a thing was possible wasn't even imagined up till then." Zovirax, which was released for use in 1982, has become the single most profitable product offered by the Burroughs Wellcome laboratories, and comes both as an ointment for direct application onto the sores and in capsule form; it may also be given intravenously in very serious cases. For an acute outbreak, a five-day course of the ointment or capsules will usually clear up the sores. Some people have frequent recurrences of herpetic infections and need to be on long-term preventive treatment with Zovirax capsules, but if this is the case, the patient must be carefully monitored by her physician for any signs of toxicity.

Interestingly, stress management seems to help decrease the incidence and severity of recurrent genital herpes. This mind-body connection has long been suspected, but one recent study, conducted by Dr. David Longo of the Geisinger Medical Center in Pennsylvania and published in the *Journal of Consulting and Clinical Psychology*, supports this theory with evidence. Twenty-nine people who were prone to frequent outbreaks of genital herpes participated in support group sessions focusing on the emotional and sexual difficulties they experienced because of the virus. In addition, half the group was given strategies for dealing with their herpes, including relaxation, mental imaging, and stress reduction techniques. At the end of six months, this group showed less depression, anxiety, and half as many outbreaks of herpes as the group who received support but no tangible strategies. Moreover, with relaxation techniques and the like, the participants' herpes episodes were comparatively short-lived and less severe than previously experienced.

Herpes infections represent an additional risk for pregnant women, because if the herpes infection is active at or near the time of childbirth, the baby can contract it in the birth canal during delivery. Consequently, if there is a history of herpes—even if the infection has not been apparent in recent months or years—it is absolutely essential to discuss it explicitly with the obstetrician or midwife well before the due date, so that appropriate action can be taken to ensure the safety of the baby—usually by means of a test administered immediately before delivery. If there is positive indication of herpes activity just before birth, a cesarean delivery is called for.

AIDS

In many respects AIDS has altered the course of modern medicine. It has also altered forever the role of sex in casual relationships, with knowledgeable heterosexual and homosexual partners both vastly more concerned about their sexual encounters. AIDS has no true cure, and the prospects of finding one in the next decade—before many people contract it and die from it—are unclear. It is truly the scourge of our times, one that has created a pervasive distress among a wide range of health professionals.

Originally called HTLV-III, the human immune deficiency virus (HIV) has grown to become a large concern in the heterosexual as well as the homosexual communities. Current data indicate that men and women who develop the antibody for HIV will, at a rate of perhaps 10 percent a year, go on to develop AIDS or AIDS-related complex (ARC), and will die.

Current studies have been following certain populations—most notably, homosexual males—since the early 1980s. Spread of the disease has prompted further studies in heterosexual communities. Conclusive results from these won't become available for several years, but it appears that AIDS will be an illness with very high mortality. We don't yet know if that mortality will ultimately be 100 percent—that is, no cure for existing cases —but indications thus far point to a death rate greater than 50 percent. That is why it has, with some melodrama, been called the great plague of our time, evoking the struggles of earlier societies to deal with bubonic plague and other serious infectious illnesses.

The "AIDS test" is not really a test for AIDS, but rather a test for the antibody to the virus. A two-part test was developed and is widely available. If both parts are positive, indicating the presence of HIV antibody, the news is not good. There are very few false-positives. Most likely a positive test, if properly done, is a positive test. In the last year, more tests have come out to detect the presence of HIV antibodies; it is likely that as these tests become more sophisticated, the incidence of false-positives will shrink to the point of negligibility.

The HIV virus infection is usually transmitted in semen. The other major route of infection is the blood. Transfusions were the way most hemophiliacs contracted HIV infections (blood has been effectively screened for several years now). Drug addicts pick it up using contaminated needles, and babies acquire it *in utero* via the mother's blood. Though there are theories that HIV may be transmitted through other body fluids such as tears and saliva, these theories have no evidence to support them and do nothing but unnecessarily incite public fears.

How does the whole issue of AIDS apply to most 35-plus women? Women whose partners are nonmonogamous, bisexual, or gay males, or who have been IV drug abusers, are certainly at high risk of HIV infection. Women who have had multiple male partners, especially if the sex has been unprotected, are also at significant risk.

Clearly, the approach to AIDS must be prevention of the infection. Though much is written about treatments, and indeed agents such as AZT do appear to improve survival, the fact is that as of this writing there is no cure. The best protection other than abstinence is mutual monogamy: no sex whatsoever outside the partnership. If that is not going to be the case, then the 35-plus woman must insist on latex condom usage, probably with a spermicidal jelly.

As advised earlier with regard to gonorrhea, outside of a long-standing monogamous relationship, you should avoid rectal sex altogether, even with a condom, because the possibility of tears and viral penetration is just too great. Also avoid unprotected oral sex, which may mean, for all practical purposes, no oral sex. It is not enough with oral sex to stop short of ejaculation, because often there is a preejaculatory fluid that can carry the infection.

Once again, if a male partner will not use a condom, dump him! And certainly don't believe him in regard to his sexual history or if he tries to make a case against condom use.

When it comes to any sexually transmitted disease, we emphasize the point: you must *insist* on condom use with your partner when long-term monogamy is not your situation. There is a lot of talk about women's liberation, but men still seem to hold the dominant role in sexual matters in this country. Sexuality too often involves a man's ejaculation and not a woman's orgasmic pleasure, nor a woman's protection from sexually transmitted diseases. Often women "let" men choose whether to use a condom or not. This is just plain crazy. Women of all ages must protect themselves; they cannot rely on men to do so. As with pregnancy, time has shown that women who depend on men in these areas—to be blunt—often get screwed twice.

35-PLUS SEXUAL SATISFACTION—AND DYSFUNCTION

The myth of sexuality is that desire declines with age; the reality is that the vast majority of sexually active women reach their peak potential for sexual fulfillment in their middle years—a level that for most remains relatively stable well into their sixties.

Sexual pleasure presumes communication with a partner about what is pleasurable and what is not—as well as spontaneity in the encounter. There's no need to get hung up on scheduling sex. Who can enjoy feeling obligated to perform? It is just as important for you and your partner to feel free to say no as it is to say yes—without holding grudges. Whether you make love once a month or every other night, what matters is that your encounters and their frequency are agreeable and satisfying for *both* of you.

With physiological maturity in your favor, you would think a rousing good sex life would follow—but as with most good things in life, it doesn't always turn out that way. One of the most common reasons for a diminished sex life is ordinary fatigue. Careers frequently peak or undergo reevaluation in the middle years, a situation that often brings with it stress, fatigue, and tensions that are usually brought home—not left behind at the office. It is an atmosphere that does little to foster sexual desire—particularly when both partners are juggling professional work with raising children. If desire for your mate is too frequently overwhelmed by your desire for sleep, or kept at bay by career worries, it's time to take stock of your situation.

Women entering menopause may also experience sexual dysfunction because of physiological changes—they may be temporary but they require attention, not just for you but for your mate, for such changes may have an effect on your partner's libido.

Midlife is a time when your spouse may be going through his own changes, too, a "midlife crisis" that can implicate his whole sense of himself as a man—his career success, his sense of purpose, his sexuality. All this may come at a time when he's experiencing anxiety over changes in his ability to perform sexually—and he may well be embarrassed or otherwise reluctant to discuss it.

These are all common but volatile elements in a sexual scenario that unfolds for many couples in the middle years—the key is to address them.

Solving Sexual Problems

In everyday clinical practice, the major categories of sexual dysfunction in 35-plus women seem to be related to decreased desire as well as decreased fulfillment with sex, which often means not having an orgasm; or having pain with sex (dyspareunia); or a common but infrequently addressed problem—decreased opportunity for sex, which includes the couples too harried by circumstances to cultivate their sexual relationships, or a partner who is either uninterested in or unable to have what is thought of as satisfactory sex.

If you tend to let your mate make the first move in sexual matters, this is a time when *your* initiative may be crucial. If you are able to communicate with your partner and can resolve the situation using your own resources, that's great. However, if your physical and your mental states seem to conspire against your sex life, and nothing seems to affect change, then seek outside advice. It really can make a difference, and there's nothing more threatening to the intimacy that nurtures your life together than for one or both partners to suffer in silence.

In getting an outside assessment of the situation, the physician or therapist you approach must be genuinely interested in sexuality and sexual dysfunction. Some general internists and family practitioners are skilled in this area, but they tend to be in the minority, and in our country, it is far more common to find solutions with a skilled, certified gynecologist, often working in concert with a sex therapist or possibly a skilled marriage counselor. Whatever route you choose, receptivity to your problem on the part of the doctor or therapist is essential, and you should feel no qualms about pursuing a solution with another professional if you don't feel confident about the quality of help you're getting, if you are not getting enough support, or do not feel the approach is suitable. Some doctors are perfectly competent to deal with all matters regarding reproductive functions, but may not be equipped to address matters concerning broader issues of female sexuality.

Discussions of sexual dysfunction in women properly begin with a careful menstrual history, followed by questions of whether sex is still actively pursued, with whom it is experienced and how often, and whether it is orgasmic. You may feel uncomfortable addressing these topics, but they should be aired openly and candidly discussed with your physician or therapist. It's the only way a realistic plan of action can be initiated.

Physiological Dysfunction

If there is a clear history of sexual dysfunction, a thorough gynecology exam should follow the initial history.

VAGINAL DRYNESS.   Although rare in premenopausal women, problems with vaginal dryness do occur and usually respond well to hormonal treatment or vaginal lubrication (the latter in the form of either general lubrication or topical hormonal preparations). Improvements with sexual performance often follow rapidly.

PAINFUL INTERCOURSE.   If there is a problem with infection or persistent discharge that has led to pain with sexual intercourse, this can also be treated effectively. Ordinarily a yeast infection is readily cured with vaginal suppositories; a bacterial infection can be treated with antibiotics.

If your gynecological examination shows a completely normal situation and there is no evidence of hormonal problems, sex therapy might be worth considering, provided it involves both partners. It is virtually impossible to succeed in therapy without mutual willingness and participation, with one's partner eager to improve the situation and willing to be part of its solution.

Sexual Fulfillment

There continue to be arguments about whether women's orgasms can really result from stimulation of the vagina, with many women maintaining that clitoral stimulation is the only thing that counts. You should be comfortable enough with your mate to guide him in the matter of foreplay; nor should he be defensive about this, although some men are. Never imagine that not having big orgasms by way of vaginal stimulation in any way marks you as frigid, a terrible word that almost never applies. Nor is orgasm the only measure of sexual pleasure. What counts in the end is whether or not the two of you are happy and comfortable with your sex life.

At the crux of sexual satisfaction is that special, intangible connection between you and your mate that fosters desire, intimacy, and sexual fulfillment—the foundation upon which your relationship rests and continues to grow. Addressing problems openly, in an atmosphere of mutual trust that is free of anger and blame, can bring welcome improvements in intimacy.

Although we strongly encourage women to take some initiative in this matter, increased possibilities for sexual fulfillment are not the sole responsibility of the female partner—not by any means. It's up to the male to do his share of the work. Male health issues very often affect female partners, and matters of sexual dysfunction certainly affect the quality of her sex life. It's appropriate to discuss some of these here.

Male Health Issues as They Relate to the 35-Plus Woman

Regardless of the status of her sex life, any woman who has a special relationship with a man—be it spouse, father, brother, or male friend about whose health she really cares—should be aware of certain health situations that may affect him and that unfortunately he may ignore. Of course, health choices like diet, exercise, and responses to illness apply to both men and women; the key issue is to clarify what those choices are—and then to make them. Ironically (and sexual politics notwithstanding), it remains somewhat more socially acceptable for women to be ill than for men—a holdover from all the generations past, when women were perceived as frail and men as tough and stoical. Many men are still so caught up in a macho attitude that they deny illness more persistently than women do, and end up getting much sicker as a result.

Just as we have encouraged patients in our clinical work to cooperate as families on pertinent medical and nutritional matters, we believe that you can make a significant difference in the health of your spouse, father, or friend by encouraging him in pursuit of the same positive health choices that you are making. Your good example may be enough to spur them on, but if you can gently persuade the 35-plus men in your life to read relevant sections of this book, so much the better.

Just as a woman is urged to get a pelvic, pap, and breast check, men from young adulthood on should do testicular self-examination on a regular basis, checking for any nodule or irregularity of the testicles and having them examined regularly by an internist or family practitioner. If necessary, the physician can make a referral to a urologist. Detected early on, testicular cancer is usually curable.

Examination of the prostate is the other genital component of a physical exam for a man. Prostate cancer occurs at greater frequency with increasing age, but a digital exam by a physician can often detect early signs of this—usually a hard or irregular prostate.

A rectal exam should also be performed whenever there's a complete physical exam. Some doctors advise that both a rectal examination (including a stool check for signs of hidden blood) and a prostate exam be done annually after the age of 40.

Lung and cardiovascular health are top priorities in all grown men, since the rates for male coronary artery disease are higher and begin at a younger age than for females. In large part, this is explained by the estrogen that protects premenopausal women, and it is one of several ways men seem constitutionally less healthy than women. Add the higher rate of smoking among men than among women, and the risk of accelerating coronary artery disease—hence myocardial infarction and death—becomes all the more potent.

Much has been written on the full extent of male sexuality and potency; however, a few trends deserve comment here.

POTENCY.   In a man, sexual arousal and performance peak in the teens and twenties, and begin to slow down thereafter. This is neither myth nor excuse; studies done on penis arousal time show a gradual, though not necessarily crucial, delay with normal aging. Paralleling the physiological events surrounding menopause, this is not a true decline in potency per se but it is a definite change. Sometimes, the delayed erection makes the male a better lover, since the tendency to "hit and run" becomes less frequent as a result. Even so, many men regard their ejaculation as the high point of the sexual encounter, and they need persistent education and encouragement to expand this vision. Given the male emphasis on ejaculation and having a hard penis for good sex, a decline in erectile ability not only can be devastating but can also initiate a cascade of events that ultimately leads to the end of intercourse.

If your partner is showing less interest, it may be because there is an erectile problem, either partial or complete. If this is the case, talk with him about it in a calm and supportive way, encouraging him to see his physician as soon as possible. Men are almost invariably reluctant to discuss potency problems with anyone—with the possible exception of a doctor, if specifically encouraged—and this reluctance may well extend to a lover or spouse. But in an office setting, much can be gained from an open discussion during the initial interview, when the doctor takes a medical history and candidly speaks of issues such as libido, erectile function, and general health, including use of medications. The latter is a very common cause of potency problems, as is alcohol use. The entire home environment must also be scrutinized, including issues such as general stress in the marriage, change in family roles, and whether you are going through menopause—a matter which can be of great, if only symbolic, importance to your mate.

Probing the specific details of this history may reveal marital or nonmarital stresses that are causing a decrease in libido; if the libido is decreased, erectile function may well decline. A few men candidly reveal that while they experience impotence with their spouses, they suffer none with another person—proof positive that they are not dealing with a physical potency problem but rather one of mental attitude.

GENERAL HEALTH.   On the physical side, the medical history might reveal symptoms of diabetes, thyroid problems, prostate problems, or vascular disease—any one of which can lead to problems with potency and sexual function. During the physical exam, then, the doctor should pay attention not simply to the genitals and prostate but to factors such as mental status and general affect (mood). Physical factors such as blood pressure and general vascular status (especially evaluating the pulses in the lower extremities, which give some hint as to the blood supply available to the genitals), will be evaluated, along with any signs of metabolic (hormonal) dysfunction.

Backing up the office visit is laboratory work that includes a complete blood count as well as general chemistries, with a urinalysis and specific checks of blood sugar, thyroid function, and levels of testosterone and prolactin.

Clearly, if medication is causing a problem, the patient should work with his doctor to change it. In most cases, a substitute usually can be found. For example, if methyldopa (Aldomet), used to treat hypertension, is causing a problem, an ACE inhibitor can be tried instead. If medication has been ruled out, the next area to explore is metabolic (hormonal) function. Diabetic control and control of an abnormal thyroid can be effectively treated with medication and, in some cases, medication and diet. Improvement of a metabolic problem may well lead to an improvement in sexual function, as overall health improves.

If examination shows a large prostate, or even signs of an infected prostate, as in prostatitis, this may be treated with antibiotics and then, if necessary, a urology referral can be made. If evidence is found of a vascular (blood vessel–related) problem—that is, if penis and genitals are not getting enough blood supply—the 35-plus male may benefit from medication and possible vascular surgery.

Testosterone—the male hormone—can be prescribed; this is an especially important option that often proves effective if impotence is partial and blood testosterone is truly low. There is usually a choice of male hormone tablets taken on a daily basis or monthly injections which give a sustained release. This treatment requires close physician follow-up, however.

OTHER SOLUTIONS.   In cases of complete impotence, when there is no erection or ejaculation at all, if there is no underlying medically treatable cause, then testosterone will rarely work. A penile implant, however, may allow the patient to have reasonably normal intercourse. Penile implants come in two basic types: the rigid form, which gives the man a fairly erect penis at all times, and the hydraulic type, which more closely simulates normal physiology. In both cases, surgery is required but, while there is some risk of infection, generally the results are good.

In addition to the option of a penile implant, there is a new treatment involving direct injection of the penis with medications, specifically a combination of papaverine and phentolamine. These are designed to allow the penis to become engorged with blood. The treatment produces an erection, but it requires very specific urological care as well as substantial patient motivation.

After ruling out possible causes for impotency, a doctor can provide a referral to a sex therapist, at least for a general evaluation. Addressing the psychological side of the problem may well bring the sought-after improvement.

Few issues are as emotionally charged for the 35-plus male as a decrease in sexual potency. Patience and a loving interest on the part of his partner are the keys to making improvements in this area. In many ways, the choice that a 35-plus male makes in seeking help for potency problems is the crucial first step toward improvement. The move itself can have an immediate positive effect on his relationship with his spouse. Without appropriate action, many relationships—including mature, long-lasting ones—can founder, sinking to levels where sexual problems become unsolvable and threaten the entire endeavor.

Although this book has focused on the many positive choices for health, and on the positive ways of responding to health problems, this focus on male problems is crucial not only for the man but for his female partner as well.

It is still very common in our society for men to perceive their impotence problems as shameful and to hide them. In essence, the man who chooses to do nothing about it will suffer—and that aspect of the problem is rarely a kept secret. By definition, sexual fulfillment involves two people, and this is an instance when you will need to take the lead—by lovingly encouraging your mate to seek attention and care.

PART FIVE

Cancer and the 35-Plus Woman— Updates and Prevention

I N MAURICE SENDAK'S BOOK *Where the Wild Things Are*, a little boy named Max bravely confronts roaring beasts with gnashing teeth and terrible eyes and terrible claws, and commands them to "Be still." Young children who know this story like to hear it again and again, reacting always with the same sequence of fear and anxiety as the coming of the beasts is anticipated, and then with supreme relief as Max not only finds the power to tame but also to control them.

Children have all sorts of real and imagined fears—of wild things lurking under the bed, wavy shadows on the wall, thunder clapping in the night —and they are lucky to find an outlet in the genius of Maurice Sendak and others like the Brothers Grimm. The fears we grown-ups must confront are no less real; we just don't have wonderful stories or reassuring adults to sidle up to for protection. We've got to confront them on our own, particularly when it comes to the collective monster known as cancer.

The AIDS virus notwithstanding, cancer seems to be what 35-plus women fear the most—an out-of-the-blue threat that can strike young and old alike. It is the rare individual who reaches her fortieth birthday without knowing someone in her generation who is battling some form of cancer. Such situations quickly bring home an awareness of mortality and a new appreciation of good health. They also cause concern. Often, when a woman makes an appointment with her doctor to discuss certain new symptoms, the underlying worry is that those symptoms are signs of a malignancy. And when the results of the visit are negative, the usual reaction is a heartfelt, "Thank God it's not cancer."

For most 35-plus women, the annual visit to the gynecologist for breast and pelvic examinations is the most regular consultation outside of visits to the dentist. Most of us feel a shiver of anxiety waiting for the results of a pap smear or mammography; this is particularly true for those women who have had any kind of hormonal treatment—which includes the use of birth control pills. Very few of us fall outside that category, since the pill has been prescribed not just for birth control but also for irregular periods and other hormonal irregularities. Because of this focus, breast cancer and cervical, ovarian, and endometrial cancers probably lead the list of women's cancer fears. But in fact the incidence of invasive cervical cancer has greatly declined, just as the survival rate for breast cancer has improved. After breast cancer, the big cancer monsters for women are actually colorectal cancer and lung cancer—the incidence of the latter rising toward the level of incidence in men.

As it is throughout this book, prevention is the main thrust here, but not all risk factors are under your control. Certainly your genetic background is not. In any cancer, early detection greatly improves your chance of survival. In this chapter we'll give you basic information on detection, diagnostic procedures, and standard treatments, along with some information on recent research; the next chapter will cover prevention strategies in some detail. Forewarned is forearmed, but it is useless and counterproductive to harbor irrational fears about cancer. What we mean to give you is a healthy respect for the beast.

CHAPTER 19

Six Cancers of Special Concern to 35-Plus Women

BREAST CANCER

OF ALL CANCERS, BREAST cancer unquestionably evokes the greatest concern, since its incidence in middle-aged women is rising. An estimated 130,000 to 140,000 new cases were diagnosed in 1988, and an estimated 40,000 deaths were predicted. The risk of developing this cancer increases from ages 35 to 40, with detection in the over-50 age group accounting for a full two-thirds of all the diagnoses made. Breast cancer is a risk that does not significantly decline after that, either. Despite hopeful new methods of detection and treatment, including ways to distinguish fast-growing tumors from slower-growing ones in the early stages and tailoring therapy accordingly, breast cancer continues to be the leading cause of death among women in their productive middle life. Theories abound as to why this is so, involving such issues as changes in life-style, diet, or timing of events in the reproductive cycle. But the puzzle of why breast cancer is on the increase remains unsolved.

In an article published recently in the *New York Times*, Dr. Melvin Konner candidly urged women to make the issue of breast cancer a feminist one—that is, to take practical measures of prevention, but also to put pressure on the government to fund areas of basic research where a cure might be found. He suggested writing to representatives in Congress to find out what they are doing, and why they are not doing more to eliminate this disease. Dr. Konner also made an analogy. If men of power in the White House and elsewhere were to get testicular cancer, and the rate were to climb to over 100,000 men annually, and if they were to undergo painful treatments and eventually one-third of them would die, we would surely see an unprecedented commitment of resources to finding a cure. Indeed, whatever the reasons for the lag in beating breast cancer, every 35-plus woman needs to become politically active and push politicians toward allotting more funds for finding a cure.

In the meantime, secondary screening remains the most effective way to save lives, through both self-examination and mammography. The fear of radiation from mammography pales in comparison with its benefits: for every 1 million 40-year-old women who have mammograms, almost 800 cases of breast cancer would be caught while only 10 cancer diagnoses might result from the effects of the mammography itself. Although routine mammograms probably increase the number of early diagnoses, 90 to 95 percent of all breast cancers are still found by self-discovery, so self-examination remains an important tool in detection.

Known Risk Factors

Breast cancer has been labeled "civilization's cancer," with changes in the life-style and dietary choices of women exerting as much influence as genetics, at least in our society. Some of the risk factors that predispose a woman toward breast cancer include:

- Family history, particularly the incidence of breast cancer in relatives on the maternal side—that is, a mother, a sister, a maternal cousin or maternal aunt
- Specific genetic factors. While the puzzle pieces continue to be moved around in trying to accurately pinpoint the major breast cancer risks, scientists are closing in on specific genetic factors implicated in the incidence of cancer; in the case of certain breast cancers, the protective, "anti-oncogene" gene or genes from chromosome 17 are absent. Studies centering on the missing genetic elements of chromosome 17, which were reported in the December 1988 issue of the British medical journal *The Lancet*, showed that while the specific gene had not been determined, it appeared to be in the same region of the chromosome implicated in colon cancer, osteosarcoma, and lung cancer—a fact that "is of particular interest in view of the extensive evidence that 'breast cancer families' commonly show, in addition, an excess of other types of tumor."
- Early menstruation, having no children or a late-in-life pregnancy, late menopause—that is, the timing of certain hormonal changes in the reproductive cycles.
- Breast cancer in an opposite breast, even if that breast has been removed via radical mastectomy; cancer in one breast statistically increases the chance of cancer in the remaining breast.

- A high-fat diet. Fat seems to play a partial role in the other causes mentioned—causes that are largely out of a woman's control—but lowering the amount of fat in the diet offers one of the most promising roads to prevention. Those who advocate a low-fat diet have much evidence to back up their claims. In fact, of all the suggested links between diet and cancer, the association between dietary fat and breast cancer comes closest to fulfilling the criteria epidemiologists look for when making inferences about causes of disease. Based on this correlation, specific dietary guidelines are given in Chapter 20.

Medical Diagnosis and Treatment

When a suspicious lesion is encountered by palpation or mammography, a biopsy is usually advised. If the biopsy is positive for cancer, surgery is required in all cases. The earlier a breast cancer is discovered and treated surgically, the more hopeful is the prognosis for survival. New evidence suggests that postoperative chemotherapy improves chances even further.

What kind of surgery is to be done is a controversial issue. Many years ago, breast surgery for cancer was always the radical mastectomy—removal of the cancerous lesion and the breast, part of the muscle structure and, under the arm, the lymph nodes nearest the breast. Generally speaking, this is no longer done; even surgeons who are considered traditional in their approach do what is called a modified radical mastectomy, which includes removal of the whole breast and dissection of the lymph nodes in the underarm, but leaves the chest muscle under the breast intact. This approach is less disfiguring than a radical mastectomy, less likely to impair lymph flow, and apt to provide greater range of motion in the arm.

In recent years, a body of data has accumulated to suggest that even less radical surgery may be adequate—specifically in instances where the breast cancer is less than 2 centimeters in diameter (less than seven-eighths of an inch) and when there are no enlarged lymph nodes in the underarm on the same side. Patient and surgeon may want to consider a segmental mastectomy, popularly called a lumpectomy, which usually involves removing about a quarter of the breast tissue (not enough to seriously disfigure the breast), with the cancer in the midst of that quadrant. Following this type of removal, postoperative radiotherapy is advised, using X-ray beams to "burn away" the cancer tissue. That's radiotherapy. Chemotherapy is when antitumor medications are used; the type and amount of drugs depend on the extent and type of the cancer.

If a lumpectomy is done, the surgeon still calls for a pathological examination of the lymph nodes under the arm on the same side, taking specimens by surgical removal in a process referred to as axillary node dissection. This is a very important step in assessing tumor spread. The combination of analyzing the actual tumor for estrogen activity as well as examining the axillary node specimens for evidence of tumor spread is a big factor in subsequent decisions about whether chemotherapy should be offered and, if so, what kind and for how long.

Increasingly, there is evidence that more women should receive chemotherapy. Some oncologists advocate that virtually all women who have had breast cancer should receive at least some type of chemotherapy, although this is certainly not yet the general practice. It is currently more likely that candidates for chemotherapy include those whose cancer has spread to the axillary nodes and those whose lab tests come back confirming a high estrogen-receptor activity.

Still, a growing number of doctors believe that aggressive chemotherapy will provide more satisfactory long-term results even in cases where it's not considered imperative. Because of its side effects, this use of chemotherapy remains controversial, at least among patients. But chemotherapy doesn't affect everyone the same way. In all cancer treatments, emotional factors play a part. In a January 1989 exchange of letters in the *New York Times Magazine,* Dr. Ezra Greenspan, Medical Director of Mount Sinai's Chemotherapy Foundation in New York, said that in his experience less than 20 percent of patients receiving chemotherapy suffer intense toxicity. He stressed that chemicals used in chemotherapy should not be viewed as "poisons" but rather as lifesaving substances, and that "the association of more positive attitudes with better drug tolerance (psychological feedback mechanisms) has been scientifically documented."

In our medical group, we use a team approach in treating breast cancer, with the primary physician continuing to monitor the patient but relying on the surgeon and internist-oncologist for specific advice, plans about chemotherapy, and follow-up, which includes annual mammography virtually forever, monthly self-exams, and periodic physician exams on the breast that remains. Strong teamwork has proved to best serve the cancer patient.

As for the outlook for breast cancer patients in general, it's a case of the older the better. Unopposed estrogen circulating to the breast—that is, estrogen that is not counterbalanced with an opposing hormone to reduce its adverse affects—is known to help carcinogens do their work. Thus women who are past menopause generally fare better than those who get cancer before menopause, when estrogen levels are normally higher. Nevertheless, anti-estrogen therapy does seem to help when the cancer occurs in postmenopausal women, however, and the anti-estrogen medication tamoxifen has been a significant addition to therapy and is well tolerated compared to many other chemotherapies.

Prevention and Early Detection of Breast Cancer

There are several positive ways a 35-plus woman can confront the risks of breast cancer; in a very real way, she can do something to help alleviate her fears. These strategies involve both detection and prevention:

- Monthly self-examinations after age 30. Set a schedule for this and stick to it. (For details write to your local chapter of the American Cancer Society for one of their excellent booklets explaining how to perform your own breast examination.)
- A baseline mammogram at the age of 35 and annual mammography after age 50, or—depending on individual considerations—annually between ages 40 and 50 as well. This is the current recommendation of the American Cancer Society, but the optimum interval for mammography is still not exactly clear; some European studies indicate that women benefit from mammograms done at two- or three-year intervals after age 40. In any case, scheduling mammography is a subject every woman should discuss with her doctor, particularly when she may be at high risk and could benefit from more frequent mammography.
- Breast feed your new baby. This strategy has proved to be good for breast health, as well as an excellent way to give a newborn a good start in life. Many more health-conscious 35-plus women have made this early mothering choice in recent years. Studies have documented the benefits of breast feeding, with women who nursed their babies exclusively on one breast showing a significant protective effect on that side.
- Eat a low-fat diet. See guidelines in Chapter 20.
- Be conservative in your intake of alcohol. Related to the same dietary guidelines of the National Academy of Science and given in Chapter 20, the question comes up as to just how much alcohol is safe, particularly when breast cancer is the issue. There is a swarm of controversy on this topic. One Harvard study concluded with a warning that as little as one drink of wine a day could put a woman at higher risk of getting breast cancer, but for various reasons (including insufficient research) that study was criticized by many and was even disputed by researchers at the Centers for Disease Control in Atlanta, which found no association at all between breast cancer and alcohol. So it seems an occasional drink, or even a glass of wine or a cocktail before dinner, is not going to cause a problem.

GYNECOLOGICAL CANCERS

Cervical Cancer

There are two types of cervical cancer: invasive (going below the mucosal lining) and *in situ*, which is superficial in depth. The difference between the two is significant, since the *in situ* variety is completely curable based on its low invasion.

Although invasive cases of cervical cancer remain at about 15,000 per year with 7,000 deaths per year, their incidence has in fact decreased by half in recent decades. But the combination of invasive and *in situ* cancers probably would equal 60,000 cases per year. The good news is that the pap smear leads to 90 percent detection of all cervical cancer. Consequently, the test can set the stage for a true cure of *in situ* cervical cancer, where the cure rate is nearly 100 percent. As for invasive cancer, the prognosis depends on how far the cancer has spread, an assessment that can only be made by an experienced gynecologist.

What are the risk factors for cervical cancer? They include:

- Sex at a young age—that is, early to mid-teen years. Women who begin their sexual experiences at a somewhat older age seem to be at less risk.
- Daughters of women who took DES—the synthetic female hormone and growth stimulant diethylstilbestrol—during pregnancy.
- Multiple sex partners. It's been shown that there's an increased risk of cervical cancer in women who have had many sexual partners, implying that there's a risk from infections, particularly papillomavirus infections. There's a strong case for monogamy or protected sex, since a promiscuous life-style seems to play a part in its occurrence, with cervical cancer being very rare among celibate women and lesbians—and very common in prostitutes.

If cervical cancer is diagnosed, a hysterectomy as a general rule is done. If the cancer is invasive, radiotherapy will probably also be used.

Endometrial (Uterine) Cancer

The incidence of this cancer appears to be rising, with approximately 40,000 new cases per year and about 4,000 to 6,000 deaths. Endometrial cancer is more common after the age of 50, and one of the clues is unexpected bleeding after menopause. However, bleeding is not always a sign of cancer and it should not cause immediate alarm. (The most common cause of postmenopausal bleeding is estrogen deficiency and its subsequent irritation and dryness.) Nonetheless, because of the risk of endometrial cancer, any postmenopausal bleeding needs immediate and thorough investigation, usually in the form of an endometrial biopsy. Regular pap smears can help with diagnosis, but they only lead to about a 50 percent detection rate because the uterus is higher up than the cervix, and uterine cancer cells don't always slough downward.

Years ago, an apparent link between long-term estrogen use in menopause and endometrial cancer was found, so that women who have had estrogen therapy may be at greater risk. As a result of this discovery, treatment is now given in the form of combined doses of estrogens and progesterones, in place of unopposed estrogen, which seems to lower the risk.

Endometrial cancer usually requires an extensive hysterectomy to hope for cure, but even an advanced tumor will shrink down from chemotherapy and radiotherapy.

Ovarian Cancer

This is perhaps one of the hardest gynecological cancers to diagnose. It is quite rare under the age of 35, but more common after the age of 45. It accounts for as many as a quarter of all gynecological cancers, with about 20,000 new cases a year and 10,000 deaths annually.

In the majority of cases, the main way to detect ovarian cancer is through careful bimanual pelvic exam—another good reason for maintaining optimum weight, since obesity decreases the value or accuracy of such an exam. Because it is often not diagnosed early, survival of ovarian cancer is only 30 to 45 percent at five years.

Treatment, as in endometrial cancer, is a complete hysterectomy, in this case with fallopian tubes and ovaries, then chemotherapy if there is evidence of spread.

Prevention of Gynecological Cancers

Incidence of the three gynecological cancers—cervical, endometrial, and ovarian—can be reduced by having regular pap smears and thorough pelvic examinations. In addition, cervical cancers can be reduced by safe sexual practices with a limited number of sexual partners (ideally, only one), to avoid the risk of infection.

Diet also has a place in avoiding gynecological cancers. In a recent cancer study conducted in Italy, researchers found that women who consumed more meat had a higher fat intake and a higher incidence of ovarian cancer than those who did not. Ovarian cancer patients also reported that they ate less fish, fewer green vegetables and carrots, and less whole-wheat bread and pasta than their healthy Italian counterparts. It was also noted that ovarian cancer was two and a half times more common in northern Italy, where cream sauces prevail, than in the southern provinces, where the cuisine is tomato-based and lower in overall fat. In this regard, the obvious inference is that the health benefit of pasta can quickly be cancelled out by ingredients that go on top and into the sauce. Tasty and popular as it is, a dish like *fettuccine Alfredo*, with its rich, creamy sauce and cheese, is extremely high in calories and fat, whereas pasta with a simple tomato *marinara*, zesty with garlic and oregano, is low in saturated fat.

COLORECTAL CANCER

Colorectal cancer tends to be somewhat gender equal, but it is a cancer of great importance to 35-plus women since 98 percent of all cases occur in people over the age of 40. There are approximately 120,000 new cases a year, and usually about 60,000 deaths per year, making it the *second* leading cause of cancer deaths in the United States. (The leading cause of death from cancer is lung disease.)

Medical Diagnosis and Treatment

Certain symptoms can give an early clue to colorectal cancer: pain, blood in the stool, sometimes a change in bowel habit. These signs warrant prompt follow-up with your physician, since weight loss or very palpable mass in the stomach or abdomen are late signs usually associated with a poor chance of survival. For that reason, as with breast cancer, the emphasis is on early detection.

One widely used detection method involves collection of a stool sample that is checked for signs of hidden, or "occult" blood, hence the name Hemoccult for the trademark of this test. The true value of this checking method remains unclear, although extended long-term studies are under way in this country to determine whether this test does in fact reduce mortality. In the meantime, while not as specific as we would like, the test provides a screening so that over the age of 50, annual Hemoccults are advised—collected properly and turned in promptly, which means within approximately one week.

If a Hemoccult is positive, follow-up is warranted, with sigmoidoscopy and an air contrast barium enema, performed by an experienced radiologist; or colonoscopy, performed by a gastroenterologist. (A colonoscopy is similar to a sigmoidoscopy except that it surveys the entire colon rather than a part of it.) Even if Hemoccults are negative, sigmoidoscopy generally is advised over the age of 50, on a three- to five-year basis, assuming previous examinations showed the area to be completely normal.

Are there high-risk groups with colorectal cancer as there are with breast cancer? The answer is yes. They include people who have a personal history of colon cancer or colon polyps, or who have a family history of polyps or colorectal cancer. If a first-degree relative has had colorectal cancer, the risk for the individual is threefold that of the general population. In this group of people with higher risk, the key is to begin screening early, and to do it frequently.

If a mass is found in the colon, either by X-ray or colonoscopy, then biopsy, sometimes via the colonoscope, is advised, followed by surgery. In this case, the treatment is primarily surgical, done by an experienced general surgeon and involving a resection of the tumor—that is, a cutting away of the cancer and some of the surrounding normal tissue, not only to remove it but also to allow for staging, a way of seeing how advanced the tumor is. Treatment for colorectal cancer may or may not require a colostomy, the diversion of stool contents to a bag, since the surgeon cannot always predict before surgery whether the colon can be reconnected after the cancer has been removed.

Once the cancer has been removed, follow-up is necessary with the surgeon and a gastroenterologist. In our group practice, we emphasize periodic colonoscopies for surveillance, which is indeed becoming the general standard in our country. In most areas, these are done by gastroenterologists.

The outlook for people with colorectal cancer is not terribly promising, with five-year survival less than 50 percent across the board, a statistic that has remained unchanged in the last two to three decades. Chemotherapy has not led to a significant change in survival rates, although studies are constantly being done. Radiotherapy rarely has a significant role, except in advanced cases. So, with nonsurgical treatment for colorectal cancer relatively ineffective, the emphasis must be on early diagnosis.

Jean Spodnik's Nutritional Advice for Preventing Colorectal Cancer

When it comes to minimizing the risk of colorectal cancer, diet clearly plays a role. Just as with diverticulosis, this form of cancer is far more common in Western populations that consume highly processed food than in underdeveloped countries where diet is primarily vegetarian. Furthermore, just as with breast cancer, reducing your fat intake is thought to lower your chances of colon cancer—a speculation that stems in part from research demonstrating that high fat intake causes greater secretion of bile acids. In their role of helping the body digest fat by emulsifying it in the stomach, bile acids combine with carcinogens that, if not efficiently eliminated, can cause cancer in the colon, or large bowel—at least as demonstrated in laboratory animals.

According to some researchers, dietary fiber minimizes the harmful effect of bile acids and thereby inhibits tumorous development. But it has not yet been determined whether an increase in dietary fiber works independently of decreased fat, or whether the two must operate in tandem for optimal anticancer effect.

In either case, dietary fiber is thought to decrease the risk of colorectal cancer in one or more ways:

- By increasing the bulk of the stool, which may dilute the concentration of cancer-causing agents
- By speeding the passage of the stool through the colon and thereby lessening the time carcinogens, or carginogenic substances and waste, can do damage; also by binding to carcinogens that might otherwise remain free to work or produce a tumor
- By none of these elaborate mechanisms at all; instead, simply by contributing to overall calorie restriction. The more low-calorie fiber consumed, the less room there is for calorie-dense foods, including foods high in fat. Tests in rats have shown that restricting calorie intake also reduces the incidence and size of tumors.

More research is needed to straighten all this out, but in the meantime, such uncertainties may not sit well with the health-conscious consumer eager to eat the right amount of fiber in the hope of preventing cancer. One thing is clear, however. According to a national survey, the average daily fiber intake of U.S. adults is only 11 grams, whereas it should be 25 to 35 grams.

Taking dietary histories all day, I get a first-hand view of what the majority of people in our country eat and how few of them include fruits and vegetables in their diet. A typical breakfast might be cereal and a glass of juice; for lunch, a quick hamburger, or hamburger and fries, or a meat sandwich—with diet soda; an afternoon snack of popcorn (not too bad because it does have some fiber), chips, or a candy bar; then dinner is a salad or cooked vegetables with the meal but never both. Clearly, fiber-rich fruits and vegetables must be increased, since a long-term diet that is high in fiber and low in fat and processed foods will almost certainly decrease the incidence of colorectal cancer.

LUNG CANCER

Fifty years ago, a health guide aimed at 35-plus women would not have listed lung cancer as a threat, either for this age group or for women at all. But in the last three decades, lung cancer has become an "equal opportunity" cancer, with increased female smoking bringing their rate of lung cancer up to that of males. There has been an almost 400 percent rise in lung cancer among women in the last four decades, causing more women who smoke to die of lung cancer than from breast cancer. Nearly 150,000 new cases (men and women) will be diagnosed each year, and there are more than 100,000 deaths per year.

Medical Diagnosis and Treatment

Early diagnosis of lung cancer is difficult. Annual chest X-rays even among smokers have not really proved useful. Diagnosis primarily involves following any unexplained, persistent symptoms carefully, particularly a cough that lasts more than three weeks. In such cases, a woman should consult her personal physician and strongly consider having a chest X-ray. If there are strong suspicions, bronchoscopy (the insertion of a flexible tube into the main bronchial tubes) may be done by a pulmonary specialist to obtain samples (washings) of the secretions of the bronchial tubes, or a biopsy of a suspicious area.

If there is a suspicious spot on a chest X-ray, and if bronchoscopy results are consistent with lung cancer, then tests must be done to assess how far the cancer has spread. In those who are candidates for surgery, a CT (computerized tomography) scan of the chest is commonly done, and sometimes even mediastinoscopy, a test whereby the center space between the lungs is examined for signs of lymph node enlargements. Surgery alone often tells the full story, and unfortunately even in patients who were thought to have no spread of disease, it often reveals so much more spread than presumed that surgical cure—removal of the cancer—is not possible. As for postoperative therapy, three-fourths of the cancers found are not really amenable to curative chemotherapy, although the remaining one-fourth who have a special small-cell type do have a good chance of response to specific chemotherapy. Unlike colorectal cancer, radiotherapy really does have a strong role in treating lung cancer. Although it is usually not curative, it can help shrink the tumor and so it is a very good palliative treatment.

If a lung cancer cannot be completely removed, the outlook is poor. Thus once again the emphasis must be on prevention. Lung cancer is mostly a one-risk disease, so that eliminating that risk—giving up cigarettes —is the key to prevention. If a woman is able to stop smoking, her risk of developing lung cancer "normalizes" by about year 12; but even by year 5, it has been halved.

The real goal for the 35-plus woman is to choose to stop smoking, not only for her own sake but also for her early to mid-teen daughters, a group in which smoking continues to increase, to serve as a positive role model. It has been shown that if women do not become smokers by the time they are 20 or 21, their risk of becoming addicted to nicotine becomes much smaller. The sooner teenagers can be persuaded that it isn't cool to smoke, the better off they will be. Quitting is tough, but it has been done by millions—in support groups, through hypnosis, and on their own.

SECOND OPINIONS

Nowhere is the value of a second opinion more apparent than in the treatment of cancer, especially in cases that are complicated or difficult to treat. In this regard, a computerized data base established by the National Cancer Institute in Maryland can be extremely useful and, in some cases, perhaps life-saving. Called PDQ (Physician's Data Query), it was set up largely at the instigation of cancer survivor Richard Bloch (cofounder of H&R Block). PDQ tells physicians where new treatments for particular cancers are being tried and what the best state-of-the-art treatments are considered to be. It makes sense to ask your doctor if he's using this before you begin any cancer treatment. The Institute has also set up a toll-free number patients can call to ask questions about their particular cancers, request PDQ printouts, and make contact with comprehensive cancer centers and second-opinion panels located in various parts of the country. The number is 1-800-4-CANCER.

CANCER, CHEMOTHERAPY, AND THE MIND-BODY CONNECTION

The subject of cancer, and breast cancer in particular, is fraught with emotional overtones, and a lot of literature has sprung up that deals with cancer and the mind-body connection—a connection that many doctors have come to view as crucial. The shared experiences of women in various phases of battling breast cancer have lent enormous support and valuable perspective to others who later develop the disease. In letters to the editor of the *New York Times Magazine* (an exchange cited earlier), a number of women and doctors responded to an article entitled "Under the Shadow of Cancer," by Eleanor Bergholz, who raised many questions about, and was reluctantly accepting of, what she describes as the toxic effects of her chemotherapy. A number of readers disagreed with her.

"Cancer treatment is not what Eleanor Berholz calls 'a sorry state,' " wrote Betty Marks. "It saves the lives of about 40 percent of those who have the disease." For Ms. Marks, an insulin-dependent diabetic who had a mastectomy and removal of two cancerous lymph nodes, choosing "the most aggressive, postoperative therapy available including a year of chemotherapy followed by lifetime maintenance on the hormone tamoxifen . . . plus Cancer Care's psychotherapy program and expert nutritional advice" has thus far proved a success. "I was not sick during my treatment," she reported, "thus I was able to work, swim, ski, jog, and spend time with the many friends who expressed their love and concern for me."

Joan R. Sovern wrote that "Not everyone becomes sick from chemotherapy and radiation." She described battling breast cancer for over five years with "brilliant and supportive doctors, a loving family and many friends to cheer me on." Her suggestions to other women in similar situations: "Everybody is frightened by breast cancer. . . . Find a doctor you trust. Do not look back. Do not focus on what may happen in the future. Rest when you need to. Return to whatever you were doing before you had cancer. Live every moment of every day."

CHAPTER 20

Cancer Prevention: Fighting Back with Diet

CAN EATING THE RIGHT FOOD cut your risk of cancer? As pointed out in connection with specific cancers discussed in Chapter 19, there is a real connection between the kind of food you eat and prevention of cancer—most notably, breast and colon cancer but undoubtedly all cancers.

Lengthy research has been done on this subject, and several reports have been published in the last decade. In 1983, the National Academy of Science's diet, nutrition, and cancer report concluded that while no special diet or special foods such as herbal teas, Laetrile, or megadoses of nutrients can cure cancer, following these six dietary guidelines very definitely helps prevent it:

1. Limit fats to 30 percent of your total daily calories. That means, for example, that in a 1,200-calorie diet, only 360 would be taken in fat (40 grams). Or of a 1,500-calorie diet, approximately 450 calories would be fat (50 grams). Using the guidelines on page 310, you can figure out how much fat you're getting from certain foods just by looking at the package label.
2. Include foods high in fiber, beta-carotene, vitamin E, and vitamin C in the daily diet. These include dark green leafy and dark yellow vegetables and cruciferous vegetables (from the mustard family) such as cabbage, kohlrabi, broccoli, Brussels sprouts, cauliflower, white turnips, and rutabagas.
3. Avoid foods that have been smoked or pickled, since they might contain nitrosamines (see page 264). These foods include sausages,

smoked fish and ham, bacon, hot dogs, bologna, and other luncheon meats.

4. Monitor your consumption of food additives and toxins.

5. Drink alcohol in moderation and do not smoke.

6. Avoid megavitamin supplements unless they have been medically advised; see guidelines in Chapter 21.

To these six points, the American Cancer Society has added one more: maintain a normal weight for your height.

The research upon which these guidelines are based is constantly being updated, yet it increasingly indicates a direct connection between food and cancer prevention. Before going on to some "anticancer shopping and cooking" strategies, let's look more closely at some of the latest findings in certain key areas.

LIMITING FAT

In July 1988, the government published its most comprehensive report on nutrition and health. Stating that overconsumption of fat and other foods was a major national problem, the surgeon general, Dr. C. Everett Koop, cited fat as the leading cause of disease and warned that it should be reduced in most people's diets.

Ironically, many of the people Koop referred to are totally unaware they are eating too much fat. We see this again and again in clinical practice, where a widespread misconception comes to light. People think that if fat can't be seen in a food, it doesn't exist. When asked what type of sandwiches a person eats, many times the response is bologna because, unlike salami, bologna is so low in fat. The reality, of course, is that 85 percent of the calories in regular bologna come from fat. All you have to do is fry it to see that. Bologna is not the only source of hidden fat, either. If you look at the list on pages 310–312, you may be surprised to see the large amounts of fat in certain foods.

INCREASING FIBER, VITAMINS, AND MINERALS

We've covered some of the studies on fiber under colon cancer in Chapter 19. As for vitamins, current studies are underway to find out more about the role of vitamin E and beta-carotene, the substance that your body turns into vitamin A. Are they instrumental in blocking the action of certain highly reactive chemicals that can alter the normal function of cells and thereby set the stage for tumors to develop?

To determine the protective properties of beta-carotene and vitamin E in warding off cancers, scientists are conducting studies known as chemo-prevention trials, in which large numbers of people are given supplemental doses of one or more substances, and then are observed over a period of several years to see if they are less likely to succumb to cancer. Some 23,000 male physicians throughout the United States are participating in such a trial, funded by the National Cancer Institute, to determine if beta-carotene supplements decrease the overall incidence of cancer; other groups are being given vitamin E.

Results of these tests will not be known until the 1990s. In the mean-time, the National Cancer Institute emphasizes that no one should inter-pret the research as a go-ahead for taking megadoses of beta-carotene, vitamin E, vitamin A, or any other nutrient, even though it is tempting to assume that if a certain vitamin or mineral is being tested, then it is merely a matter of waiting for the good news to be finalized. Such an assumption can be dangerous. Large doses of beta-carotene are relatively harmless, but too much vitamin A can cause permanent liver damage.

The mineral selenium is also being tested in a chemoprevention study, and is easily available over the counter in health food stores, but it can be toxic in large quantities.

Even vitamin C, which, like beta-carotene and vitamin E, may deacti-vate reactive chemicals—in particular, the nitrosamines described next—can cause problems, such as a predisposition to kidney stones, if taken in large supplementary doses.

MONITORING FOOD ADDITIVES

A long-standing area of cancer research involves nitrosamines, which are contained in smoked or pickled meat and fish and should be avoided.

The cancer connection actually begins with nitrate, a relatively com-mon substance found in food and water, which has been under suspicion as a cause of cancer (especially cancer of the stomach) since the mid-1970s. When *nitrate* enters the body, particularly when it is present in food that is left at room temperature, bacteria may convert the compound to *nitrite*; note the spelling; there is a big difference. Nitrite, in turn, can become attached to common organic substances to produce *nitrosamines*, which are carcinogenic.

Nitrite was originally used to preserve food, especially meat and fish, before there were refrigerators; it is still used in bacon and sausages so that the meat will look pink or red instead of gray. Generally, the practice of adding nitrite to food has declined in the last few decades, but the presence of nitrate has increased because vegetables pick it up from fertilizers in the soil; it is also found in drinking water.

Ominous as this sounds, there is no documented evidence that nitrate at the level most of us encounter it will lead to gastric cancer, since in the conversion process from nitrate to nitrite to nitrosamine, the last link is the critical one. Direct exposure to nitrosamines in your diet is actually minimal. Interestingly, studies conducted in the United States, Japan, England, and Canada have shown that groups of people with a high rate of stomach cancer have had no greater exposure to nitrates than groups with lower rates of the disease. Moreover, a 1986 study of people working in a fertilizer factory demonstrated that despite heavy exposure to nitrates, none of the workers had stomach cancer.

Direct exposure to nitrosamine-containing carcinogens is greater from inhaling cigarette smoke than it is from food, so if you don't smoke and you eat a well-balanced diet following the guidelines in this book, there's no reason to worry that nitrates in your diet will inevitably lead to stomach cancer. The key element is the conversion process, and the latest findings show that the conversion can be controlled.

Certain elements in our diet actually have been shown to cut the risk of nitrosamine conversion. Fruits and vegetables, for example, are high in vitamin C, and vitamin C is known to inhibit the formation of nitrosamines. Conversely, in regions of the world where food preservation is inadequate, bacteria contaminating the food supply may actually generate high levels of nitrosamine, thus possibly accounting for the high rates of stomach cancer in less developed countries.

Certain flavoring substances can also encourage the formation of nitrosamines, so that when intake is high, nitrosamine conversion and exposure may also be high enough to cause cancer. Such is the case with certain types of preserved fish, including the Japanese varieties known as *sanma*, *aji*, and *iwashi*, as well as with certain varieties of Japanese soy sauce and fava beans. There is a high rate of stomach cancer among the Japanese, because their basic diet is periodically low in vitamin E and the nitrosamine-inhibiting vitamin C, while constantly high in fish species prone to form nitrosamines when they are preserved with crude salt or saltpeter containing nitrate.

The American diet normally does not include these foods in quantity, but you should be aware of the risks they present. More familiar fish in this country, such as cod, haddock, bluefish, and canned sardines, demonstrate low to moderate conversion activity, and flounder and catfish show no conversion activity at all. The conclusion to be drawn here is that, compared with other countries (specifically Japan), the way nitrate interacts with the foods in our diet, combined with our relatively high intake of vitamin C, appears to work in our favor so that the incidence of stomach cancer in the United States is relatively low.

In another category altogether, bacon is one food that does not enhance anyone's chances for staying healthy. Not only is it very high in animal fat but most brands also contain nitrates or nitrites, added for color.

The typical way of cooking bacon—pan-frying—is also risky, because when the bacon is fried, the nitrates readily combine with the meat proteins to form nitrosamines. In tests at the National Center for Toxicology Research, workers found high levels of nitrosamines in bacon that was fried in a skillet temperature of 400° F.; even at a lower skillet temperature of 340° F., nitrosamines were still present.

Interestingly, bacon that was microwaved for forty-five seconds per slice —the recommended cooking time—contained no detectable levels of nitrosamines. Even when it was overcooked in the microwave for as long as seventy-five seconds per slice, only traces of nitrosamines were found. There are still reasons to avoid eating bacon, particularly because it is high in saturated fat, but if occasionally you are going to eat it, cook it in a microwave. And no matter how you cook bacon, avoid using the rendered fat, which is extremely high in nitrosamines.

ALCOHOL

Alcohol is also suspected of producing carcinogens—specifically in connection with breast cancer but also in a more general way, because it contains urethane, a by-product of the fermentation process and a potent cancer-causing agent. Urethane is found not only in wines and liquors but also in beer and table wines, some dessert wines, and bourbons and Scotches. In its report entitled "Tainted Booze," the Center for Science in the Public Interest cited the following beverages among those containing the highest levels of urethane:

- *Bourbons:* Beam's Choice Old No. 8, Virginia Gentleman, Evan Williams, Early Times, Old Taylor
- *Beers:* Golden Dragon (China), Foster's (Australia), Astra (Germany)
- *Table wines:* Calloway Temecula Sauvignon Blanc 1983, Almaden Monterey Zinfandel 1977, Carmel Samson Sauvignon Blanc 1985, Guimarra Pinot Noir, Paul Masson Rare Premium California Burgundy
- *Dessert wines:* Christian Brothers California Golden Sherry, Gallo Cream Sherry, Richards White Port, Ficklin Vineyards California Port, Paul Masson Golden Cream Sherry

In this country, the government has been slow to react to the presence of urethane in alcohol, even though it appears in about 1,000 alcoholic beverages, including more than 100 wines and liquors, at levels declared illegal by the Canadian government. Astonishingly, even with this information in hand, it took over three years for the United States to set standards for what are considered safe levels of urethane, or to specify that those at highest cancer risk are people who consume three or four drinks a day.

In January 1988, the FDA reached an accord with the whiskey and wine industry to begin voluntary reductions of urethane, but the Center for Science in the Public Interest says that the accord is only a little better than nothing, since it applies only to newly produced wines and whiskeys, and not to those already aging or on the shelves. As a result, actual urethane reduction in wine did not begin until 1989, and reductions in bourbon could take several more years because of the aging process.

As with food substances, like bacon, alcohol intake should be limited for reasons besides the risk of cancer. The American Heart Association recommends no more than two alcoholic drinks a day, but fewer than that is even better. Stomach and lung cancer are more likely to develop when alcohol intake is high, especially when the drinker is also a smoker.

AFLATOXINS

Aflatoxins are naturally occurring poisons that are caused by certain molds during the harvesting, shipping, or storing of some foods, particularly nuts, grains, and seeds. Laboratory studies have shown that the aflatoxins produced by molds cause liver cancer in animals, and they may be linked to cancers of the stomach, liver, and kidney in humans.

In the United States, commercial nuts, grains, and seeds, and the food products containing these ingredients, are monitored for safety and quality by the FDA and by the industry. To further reduce your exposure to these molds, keep nuts, grains, and seeds in dry, sealed containers. (Nuts keep best and retain their flavor if you store them in your freezer.) If such foods become moldy, throw them away.

ANTICANCER SHOPPING AND COOKING

Many of the following items may already appear on your shopping list. Whatever your present food preferences, you do not have to make all the suggested changes overnight. In any event—and especially in the case of foods like bran and vegetables from the cabbage family, which can cause gas or bloating if added in large amounts all at once—it is always best to use a gradual approach.

- Buy more fruits and vegetables, including cruciferous vegetables and others high in beta-carotene and vitamin C. Give these a larger place in your diet. Provide several servings every day and restrict or omit butter, cream, oils and fats, especially saturated fats.

- Use the high fiber list on pages 314–316 to select other vegetables, cereals, breads, and grains.
- Read all labels (see page 310) to see how much and what kind of fat has been added to a product before you purchase it.
- Choose lean meat and low-fat products.
- Select low-fat or skim-milk products and low-fat cheeses and yogurts rather than whole milk or cream products.
- Try low-fat meals such as low-fat soups, bean dishes, lean meat or fish, and mixed vegetable dishes.
- Eat salads—try them for your main course, too—but don't drown them in salad dressings containing fat or oil.
- Trim all visible fat from meats before and after cooking.
- Remove skin from poultry.
- Broil, poach, or roast meats and drain the fat from the pan before serving.
- Keep your general consumption of bacon low, if you eat it at all, and when you do eat it cook it in a microwave.
- Cut down on the amount of fat, cream, and rich sauces you add to foods in cooking and at the table; season foods with herbs, spices, or lemon juice instead.
- When eating out, avoid high-fat foods such as hamburgers, fried chicken, French fries, and fried fish.

The media will always celebrate the man or woman who obeys none of the rules and lives a long life, like the ninety-year-old senior spitfire who drinks like a fish and puffs two packs a day. But when it comes to cancer prevention, the probability of cancer is much lower in people who make positive health choices. These are the ones who do not look to high-tech solutions to save them from the consequences of self-imposed abuse. If a cancer diagnosis is made, even the very best chemotherapies can't reliably guarantee a good quality life; only in certain cases do they effect a cure. The emphasis here is necessarily on screening and prevention, in an atmosphere free of panic. This is where the greatest number of lives will be saved.

PART SIX

A Midlife Review of Basic Nutrition

THROUGHOUT THE BOOK WE have discussed the ways in which diet plays a vital role, not only in maintaining good health and optimum weight, but in the prevention or treatment of conditions such as diabetes, arteriosclerosis, hypertension, and even premenstrual syndrome. Part Six covers the details of good nutrition. Chapter 21 discusses the basics, Chapter 22 moves on to specific exchange lists and charts relevant to each of the diets described earlier in the book—providing a convenient reference section that you can use when shopping or preparing meals, and when dining out as well. (You'll even find there the calories and fat content of Whoppers and Egg McMuffins.) Chapter 23 covers food additives and contaminants.

CHAPTER 21

Jean Spodnik's Lowdown on Good Nutrition

IN MY CONVERSATIONS WITH patients about food selection, I discover how often they make unwise choices, apparently as much out of habit as anything else. Adult eating habits sometimes can be traced all the way back to prejudices acquired in childhood. You may remember a famous *New Yorker* cartoon of a child staring defiantly at her plate and saying, "I say it's spinach, and I say to hell with it!" Just as often, it was Pop who hated broccoli, so Mom never cooked it, and the vegetables that did make an appearance on the typical 1950s dinner table were often cooked within an inch of their lives.

We are also influenced by fads and advertising. Weight-reduction fads induce the dieter to follow unbalanced formulas that push one type of food instead of a variety; no doubt the old hard-boiled egg and grapefruit diet will come to mind. But today as never before an extraordinary range of wonderful vegetables and fruits is available to us, so that staying on a sensible diet need never be an exercise in boredom or sensory deprivation. Mealtime can be as adventurous as you like, even on a budget. The more exotic fruits and vegetables are likely to cost no more per serving than overpriced "convenience" and junk foods. Where once there were only Bartlett pears, now grocery stores carry Seckel, Bosc, and Comice. Now we have a variety of apples—some of them old favorites making a comeback—where we once only saw Delicious and Macs. Now we have arugula, radicchio, and red-leaf lettuce where iceberg once held nearly exclusive domain. Fresh pineapple, nectarines, kiwifruit, mangoes, papayas, melons, and berries out of season can add a sense of luxury to your meals, just as the wide array of fresh fish available in many markets and dozens of different whole-grain breads and pastas available almost everywhere can add economical variety to your menus. A balanced low-fat diet no longer means frequent return engagements of chicken, green beans, and lettuce salads.

The optimal diet for normal nutrition includes foods from the basic four food groups: grains, meats and fish, milk and milk products, and vegetables and fruits (see page 295). Choosing foods from all four groups gives you a wide and pleasing range of good things to eat, while supplying all the basic nutrients for sound health.

Except for the water we drink and the oxygen we breathe, the needs of the body can be met only by food. All foods are compounds of natural chemicals that include various nutrients. There are six classes of nutrients: carbohydrates, protein, fat, vitamins, minerals, and water. These do three vital jobs.

- Provide calories for energy—to keep internal systems going, stabilize body temperature, and fuel growth and activity
- Provide materials to make, repair, and maintain body tissue
- Provide substances that help regulate body processes

ENERGY NEEDS

The energy of food is measured in calories, which are units of heat. One calorie is needed to raise the temperature of 1 kilogram of water 1°C. To gain or lose 1 pound, during a given period of time you must eat about 3,500 more calories or 3,500 fewer calories than your body needs for energy.

After food is ingested, it is broken down in the small intestine into nutrients, which are drawn through the intestinal walls, carried into the blood, and then taken by the blood to each cell in the body. It is in the cell that metabolism occurs and where the nutrients are converted into energy.

The three nutrients that produce energy are carbohydrates, proteins, and fat. Carbohydrates are our most efficient source of energy: they are readily broken down into glucose in the blood. The blood's glucose level must stay within a certain range for you to remain healthy and, under normal circumstances, the body has a very elaborate alarm system that ensures this (see Chapter 11 for more on blood sugar). This system is vital, since blood glucose feeds brain cells, nerves, and other body tissue. Even in a fasting state, when only water is being taken, the healthy person will be able to maintain a normal glucose level from glycogen stored in the muscles and from body fat (as free fatty acids or triglycerides). As a last resort, the body will convert its own proteins into glucose.

The body protects itself by using the "cheapest" energy fuel available: carbohydrate first, then fat and protein. Although the body primarily uses stored fat for energy when there is not enough carbohydrate, it also uses protein—from food, from the blood, and also from muscle stores.

If you go on a low-calorie diet, in the initial phase you will undergo an abrupt loss of body protein, indicated by high levels of nitrogen being excreted in the urine. Over the ensuing 1 to 3 weeks of the diet the situation usually stabilizes, especially if you include plenty of protein in your weight-loss diet. A zero nitrogen balance indicates that protein is no longer being lost from the muscles.

Individual variability in the response is great, however, with some people never attaining zero nitrogen balance over the period of the diet. Continuing nitrogen losses occur more frequently in men than in women, and in those who are extremely obese. The continued loss in obese individuals may simply indicate that as body fat decreases, the need for extra muscle and tissues to support the extra weight decreases.

But it is only after a long period of fasting or starvation, as in anorexia, that real damage occurs—the body literally breaking itself down by raiding the major organs (which are made of protein) for energy.

CARBOHYDRATES

With the exception of the fiber they may contain, 100 percent of carbohydrates can be readily converted to energy by the body, making them our most efficient source of energy. There are three major categories of carbohydrate: sugar, starch, and fiber.

Sugar

All the food carbohydrates, except lactose (sugar found in milk), are formed in the vegetable kingdom, and simple sugars form the basis of all carbohydrates. Simple sugars are usually divided into two groups: monosaccharides and disaccharides. The monosaccharides—the very simplest sugars—are glucose, fructose, and galactose.

Monosaccharides

	GLUCOSE	FRUCTOSE	GALACTOSE
Food Sources	Corn syrup Honey Fruits Vegetables	Honey Fruits Vegetables	Only in digested milk sugar

The disaccharides consist of sugar made from combinations of two monosaccharides. The three disaccharides are sucrose, lactose, and maltose. Sucrose (table sugar) is made of glucose and fructose. Lactose (milk sugar) is made of glucose and galactose. Maltose consists of two glucose molecules that are formed from the breakdown of starch.

Disaccharides

	SUCROSE	LACTOSE	MALTOSE

Food *Sources*	Cane sugar
	Beet sugar
	Maple sugar
	Some fruits and
	  vegetables in
	  their natural
	  forms
		Milk
		Cream
		Whey
			Sprouting grains
			
			Partially digested
			  starch

While both monosaccharides and disaccharides are sweet, some are much sweeter than others. On a scale from 1 to 10, with 10 the most sweet, they are ranked:

Fructose	10
Sucrose (table sugar)	6
Glucose	4
Maltose	2
Lactose	0.9

Fructose occurs naturally in foods. If used in cooking it is only sweet when combined with fruit or other acid-containing ingredients. (See also the discussion of high fructose corn syrup in Chapter 11.) Of all the sugars, glucose is the most important. All digestible carbohydrates eventually break down into glucose in the blood.

The body's only form of carbohydrate storage is in the form of a polymer of glucose called glycogen. The size of the store in muscle is about 150 grams and can increase about fivefold with training and dietary manipulation, but this amount is still relatively small (see carbohydrate loading, Chapter 24). There is also glycogen stored in the adult liver—about 100 grams.

If glucose is so important to our health, why does sugar get such bad press? For healthy individuals, this comes down to three basic reasons: empty calories, cavities, and rapid fluctuation of blood sugar. A food containing empty calories is often referred to as having low nutritional density. "Nutritional density" is an attempt to evaluate the amounts of nutrients, vitamins, minerals, and protein available per number of calories in a certain food. For instance, while an orange and a piece of candy both may contain

100 calories, and both may be carbohydrate calories, the orange contains vitamin C, other vitamins, and fiber; the candy doesn't. If you eat a lot of foods with low nutritional density, you will either take in your quota of calories for the day minus the other nutrients you need, or take in empty calories plus nutritious food—and gain weight.

The latter is especially likely since, although sweets have many calories, they tend to metabolize very quickly, leaving you feeling hungry for more.

A note about brown sugar. I'm often asked if this is a nutritionally superior sweetener that contains significant amounts of iron, calcium, and phosphorus. It isn't. Brown sugar is just refined white sugar with molasses added to give it its characteristic color and flavor. You'd have to eat almost 1½ pounds of brown sugar just to get the RDA for iron, and more than 2 pounds to meet the RDA for calcium. If you decide to use brown sugar because of its taste, fine. But don't be fooled into thinking there's a nutritional bonus.

Raw sugar is a different story. Processed from sugar cane, it is "unfit for direct use as a food ingredient because of the impurities it ordinarily contains," according to the USDA.

Another sweetener I am often asked about is honey. People feel it has curative properties, and they also cite it as "natural." I always answer, "So are sugarcane and sugar beets." They all provide energy but almost nothing else. Here again, it's only a matter of taste.

Starch (Complex Carbohydrates)

Starch is formed in plants by the union of many molecules of glucose, and it is the carbohydrate found in seeds, tubers, and roots, where it is stored for future use by the plant. It has been estimated that the number of monosaccharides in the starch molecule averages between 300 and 400. These therefore are complex carbohydrates. Starch has no sweet taste and is not soluble in water, as are sugars. In the plant, starch is laid down in "granules" and when subjected to moist heat (as in cooking), starch granules absorb water, swell, and are ruptured. After cooking, the starch is more easily digested. Before starch can be used as a source of energy, however, the body must break it down into the simple monosaccharides.

Starches in the form of unrefined carbohydrates are especially wise food choices. When we refer to complex carbohydrates in this book, the emphasis is on these unrefined carbohydrates. They are economical, relatively low in calories and fat, rich in vitamins and minerals, and a good source of fiber. Some are also sources of protein. Highly processed foods, including highly processed carbohydrates, are often more expensive than their less processed counterparts, and many will lose their nutrients through processing. They will also lose much (if not all) of their fiber content. In general, the closer a carbohydrate is to its "natural" form, the more nutrients and fiber it probably contains.

Moreover, in their natural state, carbohydrates are ecologically the cheapest foods available because relatively little energy is required to produce them. Much of the world depends on carbohydrate foods for survival. They are low on the food chain. Animals eat quantities of carbohydrates (such as grasses and grains) in order to manufacture protein and animal fat. Vegetable oils are pressed from foods high in carbohydrates (corn, seeds, and olives). It takes large quantities of carbohydrate foods to support animals used for meat or to produce a small amount of oil. Thus, fats and animal proteins are, from an ecological standpoint, much more expensive to produce than plant foods.

Fiber

In the strictest sense, fiber is not a nutrient. It does not provide energy, and it is not a vitamin or a mineral, though the fibrous parts of foods may contain vitamins or minerals. Fiber is not in the usual sense digestible. By definition, fiber is "the sum of the indigestible carbohydrate and carbohydrate components of food." It can be found in vegetables, fruit, and the outer layer of grains. There is no fiber in animal products.

Fiber began to assume greater nutritional importance in the 1970s, when it was found that Africans, who had diets naturally high in fiber, had almost no incidence of diverticular disease. Westerners, on the other hand, whose diet was much lower in fiber, had relatively high rates of the disease. Fiber-rich foods provide roughage to help the digestive tract function more efficiently, but recent research indicates they may also have a beneficial role in reducing the risk of cardiovascular disease and colorectal cancer. Certain soluble fibers found in oat bran and legumes such as dried beans and lentils effectively lower blood cholesterol and may help stabilize blood sugar in diabetics. Other studies reveal that pectin—a form of fiber in many fruits and vegetables—may also help reduce blood cholesterol.

There are two kinds of fiber: insoluble and soluble. Insoluble fiber does not absorb water well. It may be softened, but it is not broken down by cooking. It increases fecal weight and provides the roughage that helps keep

Sources of Insoluble Fiber

CELLULOSE	LIGNIN	CUTIN
Soybean hulls	Wheat straw	Apple peels
Fruit membranes	Alfalfa stems	Tomato peels
Legumes	Cottonseed hulls	Seeds in berries
Carrots, celery, and other vegetables	Tannins	Peanut skins
		Almond skins

Sources of Insoluble Fiber

CELLULOSE	LIGNIN	CUTIN
Soybean hulls	Wheat straw	Apple peels
Fruit membranes	Alfalfa stems	Tomato peels
Legumes	Cottonseed hulls	Seeds in berries
Carrots, celery, and other vegetables	Tannins	Peanut skins
		Almond skins

an example. There are three types of soluble fiber: hemicellulose, pectins, and gums.

Sources of Soluble Fiber

HEMICELLULOSE	PECTINS	GUMS *
Corn hulls	Citrus pulp	Oats
Barley hulls	Apple pulp	
Oat hulls	Sugar-beet pulp	
Wheat bran	Cabbage and other foods in the mustard family	
Corn bran	Legumes	
	Alfalfa leaves	
	Sunflower heads	

* Under the category of "gums" are also ingredients frequently included in high-fiber processed foods, "natural" laxatives, and other products. These are agar (from red algae), alginate (from kelp), glycon (from yeast), gum arabic (from locust beans), gum tragacanth and guar gum (from legumes), psyllium (from flaxseed or plantains), and xanthan (from prickly ash trees).

FATS (LIPIDS)

Fat is a highly concentrated source of energy, providing over twice the calories found in the same amount of carbohydrates or protein. Fats, more correctly called lipids, are composed of the same elements as carbohydrates —carbon, hydrogen, and oxygen—but in a different form and in a different proportion (lipids have much less oxygen than carbohydrates). The typical simple lipid is called a triglyceride because it has three fatty acids. Ninety-eight percent of the lipids in food are triglycerides of some kind.

Only a small amount of fat is needed in the diet, but this small amount is important for several reasons:

1. Lipids provide essential fatty acids that help form part of the membrane around each cell in the body. They also help manufacture a

substance similar to hormones, and play a role in how cholesterol is used and excreted.
2. Lipids carry vitamins A, D, E, and K into the body. These vitamins are dissolved in fats and stored in the fat cells of the body.
3. Lipids are the primary source of energy for the heart.

Vegetable Sources of Lipids

	PERCENT OF FAT
Vegetable oils	100
Margarine	100
Nuts and seeds	45–90
Chocolate	53
Olives	89
Avocados	88
Wheat germ	15

All healthy bodies, even the very muscular and very thin, have some fat stores. It is important to keep a small store of fat in the body. When other fuel is not available, this energy "savings account" provides the needed energy. Of course, fat stores can be maintained by extra carbohydrates and protein, not just dietary lipids.

Remember that whatever regimen you may put yourself on regarding fat intake, children and adolescents *must* get at least 30 percent of their

Animal Sources of Lipids

	PERCENT OF FAT
Lard, tallow	100
Butter	81
Bacon	50–85
Hard cheeses	24–75
Beef	15–45
Egg yolk	83
Cream	11–37
Whole egg	68
Chicken	15–32
Fish	1–10
Whole milk	3–5
Low-fat milk	1–2
Skim milk	0
Whole-milk cottage cheese	4
Low-fat cottage cheese	½–2

calories from fat. A deficiency of fat in a child's diet can lead to growth retardation, sparse hair growth, poor wound healing, and increased susceptibility to infection.

Much of the fat in meat is closely combined with the flesh; this is called marbling. Thus, beef, lamb, and pork all contain fat even when the visible white fat is removed. The main sources of fat in chicken and turkey are the skin and dark meat. Poultry is usually lower in fat than beef, lamb, or pork, although duck and goose may have as much or more fat than beef. Fats in these animals may be saturated or unsaturated, and contain some cholesterol. The fat in eggs is all in the yolks and is high in cholesterol (see Chapter 8 for information on saturated fats and cholesterol). Since fat is the most concentrated source of energy, cutting down on fat is the easiest way to cut out calories.

PROTEIN

Protein not only is a source of energy but it plays an important role in the body. It is the protein portion of food that makes it possible for the body to:

1. Build new tissue in growth (during childhood and during pregnancy and lactation)
2. Replace damaged tissue and constantly dying cells
3. Maintain muscle tissue
4. Form enzymes
5. Make essential hormones, antibodies, and other glandular secretions

What distinguishes protein from carbohydrates and fats is the presence of nitrogen. In the human body, muscles, enzymes, antibodies, and hormones are all proteins and all need nitrogen. "Protein" is a general term for a combination of twenty-two compounds called amino acids. Like members of the same family, each amino acid has the same basic structure but different features and functions.

Some amino acids can be made in the body from other amino acids. Eight or nine of them, however, cannot be made by the body and must be provided in foods; these are called the essential amino acids. They must be consumed in the right amounts and in the right proportions, or they will not be well assimilated.

The two basic kinds of protein foods are animal protein and vegetable protein. Most animal proteins—such as eggs, fish, meat, milk, and dairy products—have all the essential amino acids in the right proportions, so these foods are complete proteins readily used by the body.

Vegetable proteins are different. They are found in foods such as nuts, seeds, dried beans, dry peas, tofu (soybean curd), and grains such as wheat, corn, and rice. These foods contain most of the essential amino acids, but not all of them and not in the right proportions. Some are low in one or two amino acids; these low or inadequate amino acids are called limiting amino acids. Thus, a vegetarian must combine vegetable proteins in a certain way in order to get complete or usable protein. These are called complementary proteins.

VEGETARIAN DIETS

Getting adequate protein and certain vitamins and minerals requires some planning for vegetarians.

There are two types of vegetarians: vegans, or strict vegetarians, who eat neither animal flesh nor any animal products, which rules out dairy foods and eggs, and ovolactovegetarians, who eat no animal flesh but do eat eggs and milk products (*ovo* meaning eggs and *lacto* meaning milk).

Many of our patients describe themselves as vegetarians, but when they're questioned it turns out that in addition to eggs and dairy products, they still eat poultry or fish in small amounts, but no red meat. They are semivegetarians.

It is likely that the vast majority of vegetarians in the United States belong in the semivegetarian group and use some animal flesh and dairy products, and a good many are also ovolactovegetarians. The distinction is important because nutrient intakes and deficiencies of vegans are quite different from those of ovolacto- or semivegetarians. Indeed, whereas all three types of vegetarian diets may confer health benefits, vegan diets also present the risk of deficiencies.

Plant foods contain fewer essential amino acids than do equivalent quantities of animal food, but a plant-based diet can provide adequate amounts of amino acids if proteins from unrefined grains, legumes, seeds, nuts and vegetables are combined so that amino acid deficits in one are made up by another.

For practical purposes, balancing protein does not mean you have to balance the amino acids found in each food item. A good amount of the protein requirement for ovolactovegetarians is supplied by dairy foods and eggs or egg whites; the rest can come from complementary combinations of grains and legumes.

A more precise application of complementary proteins is essential to an all-plant or vegan diet. A diet whose protein source is derived from 60 percent grains, 35 percent legumes, and 5 percent dark leafy green vegetables will generally have a desirable amino acid pattern for meeting human protein needs.

The complementary protein list that follows covers some basics, but if you are a strict vegan you will need more information on this than we can provide here, and you should be under the guidance of a nutritionist to be sure that you are getting all the nutrients you need—*especially* if you are planning a pregnancy or have any special health problems.

If you are an ovolactovegetarian or simply wish to restrict your intake of meat, the list will help you to plan meals that will meet most protein requirements and will be satisfying as well. Nuts and seeds can be part of a complementary protein, but the main complementary proteins are combinations of legumes and grains. It's interesting to note how many favorite regional or ethnic dishes combine these foods, as if taste were guided by instinct: red beans and rice, black-eyed peas and corn bread, beans and tortillas.

Note that *legumes* include soybeans, red (kidney) beans, lentils, dried beans such as pinto, speckled, navy, and lima or butter beans, dried split peas (but not fresh green peas), chickpeas (garbanzo beans), black-eyed peas, and other field peas such as crowder and purple hull. While soybeans are not as nutritionally dense as meat, they are the best source of protein among the legumes.

Wheat includes whole-wheat bread, bulgar wheat (kasha), and whole-wheat pasta.

Corn includes corn and cornmeal (corn bread, corn tortillas, corn meal mush and polenta).

Note that the complementary proteins list includes milk and cheese. While these are not vegetables and are complete proteins in themselves, adding them to rice or wheat isn't just a matter of eating some protein along with the grain; the combination will enhance the available protein in the grain as well.

COMPLEMENTARY PROTEINS (with some examples of dishes)
Rice and legumes (rice and beans)
Rice and cheese (rice casserole with vegetables and cheese)
Wheat and cheese (whole-wheat pasta and cheese)
Wheat and sesame (whole-wheat pasta salad sprinkled with sesame seeds)
Wheat, peanuts & milk (peanut butter sandwich on whole wheat, with a glass of milk)
Corn (including cornmeal products—corn bread, tortillas, etc.) and legumes (black-eyed peas and corn bread)
Beans & sesame (tofu patties sprinkled with sesame seed)

You may also combine beans and peanuts, and peanuts and sunflower seeds, though the latter combination is extremely high in fat* and should be used only on occasion, balanced out with very low-fat foods. A good

---

* Nuts and seeds are high in fat and should not be used in phase 1 or phase 2 of the 35-plus Diet. For phase 3, or the maintenance program, check serving sizes for nuts under the unsaturated fat exchange, and count nuts as part of your allotment for fats.

vegetarian cookbook will give you a lot of ideas for dishes that combine complementary proteins.

Meat Substitutes

Many meat substitutes, or analogues, as they have come to be called, are made with traditional soy products like tofu, a soybean curd; tempeh, cooked and fermented soybeans; or miso, a fermented soy paste. Others are based on modern laboratory-produced soy derivatives. You can buy meatless beef, meatless turkey, and meatless chicken—some even have a smoked taste.

Ounce for ounce, soy protein concentrates and isolated soy proteins contain as much protein as meat. Most of the oil (largely polyunsaturated) is removed, so they are virtually fat-free. Another advantage of isolated soy protein is that it contains much less of the carbohydrates that may cause flatulence.

Unfortunately, in many meat substitutes soy protein is not all you are getting. Processors generally add oils and fats, some partially hydrogenated, to these products to fake the look of beef, bacon, ham, tuna, or even luncheon meats. Some soy-based products have as much fat as lean ground beef (although they contain less saturated fat and no cholesterol), and some contain sodium in the form of MSG, soy sauce, or salt. Vitamins and minerals may be added, too, but compared to meat, many of these products remain notably deficient in iron, zinc, and other trace minerals. With all of these products, you must read the labels carefully.

For information on specific meat substitutes (analogues), see Chapter 22.

VITAMINS

Vitamins and minerals are used as "co-enzymes" in the body, assisting the body in its various functions. Each plays a unique role and is needed only in very small amounts.

The recommended dietary allowance (RDA) of a vitamin or mineral is defined by the Food and Nutrition Board, a committee of the National Academy of Sciences, as "the levels of intake of essential nutrients considered—on the basis of available scientific knowledge—to be adequate to meet the needs of practically all healthy persons." Contrary to popular belief, the RDAs are not minimums. The term that defines the real minimum amount is the MDR—minimum daily requirement—and is the amount of a nutrient that is needed to prevent true deficiency. The RDA is usually two to three times the MDR, and thus it provides a respectable margin of safety. Nevertheless, the major objective of the RDA is to define basic nutritional requirements; RDAs don't really address the potential benefit, if any, of megadoses of various vitamins.

The nutritional scientists who formulate the RDAs probably feel that evidence must clearly show that the potential benefits of vitamin megadoses outweigh the possible risks before they can recommend higher dosages. This approach is analogous to that used by the FDA in approving drugs: that safety and efficacy be proved beyond reasonable doubt before a drug is approved.

Only four fat-soluble vitamins (A, D, E, and K) and nine water-soluble substances (B_1—thiamine, B_2—riboflavin, B_3—niacin, B_6—pyridoxine, B_{12}—cobalamin, folic acid, pantothenic acid, biotin, and vitamin C) are currently recognized as vitamins. It seems that every week one hears of newly discovered "vitamins" like inositol, B_{15} (pangamic acid), and B_{17} (Laetrile). These substances are not recognized as vitamins by medical experts, because they fulfill neither of the criteria that define vitamins: (1) no dietary requirement for the compound has been demonstrated, and (2) no deficiency disease occurs if it is absent from the diet.

B_{17}, Laetrile, which has been touted as a cure for cancer, is a good example of a substance that can be downright harmful. B_{17} is derived from raw bitter almonds and apricot pits, which contain cyanide. If it is taken in large enough doses, dangerous cyanide levels can be reached. Who knows how many Laetrile recipients actually died from cyanide poisoning rather than from disease?

In promoting these unrecognized vitamins, enthusiasts often argue that the substance in question is actually a necessary nutrient—that is, an undiscovered vitamin. The total parenteral nutrition test is strong evidence refuting this idea. Many individuals have been maintained for extended periods on total parenteral nutrition (TPN). Individuals on TPN receive all their nutrients intravenously, and may take nothing by mouth for months. They receive essential amino acids, fats, and carbohydrates, as well as recognized vitamins and other nutrients. The fact that these individuals are able to survive for months without conventional food, and without the appearance of any symptoms indicating nutritional deficiencies, suggests that all vitamins essential to life have been discovered.

Although individual vitamins have special functions, as a group they help regulate and promote growth and the ability to produce healthy babies; they maintain the health of the nervous system and other body tissues; they assist the body in resisting bacterial infection; and they aid in the utilization of minerals and energy nutrients.

These functions, of course, are dependent on the presence of the other nutrients—carbohydrates, protein, fat, minerals, and water. All of these are essential to good health.

The table on pages 284–285 is a good overview of vitamin sources.

Essential Vitamins

VITAMIN	BEST FOOD SOURCES	DEFICIENCY DISEASE (SYMPTOMS)	SIDE EFFECTS OF MEGADOSE
A	Dairy products, liver,* eggs. Deep yellow vegetables (carrots, sweet potatoes, yellow squash), dark green leafy vegetables and broccoli contain beta-carotene, which is converted to vitamin A	Impaired growth and development. Poor vision (esp. night) and blindness. Dry skin, dry eyes	Increased pressure inside head, liver damage. Impaired vision, skin rashes, hair loss
D	Fortified milk, liver,* cod liver oil, fatty fish. Also made in the skin upon exposure to sunlight	Rickets (in children), osteomalacia (softening and deformity of the bone in adults)	High serum calcium and calcium deposits in body. Fatigue, headache, nausea, vomiting, diarrhea
E	Vegetable and fish oils, whole-grain breads and cereals	Rarely seen in healthy people, may occur in people with malabsorption syndrome (cystic fibrosis)	(Purported) thrombophlebitis,† pulmonary embolism, hypertension, fatigue, dizziness, gynecomastia,‡ vaginal bleeding, headache, nausea, diarrhea, intestinal cramps, muscle weakness and myopathy, visual complaints, hypoglycemia, stomatitis, chapped lips, urticaria (hives), aggravation of diabetes mellitus, aggravation of angina pectoris, disturbances of reproduction, decreased rate of wound healing
K	Green leafy vegetables, various other vegetables (peas, cauliflower), and liver.* Also made in human intestine	Bleeding problems, especially in newborns	Rarely taken in megadoses
B₁	Liver,* pork, oysters, whole-grain breads and cereals. Many breakfast cereals are enriched with	Beriberi, characterized by neurological and cardiovascular problems	None recognized presently

284

	Sources	Deficiency symptoms	Excess symptoms
B_2	Liver,* meat, dairy products, eggs, dark green vegetables, whole-grain breads, and cereals	Sore mouth, tongue, and throat, cracking skin in these locations; rash; anemia, neuropathy	None recognized presently
B_3	Poultry, meat, liver,* eggs, whole-grain breads and cereals, nuts and legumes (peas and beans)	Pellagra, characterized by rash (clematitis), dementia, and ultimately death	Flushing of the face, neck, and chest; headache; itching. Cardiac arrhythmias (heart rhythm abnormalities), low blood pressure, aggravation of peptic ulcers and liver damage
B_6	Whole-grain cereals and breads, liver,* green vegetables, bananas, fish, poultry, meats, nuts	Rash and oral lesions, convulsions	Nerve damage, which may be permanent. Depression, mouth fissures
B_{12}	Found only in animal foods: liver,* meat, fish, eggs, milk, nutritional yeast	Pernicious anemia (anemia and neurological symptoms of numbness and tingling in extremities)	None recognized presently
C	Citrus fruits, melons, tomatoes, strawberries, potatoes, dark green vegetables	Scurvy, characterized by bleeding gums, poor wound healing; loose teeth, sallow skin, irritability	Diarrhea, bloating, abdominal pain, kidney stones, risk of stomach cancer, decreased immunity to some bacteria
Folic acid	Liver,* dark green vegetables, wheat germ, legumes	Megaloblastic anemia,§ mouth lesions, possible increased birth defects	None presently recognized
Biotin	Eggs, liver,* dark green vegetables	Not known on natural diet	None presently recognized
Pantothenic acid	Eggs, dark green vegetables; in all plant and animal products, especially liver,* whole-grain cereals and bread	Not known on natural diet	None presently recognized

* Because of its cholesterol content, no more than 3 ounces of liver, once a month, should be eaten.
† Thrombophlebitis is an inflammation and blood clot in the vein.
‡ Gynecomastia is abnormally large mammary glands in the male.
§ Megaloblastic anemia is enlarged red blood cells.

Vitamin Supplements

With few exceptions, megavitamin therapy is unwarranted in the majority of situations. The value of large doses of vitamin C in preventing colds, for example, is still controversial. (See Chapter 9 for more on vitamin C.) Over a period of time, megadoses can lead to kidney stones and gout in susceptible individuals. Megadoses may also lead to a burning sensation during urination and may confound urine tests for diabetes. In the absence of more compelling evidence, megavitamin supplementation cannot be recommended.

What about taking a multivitamin? The people who need a one-a-day type multivitamin and mineral supplement are those who ingest suboptimal levels of particular nutrients. They include:

- Infants, adolescents, menstruating women, pregnant and lactating women, and the elderly
- People who do something to negatively affect their vitamin levels: alcoholics, smokers, chronic users of certain medications
- Dieters who consume less than 1,200 calories a day, strict vegetarians, and food faddists

It's apparent that these groups encompass nearly everyone except some adult males and some children. However, it is important to realize that vitamin deficiency—or even suboptimal nutritional status—may not result unless an individual exhibits two or three of the above risk factors.

Here are some guidelines for choosing a vitamin supplement:

1. Choose a balanced multivitamin with minerals, rather than one or two specific nutrients, unless it has been medically prescribed. Excessive levels of a single nutrient can disrupt the body's balance and actually alter nutrient requirements. In addition, a person is rarely deficient or suboptimal in one nutrient; usually several are involved.
2. Choose a preparation that provides 100 percent of the RDA for each recognized nutrient.
3. Avoid preparations that claim to be "natural," "organic," "therapeutic," "high potency," or for "stress." Purported benefits aren't worth the extra cost.
4. Ignore "natural" versus "synthetic" vitamin claims. They are meaningless. In fact, certain synthetic vitamin preparations are more effective than their natural counterparts (for example, folic acid and vitamin E).
5. Choose a preparation with an expiration date on it. Certain nutrients interact with others. An example of this is thiamin, which actually hastens the decomposition of both folate and vitamin B_{12}. As a result, vitamin preparations lose potency with time, and hot humid environments such as bathroom and cupboards accelerate this process.

RDAs of Vitamins for 35-Plus Women

According to the Food and Nutrition Board of the National Academy of Sciences, the current recommended daily allowances for a woman weighing 120 pounds are as follows:

RDA of Vitamins for Women

	AGE 23–50	AGE 51 PLUS	PREGNANT	LACTATING
Fat-soluble:				
Vitamin A	800 mcg.	800 mcg.	1,000 mcg.	1,200 mcg.
Vitamin D	5 mcg.	5 mcg.	10 mcg.	10 mcg.
Vitamin E	8 mg.	8 mg.	10 mg.	11 mg.
Water-soluble:				
Vitamin C	60 mg.	60 mg.	80 mg.	100 mg.
Thiamin	1 mg.	1 mg.	1.4 mg.	1.5 mg.
Riboflavin	1.2 mg.	1.2 mg.	1.3 mg.	1.5 mg.
Niacin	13 mg.	13 mg.	15 mg.	18 mg.
Vitamin B_6	2 mg.	2 mg.	2.6 mg.	2.5 mg.
Folacin	400 mcg.	400 mcg.	800 mcg.	800 mcg.
Vitamin B_{12}	3 mcg.	3 mcg.	4 mcg.	4 mcg.

MINERALS

Minerals are inorganic substances which, like vitamins, play many important roles in the body. Like fat-soluble vitamins, minerals in high doses are not easily shed by the body, and a buildup can cause serious problems. In other ways, though, minerals are very different from vitamins. Their structure is much simpler. They originally come from the soil and are not destroyed by heat, light, or oxygen. Nor can bacteria manufacture them, as they can vitamins.

Calcium, phosphorus, magnesium, iron, zinc, and iodine are sufficiently well understood to have RDAs established. Other minerals, like chloride, copper, fluoride, chromium, selenium, manganese, and molybdenum have "estimated safe and adequate daily intake" levels established. Some, like sulfur, are insufficiently understood to have either label applied to them. And several, including tin, vanadium, cadmium, and nickel, are not currently recognized as essential nutrients.

The need for mineral supplements depends on both your age and your sex, as well as other nutritional factors. Postmenopausal and lactating women should take a calcium supplement unless their diets are unusually high in calcium. Iron supplements should be taken by most menstruating women unless their diet is especially iron rich. Zinc supplements should probably be taken by most vegetarians, and should definitely be taken by vegans. Fluoride should be taken by all children, and probably most adults, unless your water supply is fluoridated.

I must emphasize that when I speak of supplementation, I am recommending the RDA of these minerals, not megadoses. The table below is a good overview of mineral sources.

Essential Minerals

MINERAL	FOOD SOURCES	DEFICIENCY	SIDE EFFECTS OF MEGADOSE
Calcium	Dairy products, green vegetables, sardines and salmon, figs, and sesame seeds	Osteoporosis, poor maintenance of muscle and nerve tissue	None recognized at this time
Iron	Beef liver,* blackstrap molasses, red meats, cooked dried beans, and fortified cereals	Anemia	Iron toxicity, the fourth most common cause of poisoning in children under five years of age
Phosphorus	Milk, fish, chicken, beef liver,* cooked dried beans, seeds, and flowers of plants	Unlikely because it is found in so many foods	Too much phosphorus leads to a loss of calcium
Magnesium	Cooked dried beans, beet greens, roasted peanuts, avocados, and bananas	Rare, except in alcoholics and in cases of malnutrition. May cause coronary vasospasm	Respiratory depression and low blood pressure
Zinc	Meat, poultry, fish, shellfish, dairy products	Stunting of growth in children	May replace magnesium. Interferes with absorption of calcium, iron, copper, and selenium. Can cause copper deficiency anemia

Essential Minerals *(continued)*

MINERAL	FOOD SOURCES	DEFICIENCY	SIDE EFFECTS OF MEGADOSE
Iodine	Seafood, seaweeds, iodized salt	Goiter and cretinism; infants born to parents deficient in iodine are mentally retarded for life	Thyrotoxicosis (too much iodine affects the thyroid as seriously as too little)
Copper	Oysters, lobster, beef liver,* fortified bran cereals, avocados, other shellfish, legumes, copper pots and water pipes	Rare. Copper helps convert iron into hemoglobin	None recognized at this time
Manganese	Tea, fruit, rice, spinach, carrots, milk, bran flakes, and whole-wheat bread	Rare	Not from food; can be toxic to miners who inhale dust
Fluoride	Fluoridated water, tea, seafood, wheat germ, potatoes, spinach	Rare	Mottled teeth and easily broken bones
Chromium	Yeast, large amounts of black pepper, beef, and some vegetables	May impair glucose tolerance	None recognized at this time
Selenium	Whole wheat, barley, garlic oats, mushrooms, seafood, meat	Has been implicated in pathogenesis of cancer	Nausea, loss of hair and fingernails. Acute poisoning can be fatal.
Molybdenum	Meat, especially lamb; cereals, buckwheat, tomatoes	Rare	High doses have led to copper deficiencies

* Because of its cholesterol content, no more than 3 ounces of liver, once a month, should be eaten.

Mineral Analysis of Hair

Hair analysis is based on the hypothesis that the body's mineral status can be determined by assaying concentrations of minerals in a hair sample. One factor that counters this theory is that hair is continuously exposed to the external environment. Since hair grows at a rate of ½ inch per month, the tip of a 1-inch strand of hair has been exposed to shampoos, conditioners, contaminants in the air, and so on, not to mention coloring or permanents, for two months or more. And that's a hair that's only 1 inch long. Since some shampoos contain zinc or selenium, this may significantly alter the hair's content of these minerals. Dyeing, bleaching, and permanents may also alter hair-mineral concentrations. It is interesting to note that natural hair-color differences can affect hair-mineral concentrations. For example, a black hair often will be higher in manganese than a white hair taken from the same animal.

The biggest problem with hair analysis, however, is that very little is known about the extent to which hair concentrations correlate with concentrations in the blood or organs. Advice given on the basis of hair analysis is likely to be worthless at best; at worst, it may lead to unsafe self-medication.

RDAs of Minerals for 35-Plus Women

The current daily allowances for a woman weighing 120 pounds are as follows:

RDA of Minerals for Women

	AGE 23–50	AGE 51–PLUS	PREGNANT	LACTATING
Calcium	800 mg.	800 mg.	1,200 mg.	1,200 mg.
Phosphorus	800 mg.	800 mg.	1,200 mg.	1,200 mg.
Magnesium	300 mg.	300 mg.	450 mg.	450 mg.
Iron*	18 mg.	10 mg.	30–60 mg.	30–60 mg.†
Zinc	15 mg.	15 mg.	20 mg.	25 mg.
Iodine	150 mcg.	150 mcg.	175 mcg.	200 mcg.

* See pages 102–103 for more specific information on iron requirements.
† For the first 3 months of lactation.

WATER AND ELECTROLYTES

Like vitamins and minerals, water and the electrolytes—sodium, potassium, and chloride—do not contain any calories or provide any energy.

But the body cannot survive without them. In fact, the healthy body could go days or even weeks without food energy, and go months or even years without certain vitamins or minerals, before it would show marked deficiencies or die. But three days is the limit that anyone can go without water.

Water makes up one-half to three-quarters of the body's weight. It is found in the cells and in blood; it bathes all the tissues; and it carries food through the digestive tract. The body has complex ways of maintaining water balance within a narrow, safe range. Similar complex patterns help equalize the water balance in areas of the body where it is needed.

Electrolytes

Water is separated and stored within two major compartments of the body: the extracellular space and the intracellular space.

Extracellular fluid includes: blood plasma; circulating fluids around each cell (called interstitial fluids); fluids in the bone and dense connective tissue; and protective compartments of fluid in the eye, body cavity, nerves, and joints.

The job of keeping intracellular fluid separate from extracellular fluid falls to the electrolytes. Electrolytes are free particles that contain a charge, or force. The most important electrolytes in body water are sodium, potassium, and chloride. Intracellular fluid is high in potassium but low in sodium and chloride, while extracellular fluid is high in sodium and chloride but low in potassium. These differences between the two help separate them from each other. Although the relative balances are rarely affected by consumption of foods high or low in these substances, a high sodium intake from foods or table salt may increase the total amount of water held in the body (water retention).

Water Loss and Electrolytes

Some of the ways that water can be lost from the body include urination, stools, breathing, perspiration, breast feeding, vomiting, diarrhea, and oozing from wounds or burns. In the first three cases, electrolyte loss is not a problem as long as you are healthy. The kidneys, which are the water filters of the body, conserve electrolytes. They only excrete what is not needed. If you drink a great quantity of fluids, the resulting urine will simply be more diluted than if you drank less.

Both sodium and potassium are lost in small amounts when you perspire, but it takes a great deal of perspiration to place a person in danger of an electrolyte imbalance. The best way to deal with excessive perspiration is to drink water in good amounts, although athletes involved in extremely strenuous exercise over a course of several hours may need Gatorade or another beverage made for this purpose. Salt tablets, however, are rarely a good idea. In women who are breast feeding, what's important is keeping up the total fluid intake; breast feeding is another normal process for which the body compensates in maintaining an electrolyte balance. High elevations (mountainous regions) and high-protein diets also increase the body's need for water.

Dangerous electrolyte loss can occur, however, with vomiting and severe diarrhea, and fluid lost through injuries. Uncontrolled, these fluid losses can quickly change the body's electrolyte balance. Severe diarrhea is especially dangerous in infants, and extensive wounds or burns on adults or children result in huge losses of water, electrolytes, and protein, and may lead to shock and even death if not treated immediately.

Although any sudden electrolyte loss poses a risk, potassium imbalance is especially dangerous. Potassium may be lost with some diuretics and laxative use. When potassium levels are too low or too high—conditions that can result from anorexia or bulimia—the heart can actually stop.

Sources for Water and Electrolytes

Water is obtained from all liquids and most foods. A small amount of water is also produced in the process of metabolism. Water isn't digested; it isn't broken down into its elements in the body. Instead it is absorbed through the stomach and diffuses freely throughout the body to maintain normal balance in all areas.

Food is the source of electrolytes. *Chloride* is found in table salt and in many foods, so deficiency in an otherwise healthy individual is unlikely. *Potassium* is the major ingredient in salt substitutes and is found in many foods from both the plant and animal kingdoms. *Sodium* is also naturally present in many foods, but a large percentage of what we ingest comes from the salt we add to them. Condiments, MSG, and spice and herb mixtures frequently contain salt; onion, garlic, and celery salts, for example, are high in sodium. Additives in processed foods and some medications contain sodium as well.

OTHER NUTRITIONAL FACTORS

While claims for "new" vitamin discoveries haven't turned up much of interest or value, research continues into known vitamins and minerals and their exact role in the body. As the vitamin and mineral charts indicate, there are a few things we still don't know. Generally, however, the role of nutrients in building and maintaining body tissues has been mapped out well enough that we have a pretty good idea of what we need to maintain normal physical health. Right now the more exciting area of nutritional research seems to be into elements that have an impact on our mental and emotional health. These nutritional elements include tryptophan, adipsin, and choline, which are food precursors for neurotransmitters; and components of fat such as the endogenous peptides, which are also implicated in mood and appetite control. These are discussed in the chapter on the brain, as well as under weight control, PMS, psychosomatic illness, and fitness.

CHAPTER 22

Making Good Nutrition Easy

THIS IS A BASIC REFERENCE chapter you'll turn to again and again. Here you will find guidelines and exchange lists for meeting basic nutritional needs, and for following all the dietary regimens called for in this book.

35-PLUS BASIC NUTRITION

You'll remember the U.S. Department of Agriculture's four basic food groups from public school days, but we repeat them here for easy reference. Foods grouped together are similar in general chemical makeup and hence contribute the same types of nutrients to the diet, although not always in the same relative proportions. No single group supplies all the essential nutrients in proper proportions to maintain health, so your daily diet should include foods from all four groups.

You'll notice that these basic food groups do not list pure sugar, butter, oils, or other pure or nearly pure fats. (Fats are included in the exchange lists, however.) Although these provide calories, and fats carry certain vitamins, these can be gotten from foods that contain a certain amount of fat: meats, fish, nuts, dairy products, and some vegetables. Pure sugars and fats provide calories without much if anything in the way of nutrients, thus the term "empty calories."

The suggested servings of these four groups roughly correspond to current dietary recommendations for carbohydrates, proteins, and fats in the normal adult diet. The 35-plus woman with no weight problems or other

Basic Nutrition

The Four Basic Food Groups

FOOD GROUP	ROLE IN DIET
Grain products—wheat, oats, barley, rice, cereals, pasta, bread and other baked goods made with flour (whole-grain or enriched preferred)	Inexpensive sources of energy and protein. Whole-grain or enriched products contain more iron, B vitamins, and fiber
Meat group—lean meats, poultry, fish, shellfish, eggs (or substitutes), dried beans, and peas	Valuable sources of protein; also furnish certain minerals (e.g., iron) and B vitamins
Milk and milk products—hard and soft cheeses, buttermilk, yogurt, kefir	Valuable sources of protein, calcium, and other minerals and vitamins
Vegetable/Fruit group—all fruits and vegetables, including potatoes, leafy green and yellow vegetables, citrus fruits, tomatoes, cabbage	Chiefly important as carriers of minerals, vitamins, and fiber. High in iron, vitamin A (beta-carotene), vitamin C

dietary restrictions should still watch her daily intake of fats, especially given the correlation between dietary fat and breast cancer. Both the American Heart Association and the American Cancer Society suggest that all adults limit their fat intake to 30 percent of total calories consumed. They recommend a diet composed of 50 to 55 percent carbohydrates; 15 to 20 percent protein, less than 30 percent fat, and less than 300 milligrams per day of cholesterol. (Note: The 35-plus diet manipulates these ratios for weight loss: see page 28.) Alcohol consumption should be limited to 50 milliliters a day—about two drinks—if consumed at all, since studies have also implicated alcohol in incidences of breast cancer.

You'll discover that a diet that is 30 percent fat is a very low-fat diet. If you can keep yourself within a range between 30 and 35 percent, you're doing pretty well. It's important, however, that children up through adolescence have at *least* 30 percent of their calories from fat in order to maintain healthy growth.

THE 35-PLUS DIET EXCHANGE LISTS

What follows are the basic exchange lists for a 35-plus metabolism diet for weight loss. To use the exchange list for weight reduction you *must* follow the guidelines described in Chapter 3. There you will find the number of servings allowed in each category for the quick start, second phase, and maintenance phase of the diet. The number of servings in each category has been worked out to maintain a precise ratio of carbohydrates, fats, and proteins; strict adherence to the ratios is essential to success.

You will notice that in some cases the size of a serving is small: one serving of meat, fish, or poultry, for example, is 1 cooked ounce. This is to make it easier to manipulate the various elements of the diet. The actual portion of lean protein in any given meal, however, varies from one to six servings: one at breakfast, three at lunch, six at dinner. This might translate

Low-Fat Protein Exchange *

FOOD	1 SERVING
Beef	
Dried or chipped, chuck, flank steak, London broil, round or sirloin steak, ground round or other 95% fat-free ground beef; lean corned beef (corned round); sirloin tip roast, tenderloin	1 ounce
Cheese	
½ to 1% butterfat cottage cheese	⅓ cup
½ to 1% butterfat ricotta cheese	¼ cup
Any skim milk cheese that is 5 grams of fat or less per ounce	1 ounce
Eggs	
2 whole eggs per week	1
Egg whites	2
Egg substitute	¼ cup
Fish	
Fish, fresh or frozen (no breading)	1 ounce
Canned salmon or tuna, packed in water	¼ cup
Clams, oysters, or scallops	5
Crabmeat	¼ cup
Lobster, out of shell †	¼ cup
Shrimp (medium) †	5
Sardines †	2 small or 1½ medium
Lamb	
Leg, leg steak, or sirloin (not shank)	1 ounce
Pork	
Fresh ham steak or center-cut ham	1 ounce
Extra-lean smoked ham, center-cut	1 ounce
Pork tenderloin	1 ounce
Poultry and Game	
Chicken, cornish hen, guinea hen, pheasant, turkey (skin removed), 93 to 95% fat-free ground turkey 95 to 98% fat-free turkey lunch meats	1 ounce
Rabbit	1 ounce
Veal	
Cutlets (not breaded), leg, loin, rib, shank, shoulder	1 ounce
Venison	1 ounce

* Poultry, fish, cheeses and cuts of meat not on this list have been omitted because they are too high in fat. Use only the cuts of meat, trimmed of all visible fat, that appear on the list. Weights given are weights after cooking.

† Lobster, shrimp, and sardines are limited, as recommended by the American Heart Association. You may use *one* of the three once a week, no more than 3½ ounces per week.

into 1 ounce of lean ham at breakfast, 3 ounces of skim-milk cheese at lunch, and six ounces of broiled chicken for dinner.

Note to nondieters: The exchange lists provide food ideas that can be a basic reference for meeting your dietary needs, as described on page 295. If weight or other health problems are not an issue, you are free to add some foods not in the diet, including choices from the lists of "forbidden foods," but use discretion and refer to the lists to become aware of how much fat and sugar you may be consuming.

Low-Fat Protein Exchange for Vegetarians

FOOD	1 SERVING
Legumes* (Only 1 serving per meal; 1 serving counts for 2 protein exchanges. The rest of the protein should be made up from low-fat cheese, eggs,† egg whites and egg substitute.) Cooked serving listed.	
Black beans	¾ cup
Black-eyed peas (cowpeas or field peas)	1 cup
Broad beans	¾ cup
Chickpeas	¾ cup
Kidney beans	1 cup
Lentils	1 cup
Lima beans	1 cup
Mung beans	⅔ cup
Navy beans	1 cup
Soybeans	¾ cup
White beans	¾ cup
Tofu (soybean curd)	5 x 5½ x 2-inch square
Cheese	1 serving = 1 ounce
½ to 1% low-fat cottage cheese	⅓ cup
or ricotta cheese	¼ cup
Any skim milk cheese that is 5 grams of fat or less per ounce	1 ounce
Eggs	
Whole eggs†	1
Egg whites	2
Egg substitute	¼ cup
Peanut butter	
Natural or fresh ground‡	1 tablespoon

* High in soluble fiber.
† Use no more than two whole eggs or egg yolks per week.
‡ Use no more than 1 serving per day because peanut butter is high in fat.

Starch Exchange

FOOD	1 SERVING
Breads	
Bagel (whole-wheat, rye, white)	½ small
Breadsticks	2 8½-inch
Dried bread crumbs	3 tablespoons
English muffin (whole-wheat or white)	½ small
Frankfurter bun	½
Reduced-calorie bun (high fiber)	1
Hamburger bun	½
Pita bread, small (whole-wheat or white)	1
Raisin bread (not frosted)	1 slice
Reduced-calorie bread (high-fiber)	2 slices
Roll (plain, white, rye, or whole-wheat)	1 small
Rye or pumpernickel*	1 slice
Tortilla, corn	1 6-inch
Tortilla, flour	½ 8-inch
White bread, including French and Italian	1 slice
Whole-wheat bread*	1 slice
Cereals—not sugar-coated	
Bran Flakes,* 100% Bran	½ cup
Bulgar or Kasha (cooked)	½ cup
Oatmeal,* oat bran (cooked)	½ cup
Cream of Wheat, Cream of Rice, Ralston (cooked)	½ cup
Cornmeal (dry)	2 tablespoons
Flour, cornstarch, tapioca (dry)	2½ tablespoons
Grits (cooked)	½ cup
Kashi,* cooked	½ cup
Kashi,* puffed	1 cup
Pasta, enriched or whole-wheat (cooked)	½ cup
Puffed Rice or Wheat*	1½ cups
Special K	1 cup
Rice (enriched or whole-wheat), barley (cooked)	½ cup
Wheat germ	2 tablespoons
Ready-to-eat cereal—others not listed ‡	¾ cup
Crackers	
Arrowroot	3
Graham*	2 squares
Matzo	1 6-inch round
Melba toast (plain, whole-wheat, rye)	4
Oyster	20
Pretzels †	25 sticks 3⅛ x ⅛ inch
Rice cakes	2
Rye or wheat wafers*	3 2 x 3½-inch
Saltines	6 2½-inch square
Legumes, dried	
Beans, peas, lentils (cooked)	½ cup
Popcorn	
Air-popped popcorn, no added fat*	3 cups

Starch Exchange *(continued)*

FOOD	1 SERVING
Brewer's (debittered) Yeast	3 tablespoons
Soup	
Canned, dried, or instant, vegetable or noodle type, half solid, half broth	1 cup
Starchy Vegetables	
Corn kernels	⅓ cup
Corn on the cob	1 small
Hominy	½ cup
Lima beans	½ cup
Mixed vegetables	½ cup
Parsnips	⅔ cup
Peas, green (canned, fresh, frozen) *	½ cup
Potato, white *	1 small
Potato, mashed	½ cup
Pumpkin *	¾ cup
Winter squash (acorn, butternut, or hubbard) *	½ cup
Sweet potato *	¼ cup

* Contains soluble fiber.
† For low-salt diets, use only unsalted varieties.
‡ See soluble fiber list for which cereals contain it.

Vegetable Exchange

Eat at least four servings a day or more, as desired.
A serving is ½ cup cooked or 1 cup raw.

artichokes	eggplant
asparagus	endive † ‡
bamboo shoots	escarole † ‡
bean sprouts	fennel
beet greens * ‡	kale * † ‡
bok choy * †	kohlrabi
broccoli * † ‡	leeks
brussels sprouts * †	lettuce §
cabbage * ‡	mixed vegetable juice (limit 1 cup) *
carrots ‡ §	mushrooms
cauliflower *	mustard greens * † ‡
celery	nori seaweed
chard *	okra
chicory † ‡	onions §
Chinese cabbage *	pea pods
collard greens * † ‡	peppers * ‡
cucumber §	pickles—fresh, dill, or sour
dandelion greens * ‡	radishes §

Vegetable Exchange *(continued)*

romaine † ‡	squash, yellow straightneck
rutabaga	string beans, green or wax
sauerkraut	tomato juice (½ cup) *
scallions	tomatoes (limit 1 to meal) * ‡
spinach §	turnip greens † ‡
squash, flat, scalloped	turnips
squash, summer §	watercress *
squash, yellow crookneck	zucchini

* Good source of vitamin C
† Good iron source
‡ Good calcium source
§ Contains soluble fiber

Fruit Exchange

Canned fruits are packed in water (no sugar added); fresh or frozen fruit has no sugar added. Drain juice if fruit is packed in its own juice.

FRUIT	1 SERVING
Apple †	1 small
Apple juice or cider	⅓ cup
Applesauce, natural	½ cup
Apricot nectar	⅓ cup
Apricots, canned	½ cup
Apricots, dried	4 halves
Apricots, fresh	2 medium
Banana †	½ small
Berries	
Blackberries †	½ cup
Blueberries	½ cup
Boysenberries	1 cup
Currants, dried	¼ cup
Currants, fresh	1 cup
Gooseberries	⅔ cup
Loganberries	½ cup
Raspberries	½ cup
Strawberries	1 cup
Cherries	10
Cranberry juice, artificially sweetened	6 fluid ounces
Cranberry juice, sweetened	¼ cup
Dates	2
Figs, dried	1 small
Figs, fresh	1 large
Fruit cocktail, canned	½ cup
Fruit punch	¼ cup

Fruit Exchange *(continued)*

FRUIT	1 SERVING
Frozen Fruit Desserts	
Vitari	2½ fluid ounces
Grapefruit, fresh * †	½ medium
Grapefruit juice *	½ cup
Grapefruit sections *	¾ cup
Grape juice	¼ cup
Grapes	12 medium
Guava *	¼ medium
Kiwifruit	2 small or 1 large
Kumquats	3
Lemons	2 large
Limes	3
Mandarin oranges, canned	¾ cup
Mango *	½ small
Melon	
Cantaloupe *	¼ small
Honeydew *	⅛ small
Watermelon	½ slice, 10 x ¾ inches or 1 cup
Nectarine	1 small
Orange *	1 small
Orange juice *	½ cup
Orange sections *	½ cup
Papaya	⅓ medium
Papaya juice	½ cup
Peach, fresh or canned	1 medium
Pear, fresh or canned †	1 small
Persimmon	1 medium
Pineapple, canned	1 large slice
Pineapple, fresh	½ cup
Pineapple juice	⅓ cup
Plums †	2 small
Pomegranate (seeds)	¾ medium
Prune juice	¼ cup
Prunes, cooked or dried †	2
Raisins †	2 tablespoons
Rhubarb (artificially sweetened)	¾ cup
Tangerine †	1 large or 2 small

* A good source of vitamin C.
† A source of soluble fiber; see pages 313–316 for lists of foods high in insoluble fiber.

Milk and Milk Products Exchange

	1 SERVING
Low-fat (1% butterfat) milk	1 cup
Evaporated skim milk	½ cup
Powdered nonfat dry, before adding water	⅓ cup
Skim or nonfat fluid milk	1 cup
Yogurt—nonfat or skim-milk, unflavored	¾ cup

Fat Exchange

	1 SERVING
Polyunsaturated Fats	
Almonds	10
Avocado	⅛ (4-inch diameter)
Brazil nuts	2
Chestnuts	3 large
Coffee creamer (Polyrich)	2 tablespoons
Cooking oil—safflower, sunflower, corn, cottonseed, soy	1 teaspoon
Filberts (hazelnuts)	5
Hickory nuts	7
Lichee, dried or fresh	6
Margarine—soft, stick dietetic, or whipped (made with safflower, sunflower, corn, cottonseed, or soy oil); first ingredient should be liquid oil	1 teaspoon
Olives	5 small
Peanuts	
spanish	20
virginia	10
Pecans	2
Pine nuts (pignoli nuts)	1 tablespoon
Sesame seed oil	1 teaspoon
Salad dressing	
regular (not bacon or blue cheese)	1 tablespoon
low-calorie	2 tablespoons
mayonnaise, regular	2 teaspoons
mayonnaise, low-calorie	1 tablespoon
Seeds	
pumpkin or squash kernels	1 tablespoon
sesame seeds	1 teaspoon
sunflower	1 tablespoon
Walnuts, English or black	5 halves
Wheat germ oil	1 teaspoon
Monounsaturated Fats	
Olive oil	1 teaspoon
Peanut oil	1 teaspoon
Rapeseed (canola) oil	1 teaspoon

Fat Exchange *(continued)*

	1 SERVING
Saturated Fats (these should be severely restricted)	
Bacon, crisp	1 strip
Bacon fat	1 teaspoon
Butter	1 teaspoon
Cashews	4
Coconut, shredded	2 tablespoons
Coconut or palm oil	2 tablespoons
Cream cheese	1 tablespoon
Cream-cheese spreads	2 tablespoons
Cream, half-and-half	2 tablespoons
Cream, heavy	1 tablespoon
Cream, sour	1 tablespoon
Cream substitute, liquid or dry (Cremora, Coffee Rich)	2 tablespoons
Lard	1 teaspoon
Macadamia nuts	3
Margarines from hydrogenated fat (regular stick)	1 teaspoon
Pistachio nuts	15
Salt pork	¾-inch cube
Suet	¾-inch cube
Vegetable shortening (Crisco or Fluffo)	1 teaspoon
Whipped topping	2 tablespoons

FOODS TO OMIT

Cakes

Candies

Cookies

Dietetic candy, cookies, cakes, ice cream

Doughnuts

Gelatin, flavored, with sugar

Honey

Ice cream

Ice milk

Jams, jellies, preserves

Molasses

Pastries

Pies

Puddings made with sugar

Soda pop containing sugar

Sherbet

Sugar

Sweet liqueurs and cordials, even if alcohol is permitted

Sweet rolls

Sweetened powdered drink mixes

Syrups

Complementary Proteins

Complementary proteins are combinations of incomplete (vegetable) proteins that together make a complete protein. These combinations include whole grains, legumes, nuts and seeds. (For more information on vegetarianism, see pages 280–282.)

GRAINS	LEGUMES	NUTS & SEEDS	COMPLETE PROTEINS
Rice	Black-eyed peas and other field peas such as crowder, cream, and purple hull	Peanuts	Rice and legumes
Wheat (includes whole wheat bread, bulgar wheat or kasha, and whole-wheat pasta)		Sesame seeds	Rice and cheese ‡
	Chick-peas (garbanzo beans)		Wheat and legumes
			Wheat and cheese‡
Corn (includes whole corn and foods made with cornmeal such as corn bread, corn tortillas, cornmeal mush and polenta)	Dried beans such as pinto, speckled, navy, lima and butter beans		Wheat and sesame †
			Wheat, peanuts† and milk‡
	Dried split peas (but not fresh green peas)		Corn and legumes
	Lentils		Beans and sesame†
	Red (kidney) beans		Beans and peanuts†
	Soybeans*		

* While soybeans are not as good a protein source as meat they are the best source of protein among the legumes.
† Nuts and seeds are high in fat and should not be used in phase 1 or phase 2 of the 35-plus diet. For phase 3, or the maintenance program, check serving sizes for nuts under the unsaturated fat exchange, and count nuts as part of your allotment for fats.
‡ Milk and cheese are not vegetables and are complete proteins in themselves, but combining them with grains enhances the protein available in the grain.

A Comparison of Meat Analogues

3.5 OUNCES	CALORIES	FAT (GRAMS)	% CALORIES FROM FAT	SODIUM (MG.)
Fantastic Foods				
Soy Deli Tofu-Tempeh Burger	268 †	17	57	144
Soy Deli Tempeh Burger	150	6	36	405
Tofu Burger Mix, tofu added	137	5	32	362
Worthington				
Meatless Smoked Turkey	234 * †	14	54	1,295
Meatless Veja-Links	208 †	14	61	450
Meatless Salami	208 * †	10	43	1,755
Meatless Tofu Garden Patties	126 * †	6	43	670
Loma Linda Foods				
Meatless Fried Chicken	330 * †	25	68	900
Meatless Bologna	280 * †	16	51	860
Meatless Sizzle Frank	230 †	18	70	480
Meatless Vege-Burger	110	1	8	180

* Not recommended because of high sodium content.
† Not recommended because of high fat content.

Low-Cholesterol, Low-Saturated-Fat Diet

FOOD GROUPS	ALLOW	AVOID
Lean meat, fish, and poultry: Limit to 6 ounces (cooked) per day. Other cuts of these meats that are allowed once a week are shown below. Try to eat fish 2 to 3 times a week.		
Beef	Dried or chipped, chuck, flank steak, London broil, round or sirloin steak, ground round or other 95% fat-free ground beef; lean corned beef (corned round); sirloin tip roast, tenderloin	Brisket, corned beef brisket, Boston strip steak, club steak, commercial ground beef or hamburger, porterhouse steak, rib steak, rib roast, T-bone steak
Fish	Any fresh or frozen fish, canned salmon and tuna (water packed), oysters, clams, mussels, scallops, and crab. Lobster, shrimp, or sardines may be used once a week (3½ ounces cooked)	Fried fish, fish in cream or cheese sauce
Lamb	Leg, leg steaks, sirloin	Breast, shank
Poultry and Game	Chicken, cornish hen, guinea hen, pheasant, turkey (skin removed), 93 to 95% fat-free ground turkey	Capon, duck, goose, all poultry skin
Veal	Cutlets, leg, loin, rib, shank, shoulder	
Cold Cuts	Turkey luncheon meats that are 95 to 98% fat free	All other luncheon or canned meats
Fattier meats: Trim all fat; eat only one time per week.		
Beef	Canned corned beef, commercial ground chuck, rib eye, rump roast	Liver or organ meats such as brains, tripe, sweetbreads, kidneys
Ham	Center cut	Hot dogs

Low-Cholesterol, Low-Saturated-Fat Diet *(continued)*

FOOD GROUPS	ALLOW	AVOID
Pork	Leg, loin chops, loin roast, tenderloin, Canadian bacon	Spareribs, sausage, ground pork, bacon
Lamb	Shoulder chops, loin chops	Breast, shank
Other foods:		
Cheese	Less than 5 g fat per ounce, ½ to 1% cottage cheese, skim-milk cheese, mozzarella, or farmer cheese (read labels)	Cream cheese, all other cheeses except those allowed
Peanut Butter	Fresh ground or natural	All hydrogenated varieties
Eggs	Egg whites, egg substitutes; no more than 2 egg yolks per week, including those used in cooking	More than 2 egg yolks per week
Milk	Skim, 1%, 1.5%, dry nonfat, evaporated skim, and buttermilk; yogurt made from skim or low-fat milk; ice milk and sherbet with 1.5% butterfat or less and no added fats	Whole milk or whole milk drinks; dry whole milk (sweet and sour); ice cream, ice milk, and sherbet containing more than 1.5% butterfat; commercial whipped toppings made with saturated fats
Fats	Avocado, (Polyrich) coffee creamer, safflower, sunflower, corn, cottonseed, peanut, soy, olive oils, sesame oil, wheat germ, margarine (soft stick, dietetic, or whipped, as long as first ingredient is liquid vegetable oil), nuts, seeds, kernels, olives, salad dressing (without cheese or bacon)	Bacon, bacon fat, coconut or coconut oil, cream cheese, cream-cheese spreads, cream (heavy, whipping, half & half, sour), (liquid or dry) cream substitute (Cremora, Coffee Rich), lard, butter, margarines made from hydrogenated fats, salad dressing containing cheese or bacon, salt pork, suet, vegetable shortening (Crisco, Fluffo), whipped topping, macadamia nuts, pistachios, cashews

Low-Cholesterol, Low-Saturated-Fat Diet *(continued)*

FOOD GROUPS	ALLOW	AVOID
Starches	All cereals; macaroni, rice, noodles, spaghetti; whole-wheat, rye or white breads; matzos, saltines, graham crackers; hard rolls, french or Italian breads; homemade baked goods made with allowed fat, milk, and eggs; plain boiled, baked, or mashed white or sweet potatoes, legumes	Commercial pancakes, waffles; biscuits, muffins, quick breads, doughnuts; variety or butter-type snack crackers; french fries, potato and corn chips; creamed, escalloped, or au gratin potatoes
Vegetables	Fresh, frozen, or canned	Buttered, creamed, or fried, unless prepared with allowed fat
Fruits	Fresh, frozen, canned, or dried fruit or juice	None
Beverages	Coffee, tea, carbonated beverages, fruit and vegetable juices, alcohol if approved by a physician	Hot chocolate mixes
Soups	Bouillon, clear broth, fat-free vegetable soup, homemade cream soups made with skim milk, packaged dehydrated soups	All others
Sweets and Condiments	Hard candies; jam, jelly, honey; sugar, syrup containing no fat; spices, herbs; cocoa; pickles, nonstick vegetable pan spray	All other candies, chocolate, coconut; cashew, macadamia, and pistachio nuts

Butter Substitutes

	MOLLY McBUTTER	BUTTER BUDS (LIQUID)
Serving	½ tsp.	1 tbsp.
Calories	4	6
Fat	0	0
Protein	0	0
Carbohydrate	1 g.	1 g.
Sodium	90 mg.	85 mg.

Cooking Tips		
DO	ADD	USE
Poach	Wine	Nonstick pots, wok
Bake	Herbs and spices	Baking pans with a
Broil	Lemon or lime juice	rack
Steam	Water, low-sodium	Steamer
	bouillon	Poacher
	Low-fat yogurt	Broiler
	Crushed tomatoes	Barbecue or gas grill

Many people believe that seafood is difficult to cook. While most of my patients are willing to order it in a restaurant, they won't try it at home. Here are some cooking tips when making fish:

1. When fixing a meal, save fish preparation until last.
2. Cook fresh fish 8 to 10 minutes per inch of thickness, in the oven or in a pan.
3. As fish cooks, it loses its normal translucent appearance and becomes opaque. Fish is done when it is opaque and its outer surface flakes easily with a fork.
4. If cooking fish still frozen, double the cooking time.
5. Overcooking can destroy the flavor and appeal of seafood.

HOW TO DETERMINE THE FAT CONTENT OF FOODS

Studies on cancer and heart disease indicate that the optimal adult diet should be no more than about 30 percent fat. The percentage of calories from fat is not ordinarily given on a food label, but by using your pocket calculator, you can very quickly determine the percentage of fat. Although the overall balance of your diet—foods containing fat combined with non-fat fruit, vegetables, and grains—is what's important, a range of 30 to 35 percent fat in any given food item is considered acceptable and a good rule of thumb.

Of course you may use unsaturated margarine and mono- or polyunsaturated oils and salad dressings in small amounts, even though they are 90 to 100 percent fat.

By law, calories per serving, along with nutritional analysis showing grams per serving of protein, carbohydrates, and fats, should appear on the label of all prepared or processed foods. Even candy bars and snack foods will have such labels. You can determine what percentage of calories comes from fat as follows:

- Carbohydrates and proteins each supply 4 calories per gram, while fat supplies more than double, at 9 calories per gram.
- By multiplying the number of grams per serving by the number of calories per gram, you can determine the calories per serving from fat.

For example, a label may show:

Calories per serving: 117	
Nutritional analysis per serving:	
protein	10 grams
carbohydrates	8 grams
fat	5 grams

Multiply each nutrient by the calories per gram:

$$10 \text{ grams protein} \times 4 = 40 \text{ calories}$$
$$8 \text{ grams carbohydrates} \times 4 = 32 \text{ calories}$$
$$5 \text{ grams fat} \times 9 = \underline{45} \text{ calories}$$
$$117 \text{ total calories}$$

You get 40 calories from protein, 32 calories from carbohydrates, and 45 calories from fat—for a total of 117.

To determine what percentage of fat makes up the total calories, divide the number of fat calories by the total calories:

$$45 \div 117 = 38\%$$

Calorie and Fat Content of Some Foods which May Not Be Labeled

FOOD	TOTAL CALORIES	CALORIES FROM FAT	PERCENT OF CALORIES FROM FAT
Twinkie, 1	163	54	33
Iced cake doughnut, 1	184	71	39
Raised doughnut, 1	263	135	51
Toll House frozen cookies (no nuts), 1	47	23	49
Homemade chocolate chip cookies, Toll House recipe (no nuts), 1 small	46	27	59
Dairy Queen soft serve ice cream with cone, 1 small	110	26	24
Haagen-Dazs Ice Cream, Vanilla, ½ cup	273	153	56
Cheesecake, ⅛ of 8″ cake	414	251	61

Calorie and Fat Content of Some Foods
which May Not Be Labeled *(continued)*

FOOD	TOTAL CALORIES	CALORIES FROM FAT	PERCENT OF CALORIES FROM FAT
M&M Plain, 1 oz.	142	53	37
M&M Peanut, 1 oz.	143	64	45
Hershey Bar, 1.5 oz.	220	117	53
Reese's Peanut Butter Cup, 1	86	47	55
Chocolate Chips, ½ cup	430	256	60
Burger King french fries, small order	210	92	44
Burger King Chicken Sandwich, 1	475	240	51
Burger King Whopper, 1	630	324	51
McDonald's Quarter-Pounder, 1	424	195	46
McDonald's Fish Sandwich, 1	432	225	52
McDonald's Bic Mac, 1	563	297	53
McDonald's Chicken McNuggets, 6 pieces	314	171	54
Kentucky Fried Chicken, regular recipe, wing and rib (breast)	603	288	48
Kentucky Fried Chicken, regular recipe, leg and thigh	643	315	49
Kentucky Fried Chicken, extra-crispy, wing and rib (breast)	755	387	51
Kentucky Fried Chicken, extra-crispy, leg and thigh	765	398	52
Cheese Pizza, ⅛ of 14″ pie	184	94	51
Deluxe Pizza, ⅛ of 14″ pie	278	173	62
Quiche Lorraine (⅙ of 9″ pie)	543	351	65
Eggs Benedict (2 eggs)	465	324	70
Cheese omelette (2 eggs)	379	288	76
Egg McMuffin	352	297	84
Bagel (water), 3″ diameter	165	8	5
Small baking powder biscuit (2″), homemade (no butter)	103	45	44
Flaky fast-food biscuit (3–3½″), large (no extra butter)	180	90	50
Croissant, 1	100	54	54
1 percent milk-fat cottage cheese, ½ cup	83	9	11
Part-skim Mozzarella, 1 oz.	78	43	55
Sharp American cheddar, 1 oz.	90	63	70
Bleu cheese, 1 oz.	100	72	72
Brie, 1 oz.	90	63	75

Calorie and Fat Content of Some Foods
which May Not Be Labeled *(continued)*

FOOD	TOTAL CALORIES	CALORIES FROM FAT	PERCENT OF CALORIES FROM FAT
Round steak, trimmed, cooked, 5 oz.	270	75	28
Porterhouse steak, trimmed, cooked, 5 oz.	320	140	44
Cooked pork sausage, 3 oz.	231	172	74
Pepperoni, 1 oz.	139	115	83
Crisp bacon, 2 slices	85	72	85
Bologna, 1 oz.	85	72	85
Salami, hard, 1 oz.	193	180	93

Cholesterol Content of Some Foods in 3½-Ounce Cooked Portions

	CHOLESTEROL (MG.)	SATURATED FAT (GRAMS)
Fruits, grains, vegetables	0	0.0
Scallops	42	0.0
Oysters	55	0.0
Clams	65	0.0
White fish, lean	65	0.0
Tuna, white water pack	56	0.0
Extra lean ham (5% Fat)	53	4.8
Chicken or turkey, light meat, no skin	80	2.0
Extra lean beef	85	1.0
Chicken/turkey, dark meat, no skin	95	4.4
Pork tenderloin	93	2.1
Lobster	100	0.0
Crab	100	0.0
Lamb (leg)	85	0.6
Veal	120	0.8
Shrimp	150	0.0
Egg yolk	220	5.0
Beef liver	440	0.1
Beef kidney	700	0.5

Cholesterol Content of Some Foods *(continued)*

DAIRY PRODUCTS	CHOLESTEROL (MG.)	SATURATED FAT (GRAMS)
8 oz. skim milk	6	0.006
8 oz. 1% butterfat milk	8	1.1
3½ oz. 1% butterfat cottage cheese	10	1.0
3½ oz. 1% ricotta cheese	10	1.0
1 oz. Weight Watchers sharp cheddar or swiss	8	2.0
1 oz. Borden Lite Line American or Swiss	10	4.0
1 oz. Kraft Light 'n Lively American or Swiss	15	4.0
1 oz. Dorman's Light Natural Lo-Cholesterol cheese	3	5.0
1 oz. mozzarella (part skim)	15	5.0
1 oz. American processed cheese	18	7.0
1 oz. Swiss	24	7.0
1 oz. Muenster	27	9.0
1 oz. cheddar	30	9.0
8 oz. no-fat yogurt	0	0.0
1 egg white	0	0.0

Sources of Dietary Fiber ‡

This list is arranged according to food groups, with soluble fiber content indicated whenever it is significant and information is available.

FOOD SOURCE	SERVING	INSOLUBLE FIBER (GRAMS)	SOLUBLE FIBER (GRAMS)
Cereals †			
All-Bran with Extra Fiber	⅓ c.*	13.0	—
Fiber-One	⅓ c.*	13.0	—
100% Bran	½ c.*	9.1	2.2
All-Bran	⅓ c.*	8.6	1.7
Bran Buds	⅓ c.*	7.7	1.5
New Morning Oatios with Oat Bran	1 c.	6.0	2.0
Corn Bran	⅔ c.*	5.9	1.2
Natural Bran Flakes	½ c.*	5.0	—
Bran Chex	⅔ c.*	5.0	1.0

Sources of Dietary Fiber ‡ *(continued)*

FOOD SOURCE	SERVING	INSOLUBLE FIBER (GRAMS)	SOLUBLE FIBER (GRAMS)
Cereals†			
40% Bran Flakes	¾ c.*	4.3	—
Raisin Bran	¾ c.*	4.0	—
Shredded Wheat 'n Bran	⅔ c.*	4.0	—
Shredded Wheat	⅔ c.*	3.3	—
Post Toasties	1 c.	—	1.5
Kellogg's Corn Flakes	1¼ c.*	1.0	—
Puffed Wheat	1 c.	0.3	1.0
Cheerios	1¼ c.*	1.0	1.0
Total	1 c.*	2.5	—
Wheat Chex	⅔ c.*	2.5	—
Wheaties	1 c.*	2.5	—
Grape-Nuts	¼ c.*	2.2	—
Grape-Nuts Flakes	⅞ c.*	0.5	—
Nutri-Grain	1 oz.*	2.1	—
Fortified Oat Flakes	⅔ c.	1.5	1.3
Oatmeal (regular or quick)	¾ c. cooked	1.6	1.4
Ralston	¾ c. cooked	0.6	—
Wheatena	¾ c. cooked	3.0	—
Grits, regular or quick	¾ c. cooked	0.1	—
Other Grains			
Wheat Bran	⅓ c.	6.4	1.7
Wheat Germ	¼ c.	5.5	1.3
Oat Bran	⅓ c.	4.2	2.0
Popcorn, air popped	3 c.	4.8	0.8
Graham crackers	2 squares	2.8	0.5
Oat bran muffin	1 medium	4.0	2.0
Bran muffin	1 medium	2.5	—
Corn bread	1 small piece	—	0.8
Oroweat Bran'nola Natural with Bran	1 slice	2.5	—
Less Reduced Calories	1 slice	2.4	—
Roman Light	1 slice	2.3	—
Arnold Honey Wheat Berry	1 slice	2.0	—
Pepperidge Farm Honey Wheat Berry	1 slice	1.9	—
Oroweat Bran'nola Country Oat with Bran	1 slice	1.9	—
Pepperidge Farm Seeded Rye	1 slice	1.7	—
Pumpernickel bread	1 slice	—	0.5

Sources of Dietary Fiber ‡ *(continued)*

FOOD SOURCE	SERVING	INSOLUBLE FIBER (GRAMS)	SOLUBLE FIBER (GRAMS)
Rye bread	1 slice	1.0	0.4
Whole wheat crackers	5	—	0.4
Saltines	6	—	0.3
Whole wheat bread	1 slice	1.6	—
Whole wheat spaghetti	½ c. cooked	2.5	—
Enriched spaghetti	½ c. cooked	0.8	—
White bread	1 slice	0.6	—
Brown rice	½ c. cooked	1.0	—
White rice	½ c. cooked	0.1	—
Legumes			
Chick peas	½ c. cooked	6.0	2.5
Kidney beans	½ c. cooked	5.8	2.1
Pinto beans	½ c. cooked	5.3	2.0
Split peas	½ c. cooked	5.1	—
Navy (white) beans	½ c. cooked	5.0	1.4
Lima beans	½ c. cooked	4.9	1.3
Lentils	½ c. cooked	3.7	0.9
Vegetables			
Sweet potato, with skin	1 large	4.2	—
Peas, green	½ c. cooked	4.1	1.1
Brussels sprouts	½ c. cooked	3.9	—
Corn	½ c. cooked	3.9	—
White potato baked with skin	1 medium	3.8	1.9
Parsnips	½ c. cooked	2.7	—
Carrots	1 large raw or ½ c. cooked	2.3	1.8
Collards	½ c. cooked	2.2	—
Broccoli	½ c. cooked	2.2	—
Asparagus	½ c. cooked	2.1	—
Green beans	½ c. cooked	2.1	—
Spinach	½ c. cooked	2.0	0.5
Squash (winter)	½ c. cooked	1.9	—
Squash (summer)	½ c. cooked	0.6	0.3
Cabbage, red or white	½ c. cooked	1.4	—
Cauliflower	½ c. cooked	1.1	—
Cabbage, red or white	½ c. raw	1.0	—

Sources of Dietary Fiber ‡ *(continued)*

FOOD SOURCE	SERVING	INSOLUBLE FIBER (GRAMS)	SOLUBLE FIBER (GRAMS)
Tomato	1 medium raw	1.0	0.2
Bean sprouts	½ c. raw	0.9	—
Mushrooms	½ c. raw	0.9	—
Eggplant	½ c. cooked	0.9	—
Bell pepper	½ c. raw	—	0.4
Radishes	10 medium	—	0.3
Onions	½ c.	—	0.8
Zucchini	½ c. cooked	0.5	—
Lettuce, head	½ c. raw	0.3	0.2
Celery	½ c. diced or 1 stalk	0.3	—
Cucumber	½ medium	0.3	0.2
Fruits			
Blackberries	½ c.	4.5	0.6
Prunes	3 dried	3.7	1.0
Apples	1 medium	3.5	0.8
Raisins	¼ c.	3.1	0.8
Strawberries	1 c.	3.0	0.9
Oranges	1 medium	2.6	—
Bananas	1 medium	2.4	1.2
Pear with skin	1 medium	2.3	1.4
Plums	3	1.2	0.7
Blueberries	½ c.	2.0	—
Dates	3 medium	1.9	—
Peach	1 medium	1.9	0.6
Grapefruit	½ medium	1.7	0.4
Cantaloupe	¼ small	1.4	—
Apricots	5 dried halves	1.4	—
Cherries	10	1.2	—
Pineapple	½ c.	1.1	—
Grapes	12	0.5	—
Watermelon	1 c. cubed	0.4	—

* This dry measure equals 1 ounce.
† Note: Granolas and other cereals which may be high in fiber do not appear on this list because of high fat and/or sugar content.
‡ Note: Fiber figures may differ slightly from other sources because methods for analyzing dietary fiber have not been standardized.

Dietary Sources of Calcium

Highest sources of calcium are milk products, certain fish and certain vegetables. Food groups are listed in alphabetical order.

	SERVINGS	CALORIES	CALCIUM (MG.)
Beans and Tofu *			
Chick-peas cooked	½ c.	195	47
Navy beans, cooked	½ c.	143	69
Pinto beans, cooked	½ c.	131	48
Tofu †	4 oz.	86	154
Breads and Cereals			
Bread, Hollywood dark	1 slice	70	50
Cream of Wheat, instant	1 package	100	150
Regular oats, instant	1 package	110	100
Cheese			
Cottage cheese, 2% butterfat	1 c.	205	160
Cottage cheese, 1% butterfat	1 c.	80	210
Mozzarella, part-skim	1 oz.	80	210
Ricotta, part-skim	½ c.	170	285
Ricotta, 1% butterfat	½ c.	80	140
Low-fat diet cheese	1 oz.	60	158
Dairy Desserts			
Ice cream, regular	½ c.	145	90
Ice milk	½ c.	93	90
Sherbet	½ c.	135	50
Fish			
Mackerel, canned Pacific	4 oz.	204	300
Oysters, canned	4 oz.	103	100
Salmon, canned, pink	4 oz.	160	220
Salmon, red, canned	4 oz.	170	259
Sardines, oil pack	4 oz.	233	500
Shrimp canned	4 oz.	133	130
Milk and Yogurt			
Buttermilk	1 c.	100	290
Evaporated milk, skim	1 c.	200	740
Low-Fat, 1% butterfat	1 c.	105	310
Non-fat dry powder	2 tbs.	31	105
Skim	1 c.	85	300
Whole	1 c.	150	290
Dannon yogurt, non-fat or	1 c.	130	430
low-fat, plain	1 c.	150	430
Dannon yogurt, flavors, vanilla, etc.	1 c.	200	395
Dannon yogurt, low-fat, fruit on bottom	1 c.	260	330
Kefir plain (yogurt milk)	1 c.	160	350

Dietary Sources of Calcium *(continued)*

	SERVINGS	CALORIES	CALCIUM (MG.)
Vegetables			
Bok choy, fresh cooked	1 c.	25	250
Broccoli, fresh cooked	1 c.	40	140
Greens, collard, fresh cooked	1 c.	65	360
Kale, fresh cooked	1 c.	40	160
Dandelion greens, cooked	1 c.	35	150
Mustard greens, cooked leaves	1 c.	32	190
Turnip greens, fresh cooked	1 c.	30	250
Other Sources			
Plus Calcium Citrus Hill Orange Juice	6 oz.	60	160
Minute Maid Calcium Fortified Orange Juice	6 oz.	60	160

* Beans contain phytates that may also inhibit calcium absorption.
† The calcium in tofu may vary, depending on what is used to coagulate the soybean.

Low-Sodium Diet for Hypertension

	CHOOSE FROM THIS FOOD GROUP	AVOID THESE FOODS
Beverages	2 cups milk a day allowed (milk is moderately high in sodium) Carbonated beverages Fruit juice Coffee, tea Unsalted vegetable juice	Buttermilk may contain added sodium Powdered mixes for soft drink, like Kool-Aid, read label Regular vegetable juices Cooking wines or sherries
Breads	All, except those listed to avoid	Bread, rolls and crackers with salted tops, salted potato chips, salted popcorn, pretzels, pancakes, muffin and bread mixes, highly processed and almost instant are very high in sodium.
Cereals	Cooked cereals and dry; the less processing done to a grain or cereal, the less sodium it contains	Instant hot cereals have salt added. For dry cereals and hot that list sodium content, anything over 200 mg. per serving to be avoided.
Fats	All, except those listed to avoid	Bacon, bacon fat, salt pork. Read labels of bottled salad dressing. Is salt among first three ingredients?

Low-Sodium Diet for Hypertension *(continued)*

	CHOOSE FROM THIS FOOD GROUP	AVOID THESE FOODS
Meat and Meat Substitutes	Fresh meats, poultry, fish No-salt-added cheeses (some of these are low in sodium but others contain more— should be well under 100 mg. sodium per ounce) Dried beans	Meat prepared in brine, smoked meats, corned beef, bacon or dried beef, luncheon meat (regardless of whether it is turkey luncheon meat), frankfurters, salt pork, sausage, kosher meats, ham, smoked or salted fish, dried fish, anchovies, cod, caviar, sardines, cheese, salted peanut butter, pizza, gravy, meat sauce. Read label on so-called "lite" lunch meat. How much is sodium really reduced?
Starches	Dry pasta, dry plain rice, fresh potatoes	Canned pasta, rice, potato dishes or frozen dinners containing starches or processed starch dishes like Noodle Roni, Raman Noodles, Tuna Helper, etc.
Seasonings	All spices and herbs, fresh onion and garlic, onion and garlic powder, vinegar, gravy prepared with low sodium soup base, cream gravy, flavoring such as vanilla, rum, mint, etc. Fresh lemon or lime juice, wine or liquor, Baker's compressed or dry yeast, cream of tartar, calcium saccharin, Nutra-Sweet (Equal). You can now find combinations of herbs in local grocery stores, put out by the American Heart Association or you can make your own. Also sliced tomato takes place of ketchup very nicely. Ask your doctor before using any salt substitute. These preparations usually contain potassium, which can be harmful to people with some medical conditions.	Salt, ketchup, BBQ sauce, chili sauce, celery products, garlic salt, bouillon cubes, monosodium glutamate (MSG). Accent, meat extracts or tenderizers, horseradish, prepared mustards, olives, pickles, relishes, soy sauce, worcestershire sauce, sodium saccharin.

Low-Sodium Diet for Hypertension *(continued)*

	CHOOSE FROM THIS FOOD GROUP	AVOID THESE FOODS
Soup	Low-sodium bouillon cubes (less than 5 mg. sodium per cube), low-sodium canned soups, homemade soups made with allowed ingredients.	Regular bouillon, broth or consommé canned, regular canned soup, dried or instant soup mixes.
Nuts	Unsalted nuts in shell, fresh or shelled	Salted nuts
Fruits and Vegetables	All fresh, frozen or canned fruits All fresh, low sodium canned, frozen vegetables	Candied cherries or maraschino cherries Canned vegetables, pickled vegetables like cucumber, cauliflower, pepper, sauerkraut etc.

Salt Substitutes

BRAND	SODIUM PER TSP. (MG.)	POTASSIUM PER TSP. (MG.)
Nu-Salt	0.17	528
No Salt	less than 0.10	2,502
Seasoned No Salt	less than 0.05	1,332
Morton Salt Substitute	trace	2,800
Morton Lite Salt Mixture	1,100	1,500
Adolph's Salt Substitute	less than 0.05	2,480

Caffeine Content of Popular Beverages and Foods

	CAFFEINE RANGE (MG.)
Chocolate/Cocoa	
milk chocolate, 1 oz.	1–15
dark chocolate, semi-sweet, 1 oz.	5–35
baking chocolate, unsweetened, 1 oz.	26
chocolate flavored syrup, 1 oz.	4
cocoa, 6 oz.	6–42
cocoa beverage, from mix, 5 oz.	2–20
chocolate milk beverage, 8 oz.	2–7
Coffee (5 oz.)	
brewed, drip method	60–180
brewed, percolator	40–170
instant	30–120
decaffeinated, brewed	2–5
decaffeinated, instant	1–5
Tea (5 oz.)	
brewed, U.S. brand	20–90
brewed, imported brands	24–110
one-minute brew	9–33
three-minute brew	20–46
five-minute brew	20–50
instant	25–50
iced tea, 12 oz.	67–76
iced tea, canned, 12 oz.	22–36
Soft Drinks (12 oz.)	
Mountain Dew	54.0
Coca-Cola	46.8
Diet Coke	45.6
Dr Pepper	39.6
Sugar-Free Dr Pepper	39.6
Pepsi Cola	38.4
Diet Pepsi	36.0
RC Cola	36.0
Diet Rite	36.0
Canada Dry Diet Cola	1.2
Tab	45.6
Pepsi Light	36.0

CHAPTER 23

Food Safety and Food Labeling

THE FEDERAL FOOD AND Drug Administration keeps tabs on hundreds of additives and food substitutes like artificial sweeteners; additives that are considered safe for public consumption appear on an FDA "Generally Regarded as Safe," or GRAS, list. Contaminants, both natural and man-made substances like pesticides, are regulated by the Environmental Protection Agency, which tests for ninety different pesticides as well as for PCBs, other industrial chemicals, and selected chemical elements naturally found in the diet. Tolerances in both cases are determined by tests on laboratory animals, as well as by observation of the clinical symptoms and blood levels of people who accidentally receive large doses.

Several things are worth noting here. It seems that the FDA moves slowly when it comes to addressing potential problems: as Marian Burros pointed out in a *New York Times* article, it was back in the 1970s that the FDA first dealt with the question of safe levels of aflatoxins in foods, a matter which stirred public concern again when heat and drought conditions caused high levels in the 1988 midwestern corn crop. The FDA also first considered a ban on antibiotics in animal feed in the 1970s. Both questions remain open. The contamination of natural bodies of water by PCBs—polyvinyl chlorides found in industrial wastes—and by other pollutants has led the EPA and various state and local governments to ban fish taken from particular rivers, lakes, and shorelines. These matters of public health and safety quickly become political issues that can have a hard effect on local economies. Worse, various forms of pollution have taken a terrible toll on great natural resources like the Chesapeake Bay and the Great Lakes —situations that may take decades or more to reverse.

But as far as food safety goes, just as the recommended daily allowance of vitamins allows a generous margin for error, so do methods of testing food safety. Several times a year the FDA does what it calls a total diet study, in which the country is divided up into four regions. In each the FDA tests drinking water and a "market basket" of more than 120 different foods, divided into categories such as poultry, meat, fish, vegetables, and so on. Separate tests are done on the typical diets of three segments of the population: infants, toddlers, and adults, the latter represented by the typical diet of 16- to 19-year-old males, because they consume the most food—usually well over 3,000 calories a day. Overall the tests have shown American diets to have levels of contaminants comfortably under what's considered to be safe—the United States generally does better in this respect than most other industrialized countries.

As for additives, no new additive can be introduced to foods without rigid and extensive testing, which may last for years. The 1938 Food, Drug and Cosmetic Act was beefed up considerably in 1958 and 1960, when lawmakers shifted the burden of proof regarding safety from the government onto the manufacturers. The Delaney Clause added that a substance which in any dose causes cancer in man or animals couldn't be added to food. It was this clause, and the fact that the government periodically reviews existing additives, that led to the compromise 1977 warning on saccharine, because some studies suggested it caused bladder cancer in rats.

Finally, rats used in testing for additives and contaminants have been *specifically bred* to be prone to cancerous tumors, or susceptible to seizures or other maladies under scrutiny.

"NATURAL" AND ORGANICALLY GROWN FOODS

There's no legal definition of a natural food, although it is taken to mean that no artificial substances or preservatives have been added. Organically grown foods are assumed to be grown using only natural fertilizers (such as cow manure) and no pesticides. With certain produce you may feel better buying organically grown products, but in truth they may still have chemical residues in them, for these substances travel on the wind and in water, and may stay in the soil for decades. "Natural" foods are, however, almost always more expensive—sometimes costing twice as much (or more) than their ordinary counterparts.

As for organic fertilizers, plants turn these into chemical components before using them, in any event. Man-made fertilizers can be applied to replace specific nutrients missing in the soil—as determined by soil tests. If natural fertilizer, such as cow manure, is used, it's possible that the resulting crop will be low in a specific nutrient. If the cow manure is gotten from local sources, which is likely, and the animals have been feeding on local plants and grains, then anything missing from the plants will be missing from the fertilizer.

In some instances, foods touted as natural can be less wholesome than what they replace. This is particularly true with snacks. As is the case with granolas, calorie content given for these foods can be misleading. What appears to be one serving often turns out to be two and a half, and you have to do your own multiplying to find out the total calories in one package. One particular brand of "natural" snacks, made of peanuts, cocoa, and carob, turned out to have twice the calories and fat of its conventional counterpart—M&Ms—at twice the expense. Furthermore, natural snacks are just as likely to contain saturated fats as snacks found in another part of the supermarket.

Other "health foods" can be just as disappointing. Is honey nutritionally superior to white sugar? They're both made of fructose and glucose, and honey actually has more calories than sugar—64 per tablespoon as opposed to 46 for sugar. The mineral content in honey is so minute it's nutritionally insignificant, and because it's sticky, it may be worse for your teeth. How about raw milk? There's nothing nutritionally superior about it, and even if it comes from cows regularly examined by the state board of health, the possibility of disease-carrying bacteria in the milk is certainly higher than in pasteurized milk, which is simply milk that's been heat-treated.

THE ROLE OF ADDITIVES

Many additives are used to retard food spoilage, which is essential given our urban life-style, wherein much of the food we eat comes from hundreds if not thousands of miles away. Many additives occur naturally in other foods: calcium propionate, which is used to keep bread fresh, occurs naturally in Swiss cheese. Salt and sugar are still the most prevalent preservatives, and these have been in use for centuries. The addition of vitamins like B, C, and D to many foods has over the years dramatically reduced the incidence of deficiency diseases like rickets, pellagra, and scurvy. Other additives include some that improve the color or texture of a food or that help improve processing. Naturally occurring ingredients like lecithin (from soybeans) and carrobean (from the locust tree) make foods like ice cream smoother and help prevent separation. By law all additives have to be listed on food labels. These are listed in order of weight, from the highest content to the lowest. But sometimes 90 percent of a listing will be devoted to substances that make up only 1 percent of the product, giving the false impression that a product is more additives than anything else.

What about chemicals, anyway? Let's look at the chemical components of one particular food: in addition to starches, sugars, cellulose, and pectin, it contains amyl acetate, anisyl propionate, ascorbic acid, citric acid, malic acid, phosphates, succinic acid, and various vitamins. This is what is found *naturally* in a chilled melon. Acetaldehyde, acetone, butanol, diacetyl, isoprene, dimethyl sulfide, and methyl acetate are some of the chemicals occurring naturally in coffee, while tea contains benzyl alcohol, butyl alcohol, geraniol, hexyl alcohol, isoamyl alcohol, and phenyl ethyl alcohol.

Most of our concerns about food additives are unfounded. The National Academy of Science reported in 1982 that there was no evidence the use of additives had contributed to the overall risk of cancer in the population, nor, according to a five-year study by the Nutrition Foundation, is there any evidence that additives cause hyperactivity in children.

ALLERGIES AND ADDITIVES

Some additives, however, are cause for concern, among them substances that can cause allergic reactions in susceptible individuals. All of these must be listed on food labels, so read carefully. The three most common culprits include:

MONOSODIUM GLUTAMATE.   MSG dilates blood vessels and causes flushing, headaches, and real discomfort in susceptible people; it can also cause life-threatening attacks in asthmatics, and should be avoided by those whose sodium intake is restricted. It's used in processed foods and can be bought in the spice section of the store; Accent is also mostly MSG. MSG is found in a lot of Chinese food, but many restaurants will leave it out at your request.

SULFITE PRESERVATIVES.   These have been used to preserve fresh vegetables in supermarkets and in restaurants to keep salad greens looking fresh. They can cause acute, life-threatening attacks in asthmatics who are susceptible, usually within an hour of ingestion. In most states use of sulfites has been banned, but if you have any doubts about what you're getting, ask the grocer or restaurant manager.

TARTRAZINE.   This is an FD&C approved color—yellow #5—found in all sorts of foods, beverages, drugs, and cosmetics. It's been estimated that 50,000 to 100,000 people in the United States are sensitive to it. Symptoms can include hives, swelling of the face and lips, a runny nose, and also asthma attacks. If you can't tolerate aspirin, you may not be able to tolerate tartrazine—about 15 percent of those who can't tolerate aspirin are tartrazine-sensitive.

HAZARDOUS ADDITIVES AND CONTAMINANTS

There are other additives and contaminants that pose broader health risks. Carcinogens found here are also discussed in Chapter 20; artificial sweeteners are discussed later in this chapter.

AFLATOXINS.   These are potent carcinogens that may develop naturally in peanuts, other nuts, and corn. The government monitors the level of aflatoxins, but if any of these foods look or taste "off," or get moldy, throw them out.

ANTIBIOTICS.   A shocking 40 percent of all antibiotics used in this country goes into feed for livestock. Most of these are subtherapeutic doses, since for some reason antibiotics, among other things, enhance weight gain in animals. Animals are also fed therapeutic doses in the presence of specific diseases, although the U.S. Department of Agriculture requires a waiting period before these animals are slaughtered. This helps resolve some of the residue problem, but there are still troubling questions to consider.

One is that resistant strains of bacteria may actually flourish in treated animals; another is the question of what long-term consumption of meats from these animals, even with very low residues, may do to us. Antibiotics that kill helpful bacteria actually increase the presence of salmonella bacteria, a contaminant that can be a problem in poultry and eggs.

The problem is magnified in people who take a lot of prescribed antibiotics, and may be worse for those who "save" pills for later and take them at the first sign of a sore throat or cold. This kind of broad use may make you more susceptible to salmonella and may actually accelerate the development of resistant strains of bacteria: just as a vaccine gives humans immunity to certain diseases, so may antibiotics in lower-than-prescribed doses "vaccinate" microorganisms against antibiotics.

The government says that antibiotics used on livestock shouldn't cause any problems, but an independent body, the American Council on Science and Health, contends that just because no epidemics have broken out among those with close exposure to animals, it's no guarantee that long-term effects won't be serious.

DAMINOZIDE (ALAR).   This chemical, used particularly in apples to control the ripening process and set the color, has been declared a carcinogen by the EPA, and by the time this book sees print it will probably have been banned in the United States. Granny Smith apples, which are not sprayed with daminozide, are a way to go with apples if you're still concerned about its use. Other chemical residues, including some pesticides that are banned in this country, are likely to be found in imported fruit in higher quantities than in domestic, but with more public focus on this problem the situation may improve.

The National Resources Defense Council, a watchdog organization that doesn't always toe the government line, does not suggest we should reduce our consumption of fruits and vegetables, but does offer some suggestions about reducing exposure to residues. While systemic substances like daminozide won't be affected by washing, it suggests that others may be reduced by washing fresh fruits and vegetables in a weak solution of Ivory or other dishwashing liquid and water, rinsing thoroughly afterward. (This doesn't seem like a good idea in the case of leafy greens or mushrooms, however, and you should wash and rinse quickly—never leave any produce standing in soapy water.) With produce that has been waxed, peeling is more effective, although you're going to lose some nutrients with the peeling.

MERCURY. Safe levels of mercury in fish—0.5 parts per million— were established by the FDA in 1969; this tolerance applies to all fish in interstate commerce.

PARASITES. Parasites such as trichinosis in pork and others in raw fish are effectively killed by cooking. Eating raw or undercooked fish and meats is a health risk, although farm-raised fish and shellfish are usually safer to eat than those harvested in the wild. If you're bent on eating sushi, you can kill any parasites by freezing the fish before thawing and preparing it.

PCBs. Polyvinyl chlorides have been banned in this country, but the disposal of industrial wastes into many of our rivers and lakes has left a deposit of PCBs and other pollutants that is enough to cause bottom-feeding fish, and in some cases all fish, to be contaminated; shellfish along some ocean shorelines have also been affected. In 1988 the EPA advised that fish caught along certain parts of the Wisconsin shore of Lake Michigan should not be consumed because of the level of contaminants from industrial wastes, and also recommended that fish caught from the Lorain River, which empties into Lake Erie, not be eaten.

SALMONELLA. Salmonella contamination is of particular concern in eggs and chicken, and as we've discussed, the consumption of low-level antibiotics in meats increases our susceptibility to infection. Handle raw chicken carefully, making sure you wash your hands and any utensils and cutting boards with soap before handling other foods. It's wise not to use a wooden cutting board unless it's used exclusively for meats that are to be cooked, as it is extremely difficult to get these entirely clean. Most important, make sure that chicken and eggs are cooked thoroughly. You're running a risk if you eat soft-cooked eggs, but in any event don't feed underdone eggs or chicken to infants or the elderly, as they are most at risk.

SODIUM NITRITE.   Sodium nitrite is added to meats such as bacon, sausage, and hot dogs. When it comes into direct contact with heat, it forms nitrosamines, which are carcinogenic (see page 264 for safe cooking). Bacon processed without nitrite won't have the pink color of other bacon; this doesn't affect the taste, but the increased salt content ordinarily found in it does. You also need to take extra care in storing it, freezing any portion you won't be eating in a short time.

FOOD IRRADIATION

Food irradiation is not exactly a new phenomenon: the Institute of Food Technologists in Chicago recently reported that between 1958 and 1981 twenty-four countries approved irradiation treatments for some forty different foods. The FDA has been cautious about it, however, and did not approve it until late 1985. In the irradiation process, foods are exposed to gamma rays from radioactive cobalt 60. This kills bacteria, viruses, molds; it can also prevent potatoes from sprouting and kill parasites like the one that causes trichinosis. Whole foods that have been irradiated must bear an international symbol called the RADURA:

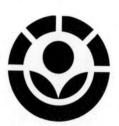

Presently it must also bear the label "Treated by Irradiation," but the FDA may eventually drop this. The requirement of the logo, however, is permanent, although manufacturers who use an irradiated ingredient—such as a spice—in a prepared food don't have to tell you so on the label.

Many people are alarmed at this whole idea, and it's easy to understand why. But irradiated foods in no way expose the consumer to any radioactivity. Opponents of irradiation claim that the government is promoting it because it's a way to use by-products of the nuclear weapons industry, but cobalt 60 is not one of these. Cobalt 60 is the same element used in cobalt treatments, although in these the dose is much stronger than what is used in food irradiation. Does irradiation destroy any nutritive content? Tests have shown it doesn't.

Food irradiation may have many potential benefits. Proponents say that it will reduce our dependence on pesticides, which have a significant impact on the ecology, and will reduce the use of other preservatives such as nitrites, at the same time that it reduces spoilage. They claim that irradiation can have a significant impact on the world food supply by preventing post-harvest losses, which in turn can improve public health in developing countries. Food irradiation hasn't been widespread in this country up to this point, but chances are the practice will increase in the near future.

ARTIFICIAL SWEETENERS

These are additives that Americans have been consuming in increasing quantities: In the last decade consumption has more than doubled. In 1986 alone, Americans spent an estimated ten billion dollars on artificially sweetened foods and beverages.

Saccharine has been around for a long time. When the FDA attempted to ban it in the 1970s, there was a great outcry from diabetics and others because at the time there really weren't any other sweeteners on the market. Cyclamates were banned in 1970 because it was found that rats given large doses had an increased incidence of bladder cancer. Though saccharine is said to pose the same risk, it remained on the market while cyclamates stayed banned. The AMA's main comment on saccharine has been to suggest that it not be used by pregnant women.

Aspartame, marketed as NutraSweet or Equal, is the largest selling artificial sweetener today. It was first approved for use in 1981, and by 1986 it was permitted not only in carbonated beverages but in Popsicle-type bars, fruit juices, instant tea, and breath mints. In 1987 the NutraSweet company submitted petitions to the FDA for allowing the use of a more stable version of aspartame, which won't be destroyed in cooking, in baked goods and mixes.

Aspartame is basically two amino acids—phenylalanine and aspiric acid. It's metabolized in the same way as something that contains protein. It does provide calories—about 4 per gram—but because it's 200 times sweeter than sugar it is used in amounts too small to make much impact on your total caloric intake. Though some adverse reactions have been reported, there has been little substantiation of them except in the case of those with phenylketonuria (PKU), a genetic disease wherein an individual can't metabolize the amino acid phenylalanine. Aspartame may also trigger migraines in susceptible people. As for other risks, the FDA has set the acceptable daily intake at 50 milligrams for each kilogram of body weight: this means that a 132-pound adult would have to drink more than eighteen cans of aspartame-sweetened soft drinks in a day to go above acceptable levels. Further studies on aspartame and its affect on memory, concentration, and coordination are being conducted by the Mayo Clinic.

Meanwhile other artificial sweeteners are in the wings. One, Acesulfam K, was approved by the FDA in 1988 for use in certain foods. It is a potassium ash, with a greater intensity of sweetness and greater stability than aspartame, and it may be cheaper to produce. Marketed under the name Sunette, it is already available in twenty countries. Questions about the product's safety—the possibility that it is carcinogenic and raises cholesterol levels in diabetic rats—have been raised, but the FDA has concluded that in both instances the rate of incidence was no higher than expected under normal circumstances.

Two other sweeteners have been developed by major pharmaceutical companies: Alitame (Pfizer & Co.) is a noncaloric dipeptide (a protein) that's 2,000 times sweeter than sugar; Sucralose (Johnson & Johnson) is 600 times sweeter than sugar.

FAT SUBSTITUTES

Aside from butter flavorings, there are no fat substitutes on the market now, but two are waiting in the wings: Procter & Gamble's Olestra and Simplesse from the NutraSweet company.

Olestra is a sucrose polymer that is not digested at all and therefore has no calorie content. Partly to ensure that fat-soluble vitamins will remain in the diet, it may be used primarily in combination with fats like shortening and oil. The Center for Science in the Public Interest has asked the FDA not to approve the use of Olestra, saying that Procter & Gamble's testing is flawed and that the substitute causes cancer, liver damage, and other serious problems in test animals. But the company has submitted thirty-five volumes of research on their product, which it says verifies that problems showing up in tests were well within normal ranges.

Simplesse, developed by the NutraSweet company, is a processed protein made from egg whites and milk protein that could be available in late 1989 or early 1990. It is a microcurd; that is, the protein is formed into tiny spheres that give the smoothness and sensation of fat. Because it's a protein it will break down in cooking, so its main use would be in such things as salad dressings, mayonnaise, ice cream, butter, and cheese spreads. Even though Simplesse contains calories, it would still significantly reduce them in these foods: In a premium ice cream, which is 12 to 14 percent butterfat, 4 ounces is 280 calories, but made with Simplesse it would be about 130. A tablespoon of mayonnaise is 100 calories; 30 if made with Simplesse; cream cheese is 100 calories an ounce, but with Simplesse it would be about 45. Clearly Simplesse can help reduce total dietary fats, but it will only be part of the answer for most people.

FOOD LABELING

Throughout this book we've stressed the importance of reading food labels. Here are some to watch for. Some of them have legal definitions; some do not.

ENRICHED OR FORTIFIED FOODS.   These have certain nutrients added that may or may not have been in the food in the first place. In the case of refined grains, for example, B vitamins that have been lost in processing are put back in. Adding iodine to salt has all but eradicated the common goiter.

IMITATIONS AND SUBSTITUTES.   What we have called sugar and fat substitutes are not literally substitutes. A food substitute is a product nutritionally equivalent to the food it imitates. Nondairy whipped toppings are usually substitutes. Even if they are slightly lower in calories than real whipped cream, most simply substitute tropical oils, which are saturated, for butterfat. Egg substitutes, on the other hand, supply the same amount of protein as real eggs, but without the fat and cholesterol. *Imitation* on a label means that a product resembles another food but is nutritionally inferior to it.

DIETETIC.   This is a legally defined term but it can be misleading. All it means is that one ingredient has been changed or restricted in the product: this could be salt or sugar. It doesn't necessarily mean that the food is low in calories or otherwise good for you. Here again be careful to read the whole label.

SUGAR-FREE OR SUGARLESS.   This is another label that can be misleading, as it indicates a food that doesn't contain table sugar (sucrose), but it may include honey, corn syrup, fructose, or sorbitol, and the latter contains calories just as the others do. Other sugars appear on food labels as dextrose, dextrins, glucose, high fructose corn syrup (discussed in Chapter 11), and molasses.

LIGHT OR LITE.   These terms have no legal definition. They are often used to indicate foods that are lower in calories or, in the case of salt substitutes, lower in sodium. Here, reading the label is the only way to discover what the word refers to, since "light" can also be used to describe texture, color, or taste.

REDUCED CALORIE.   These are foods with one-third fewer calories than what are found in the foods they resemble, as in reduced-calorie salad dressings.

LOW CALORIE.   Refers to foods that contain 40 calories or less per serving.

LEANER.   Used only to describe meat products. It means that the meat has 25 percent less fat than the standard product.

LEAN.   A meat product that is no more than 10 percent fat.

EXTRA LEAN.   A meat product that is no more than 5 percent fat.

UNSALTED.   Foods processed without added salt. The food in question may be naturally high in sodium, however, and other forms of sodium may have been used in processing. The word sodium in any combination is telltale here.

REDUCED SODIUM.   Products that have 25 percent less sodium than what is usually found in the standard counterpart.

LOW SODIUM.   Refers to products with 140 milligrams or less per serving.

VERY LOW SODIUM.   Refers to products with 35 milligrams or less per serving.

SODIUM FREE.   Refers to foods with less than 5 milligrams per serving.

COMMON FOOD ADDITIVES

Fortified foods may include added vitamins or minerals; these are listed in Chapter 22.

Colors and Flavors

Acetic acid is a key ingredient in vinegar.
Adipic acid gives a mild tartness to food.

Annato extract is a natural yellow-orange color derived from plant seeds.

Beet extract provides a natural deep red color.

Caramel is a coloring produced by browning sugar.

Carotenoids are natural food colors (light yellow to dark red) extracted from carrots and other plant and animal sources. When combined with protein, they produce greens and blues.

Disodium guanylate is a flavor enhancer used in meats and meat-based foods.

FD&C indicates a synthetic color certified by the Food and Drug Administration for use in foods, drugs, and cosmetics.

HVPC stands for hydrolized vegetable protein, made by processing protein from vegetables like soybeans. It is used as a flavor enhancer.

Maltol is a sugar derivative that is used to intensify berry flavors.

MSG is monosodium glutamate (see Allergies and Additives, page 325).

Phosphates are minerals used to control tartness.

Sorbitol is a sweetener found naturally in some fruits; while it doesn't promote tooth decay, it is not low-calorie (see sugars and artificial sweeteners for other additives used to sweeten foods).

Titanium dioxide is a mineral-derived, pure white coloring agent that produces an opaque look in soft drinks.

Turmeric, found frequently in curry and chili powders, is an herb used for coloring and flavor.

Preservatives

Benzoic acid controls mold.

BHA (butylated hydroxyanisole) and *BHT* (butylated hydroxytoluene) are used to prevent rancidity in dry foods.

Calcium propionate occurs naturally in cheese; it's used to retard mold in baked goods.

Calcium sorbate controls surface mold on cheese, syrups, margarine, and mayonnaise.

Citric acid, found naturally in citrus fruit, is used to keep cut fruits from turning brown.

EDTA (ethylene diaminetetracetic acid) prevents color changes in bottled salad dressings, sauces, gravies and canned vegetables.

Lactic acid is produced naturally in the fermentation of pickles, sauerkraut, cheese, buttermilk, and yogurt. It controls mold and is also added to cultured milk products to increase acidity.

Metabisulfite has the same function as *sulfur dioxide* (see below).

Potassium propionate has the same function as *calcium propionate* (see above).

Propionic acid has the same function as benzoic acid.

Propyl gallate prevents rancidity in cereals, snacks, and pastries. It is not as stable under high temperatures as BHA or BHT.

Sodium benzoate has the same function as benzoic acid.

Sodium chloride is table salt.

Sodium nitrite inhibits growth of botulism in cured meats, fish, and poultry. It works best in combination with vitamin C. (See Hazardous Additives and Contaminants, page 328.)

Sodium propionate has the same function as *calcium propionate* (see above).

Sodium sorbate has the same function as *sorbic acid.*

Sorbic acid controls surface molds on cheese, syrups, margarine, and mayonnaise.

Sulfur dioxide inhibits browning in fresh and dried fruits and prevents undesirable color changes when wine is exposed to the air.

Tocopherols inhibit rancidity in fatty foods. One of the tocopherols is vitamin E.

Other Additives

Calcium silicate is an anti-caking agent added to powdered foods, table salt, and baking powder.

Carob bean gum is a natural vegetable gum made from the pods of the carob (locust) tree; it serves as a stabilizer and texturizer.

Carrageenan comes from seaweed; it improves the consistency and texture of chocolate milk, frozen desserts, puddings, and syrups.

Glycerides (monoglycerides and diglycerides) are derived primarily from vegetable oils and are the most common emulsifiers.

Glycerine is a moisture retainer often added to flaked coconut and marshmallows.

Guar gum is a common vegetable gum used to thicken gravies, snacks, and pet foods.

Gum arabic is a vegetable gum that stabilizes flavor in dry-mix products.

Lecithin is an emulsifier that occurs naturally in eggs and soybeans.

Modified food starches, derived from cereal grains and potatoes, are used to stabilize, thicken, or add texture to pie fillings, gravies, and sauces.

Monocalcium phosphate removes the residual soapy taste that baking soda can leave in baked goods.

Pectin occurs naturally in most fruits, especially in apples; it gives body to jams, jellies, and preserves.

Propylene glycol improves texture by retaining moisture in foods.

Sodium alginate is a stabilizer and thickener used to keep cocoa from separating from chocolate milk and cocoa butter from separating from other chocolate products, which can give them a grayish color.

PART SEVEN

Keeping Fit Forever

Many OF US REMEMBER junior high and high school as the years under the Kennedy administration, when the race for space filtered down into the schools as a great push toward the hard sciences, and a mandate for physical fitness meant an invasion of physical education classes by the Royal Canadian Air Force. High school coaches lined up thousands of adolescents to administer the air force physical fitness tests: 50 sit-ups were among the minimum requirements for girls, who were spared the pushups and only had to do a fraction of the chin-ups required of the boys. Mostly, the kids who passed with flying colors were the ones we knew as jocks. Thousands of the rest of us—of both sexes—flunked.

Jane Fonda tells the story of how, in her forties, she mastered a blackflip during the filming of *On Golden Pond*. Challenged by Katharine Hepburn, who was then in her seventies and who was an excellent diver in her youth, Fonda weathered bruises and bellyflops until finally she managed a passable dive. When Hepburn asked her how she felt, she replied "Just terrific!"—terrific in finding the motivation to stick to something and conquer it. She is doubtless the most visible example among many women who have discovered in midlife that a regular exercise program can actually put you in better shape now than you ever were in your twenties—and maybe even in your teens. With a flexible and sensible fitness plan, even a dedicated couch potato can discover the rewards of a regular exercise program: new stamina and flexibility, increased energy and alertness, glowing skin, and a stronger, firmer, shapelier body.

CHAPTER 24

Changing a Sedentary Life-style

MOTIVATION COMES FIRST. Olympic gold-medal winner Florence Griffith-Joyner began her training program during lunch breaks and weekend time off from her job in a bank. As she says, "You've got to want it." Of course most of us are willing to leave the medal-winning to top athletes who deserve tangible recognition for their superb commitment and performance, to concentrate instead on reaping the fundamental personal rewards of a long-term fitness program. Such a program will not only extend your shot at a long and healthy life, it will significantly improve your quality of life—right now.

If what you find here produces a glimmer of motivation to change your sedentary life-style, chances are that once you experience how good it feels to get into better shape, your commitment will quickly follow. If you've been sedentary for the last year or more, and especially if you are overweight or smoke cigarettes, start with Level 1 Fitness. If you're moderately active, we'll show you how to gradually increase your level of fitness and performance, and list some sources for more serious fitness training. If you're one of the jocks who did all 50 sit-ups in high school and are now running 6-minute miles, bravo! In this chapter you'll find a special section on nutrition for women who participate in strenuous sports, information on appropriate cardiopulmonary target rates for your age group, and notes on cross-training and sports injuries.

Revving up for Physical Fitness

Much of the motivation for our lifelong fitness plan comes from previous chapters—from what you see of your body in the mirror and what is going on inside it at this pivotal time in your life. In nearly every discussion of specific situations and areas of the body, in both prevention of problems and specific health guidelines, physical exercise was prominently showcased:

- *Ideal weight and weight gain:* Exercise increases basal metabolism and helps burn calories (see chart on page 342). And except for the proverbial lumberjack—the person daily involved in prolonged, strenuous activity—exercise does not increase appetite. By temporarily raising blood-sugar levels, exercise actually reduces the tendency to overeat, not only metabolically but by easing the mind-body tensions and boredom that lead so many of us to head for the kitchen.
- *The skin:* Exercise will give you better color and firmer-looking skin because it improves circulation and underlying muscle tone—hence skin tone and elasticity.
- *Blood circulation and the heart:* Exercise can reduce the risk of a heart attack by improving the strength of the heart so it works more efficiently, pumping the same amount of blood in 45 to 50 beats per minute that the sedentary person's heart pumps in 70 to 75 beats. It also helps reduce the risk of high blood pressure; lowers blood cholesterol (at the same time increasing HDL—the good cholesterol), and reduces the craving for abusive substances. Inactive people have one and a half to two times the risk of having a heart attack than people who exercise; and the risk of dying immediately after a heart attack is three times greater for the inactive person than for the physically active.
- *The digestive system:* Physical exercise stimulates peristalsis, helping to keep the 35-plus body regular. By keeping weight down, exercise helps prevent digestive problems that typically occur in overweight people, such as heartburn and esophagitis.
- *Muscles, joints and bones:* Exercises that are loadbearing—walking, running, racquet sports—are an important factor in preventing osteoporosis, since they increase and sustain calcium content in the bone. Stretching keeps joints and muscles supple and resilient, and it expands your range of motion to an optimum for sports and other physical activities. Muscle strength and stamina increase, also increasing your capacity for physical work.
- *Endocrine glands:* By helping keep weight down, exercise reduces the risk of diabetes. It also decreases the diabetic's insulin requirements (see page 145).

- *The brain:* Regular exercise helps keeps the brain nourished, has a good effect on neurotransmitters (producing endorphins and raising the level of serotonin in the brain), and counters stress, anxiety, and depression. Regular exercise actually decreases fatigue—countering the presence of triglycerides in the blood. At the same time it promotes relaxation, alleviates tension, and improves the ability to fall asleep.

PHASE ONE: AEROBICS FOR THE HEART AND LUNGS

Somewhere along the way to molding the perfect body on the trendiest exercise machines, to buying the snazziest warm-up suits and athletic shoes, to cooking "spa cuisine" that may cost more per meal than many would spend on a week of "normal" food, the long-term goals of exercise have been lost. Short-lived food fads and trendy workouts eventually fall by the wayside. At 35-plus, long-term fitness begins with stepping back and assessing what your body really needs from exercise, finding a life sport (or two) that meets those needs, and sticking with it because you really enjoy it.

Your primary life sport should be aerobic—an activity that exercises the heart and lungs as nature intended, giving them the kind of regular, healthy workout that was shelved when sedentary work and motorized transportation took over our lives. Properly done, aerobic exercise supplies your body with the maximum amount of oxygen it can use, slowly and comfortably bringing your heart rate up to its target zone, or maximum rate of performance, for twenty to thirty minutes at its peak, and then slowly letting it return to normal. To do aerobics, you do not have to work out with a roomful of women in colorful tights; this route may be too strenuous, especially if you have back or joint problems that might be exacerbated by relatively high impact exercise. Barring that, if an aerobics class appeals to you, by all means, join one: the instruction is often excellent and the camaraderie and coaching can help keep you motivated. But the activities listed here provide ways of getting a good aerobic workout that may be more convenient and interesting.

In addition to improving the performance of your heart and lungs, and burning off calories, aerobic exercise helps to balance the ratio of muscle to fat—taking off inches in addition to pounds. Isometric exercise, including those using weights or resistance machines, is a good supplement to aerobic exercise, but it is not a substitute—it won't give your heart and lungs the workout they need. Isometric exercise has its place: it further strengthens and shapes muscles and may help counteract osteoporosis (more on isometrics on page 355). Sprinting, bowling, and baseball aren't really good aerobic workouts, either; in these the heart works in fits and starts. Aerobic exercise is necessary for cardiopulmonary health, and it is also the most efficient form of exercise for weight loss and maintenance. If you have any doubts about this, think about the physiques of sports stars. You've seen some chunky baseball and football players—not to mention wrestlers—but have you ever seen a fat swimming champion or long-distance runner? Exercise combined with weight loss has another happy effect. As you exercise, you lose weight; and as you lose weight, exercise becomes easier. It's just as much of a burden to get around carrying 10 or 20 extra pounds of body fat as it is to get around lugging 10 or 20 pounds of groceries while they're still in the bag.

Exercise and Weight Control

In order to lose 1 pound in a given time period, you must burn off 3,500 more calories than you take in. The American Heart Association (we refer to their guidelines often in this chapter) presents a sampling of average calories spent per hour by a 150-pound person doing the following activities:

AEROBIC ACTIVITY	CALORIES BURNED PER HOUR
Walking, 2 m.p.h. (30-minute mile)	240
Walking, 3 m.p.h. (20-minute mile)	320
Walking, 4½ m.p.h. (13.3-minute mile)	440
Swimming, 25 yds./min.	275
Swimming, 50 yds./min.	500
Bicycling, 6 m.p.h. (10-minute mile)	240
Bicycling, 12 m.p.h. (5-minute mile)	410
Jogging, 5½ m.p.h. (10.9-minute mile)	740
Jogging, 7 m.p.h. (8.6-minute mile)	920
Jumping rope	750
Running in place	650
Running, 10 m.p.h. (6-minute mile)	1,280
Cross-country skiing	700
Tennis (singles)	400

Body weight has an effect on the number of calories burned, because the heavier the body mass, the more exertion is required to move it. Using the sampling above, a person who only weighs 125 pounds reduces the number of calories burned per hour by one-sixth; a person weighing 100 pounds reduces them by one-third, while a person weighing 200 pounds increases them by one-third.

Picking up the pace or increasing the level of exertion does increase the number of calories expended per hour, but once the heart reaches its peak performance level—that is, its maximum capacity for utilizing oxygen, the best and safest way to burn off calories is to exercise longer. Pushing yourself too hard is likely to backfire, too. If exercise is more chore than pleasure, and if you subject yourself to unnecessary muscle strain and injury, it's going to be tough to stick with it.

Obviously, as you lose weight it will take less energy (fewer calories) to move your body around—the paradox of the "conditioning effect." But as you become stronger and more muscular, you'll be able to exercise harder with less effort. And as we've seen, not only is muscle more compact pound for pound than fat, it also requires more energy to maintain than fat tissue does. All this points to an eventual weight stabilization—an optimum balance between calories taken in and calories expended—that is one of the great rewards of a successful exercise program.

Some Things to Consider

If you are new to exercise, now is the time to choose a life sport that meets aerobic standards. What you choose depends on a number of factors:

- *Level of fitness.* Walking and swimming are less strenuous starter sports than jogging or jumping rope, and some seemingly active sports—baseball, softball, bowling, volleyball, football, and golf (with a cart or on foot)—do not actually meet aerobic standards, although they are enjoyable for other reasons and can help strengthen muscles or develop coordination. If you don't want to trade in your present sport for another one, just add a walking or jogging program; it may be easy to fit it in right before or after your game.
- *Social motivation.* Do you like solitude or socializing? Choose a life sport that reflects your preference and enhances your commitment. Some women prefer team sports or an activity like singles tennis that requires a partner; others prefer hiking, biking, or rowing.
- *Indoors or out.* Choose a sport that not only gives pleasure but is practical for the area in which you live. Bad weather and seasonal changes may present a serious challenge to your resolve if you don't anticipate them. If you ride a bike outdoors during the spring, summer, and fall, you may want to invest in a stationary bike for bad-weather days. Or choose another form of exercise altogether; variation helps defray boredom and balances out muscle strength.
- *Your daily schedule.* If you have room in your schedule to fit in three trips a week to the local gym or tennis court, great. However, if time (and money) is a factor, you may prefer to invest in nothing more than a new pair of walking or running shoes, and get out for a brisk half-hour walk or run three mornings a week or after work. Inconvenience and boredom can be big deterrents to exercise; if one is a greater obstacle to you than the other, choose your sport accordingly.

Sports That Meet the Criteria for Aerobic Conditioning

If you regularly engage in one of the following sports at least three times a week, at the given level of performance, you are getting exercise that meets the minimum requirements for aerobic conditioning. If you're starting out, you'll need to work up gradually to maintenance levels. The American Heart Association divides sports into very vigorous and moderately vigorous categories.

- *Very vigorous sports.* These need to be performed at peak level for at least fifteen minutes (not counting essential warm-up and cool-down times), at least three times a week. They include cross-country skiing, uphill hiking, ice hockey, running, jogging, running in place, jumping rope, rowing, and (at adequate levels of resistance) stationary cycling.
- *Moderately vigorous sports.* These need to be done at a brisk pace for at least thirty minutes (not counting warm-up and cool-down), at least three times a week. These include brisk walking, swimming, bicycling, downhill skiing, basketball, calisthenics, field hockey, handball, racquetball, soccer, squash, and singles tennis. Note that swimming and bicycling may be very vigorous or only moderately vigorous depending upon your speed and (for the latter) the terrain.

Determining Your Target Zone

By reaching your peak performance, we mean exercise that brings your pulse rate and respiration up to a level called your target zone. In cardiovascular exercise, pacing is all important. You can determine how hard to exercise by keeping track of your heart rate, or pulse. Your maximum heart rate is an age-derived value that is for most people a safe upper limit, a ceiling of sorts. Your best activity level—the target zone—is 60 to 75 percent of this maximum. Exercise that brings the heart rate above 75 percent is neither necessary nor predictably safe. Exercising below 60 percent gives your heart and lungs little conditioning. The table below, part of a chart appearing in guidelines published by the American Heart Association, shows average rates for ages 35 to 55.

AGE	TARGET ZONE 60–75%	AVERAGE MAXIMUM HEART RATE (100%)
35 years	111–128 beats per min.	185
40 years	108–135 beats per min.	180
45 years	105–131 beats per min.	175
50 years	102–127 beats per min.	170
55 years	99–123 beats per min.	165

Keep your heart rate at the low end of your target zone (60 percent) when beginning a new exercise program. As your strength increases, you can move toward the higher end (75 percent). Remember that you don't have to exercise at any higher rate to stay in optimum shape—and indeed you shouldn't.

Your Resting Pulse

The maximum predicted heart rate is arrived at by subtracting your age from 220. In other words, if you are 43 years old, your maximum predicted heart rate is 177. As currently used, this is a fairly crude value, since it is not adjusted for gender or weight, but it is a useful rule of thumb for estimating your target zone. Consistently pursued exercise that brings your heart rate to this target zone for a sustained period will result in good heart-lung fitness, including a *lower* heart rate when your body is at rest. A normal heart rate is between 60 and 100 beats per minute, and a rate at the lower end of this range is generally a good health sign. Over a period of several months, a consistent walking or jogging program should lead to a decrease in the resting heart rate—a pulse in the mid-70s, or even in the 60s or 50s. The more rigorous the aerobic exercise, the lower the resting heart rate will become over time.

Taking Your Pulse

1. Warm up your body for five minutes before beginning your exercise.
2. Begin the brisk part of your activity, and keep to it at a comfortable pace for a minute or two.
3. Stop moving (or slow down), and *immediately* place the tips of two fingers on one of the carotid arteries in your neck, to the left or right of your Adam's apple. Using a watch with a second hand, count your pulse for fifteen seconds and then multiply by 4—this gives you your heart rate in beats per minute.
4. Compare this rate to your recommended target zone. If it is below the target zone, continue your exercise at a slightly brisker pace; if it is above, slow down.

   Check your pulse several times during your first exercise sessions until you get a sense of your limits. Thereafter, check your pulse at the end of the peak-performance portion of each session; as time goes by you'll need to adjust your pace upward. But slow down and take your pulse any time you sense that you're overexerting yourself.

Two Approaches to Fitness

Walking or jogging is a good and uncomplicated way to start an exercise program, and for those who choose to go this route we present two programs. Choose a plan geared to your age and fitness level. We believe that the 35-plus woman who has no prior exercise history, who is sedentary, overweight, or has not yet shed poor health habits such as smoking, should try the gradual plans for walking and jogging, taken from the American Heart Association's booklet "Exercise and Your Heart." We call these plans Level 1. If you have been moderately active, are a nonsmoker, and have no health risks, a slightly accelerated program, which we call Level 2, is a reasonable approach. You should review any new exercise plan with your doctor before getting started, but if you are over 55 or have any heart, respiratory, or other serious health problems, you *must* consult your physician before beginning an exercise program.

Obviously, a jogging program is more vigorous than a walking program. In a given period of time, jogging burns more calories and gets you up to your target rate faster than walking does. But a brisk walking program can provide you with a very good workout, and it is a low-impact way to exercise, putting significantly less stress on your ankles, knees, feet, and spine. You may find that walking is simply more pleasurable than jogging, and a walking program can be carried out in situations where you couldn't or wouldn't want to jog—in the city, for example, or on the way to work, or in the course of running errands. To be effective, however, walking must be brisk, and you must wear appropriate shoes.

Warming Up

Whether you walk or jog, or choose Level 1 or Level 2, each session always begins with a warm-up. The warm-up loosens you up and helps prevent muscle strain and injury. Begin with stretching exercises, done in the clothes you'll walk or jog in—loose-fitting clothes appropriate to the temperature and humidity—and shoes designed for the purpose. Use the following guidelines or your own exercises, but be sure they include a range of motion for the neck, torso, shoulders, arms, and, most important, stretching for the thighs and calves and a range of motion for the ankles.

1.   An adequate warm-up begins with the neck and head. Slowly and gently move your head in a circle, circling first to the left several times, then repeating the rotations to the right. Do this *slowly*. Move on to the shoulders and arms. Arms straight out to either side, make repeated small circles from front to back, keeping your elbows straight and moving your arms from the shoulders; then reverse direction, circling the arms from back to front. Repeat for a count of 10 in each direction.

2. Keeping your arms straight and at chest height, swing them forward until your hands meet in front of you, your chest thrust back. Then swing the arms back, thrusting your chest forward, as far as is comfortable; alternate at a fairly brisk pace and repeat for a count of 10.

3. Next, with your arms still loosely outstretched, gently twist and rotate your torso to the right, then back to the left, for 12 or so repetitions.

4. Finally, work on the legs. Stretching and warming up muscles and joints in the legs and ankles will help prevent injury and keep you from stiffening up during exercise. Stretching the calf muscles and hamstrings is especially important in preventing painful shin splints. To stretch the hamstrings and calves, stand at arm's length from a wall with your hands flat against it at chest height, keeping your elbows straight. Bring your left leg slightly forward, bending it at the knee and shifting your weight to that foot,

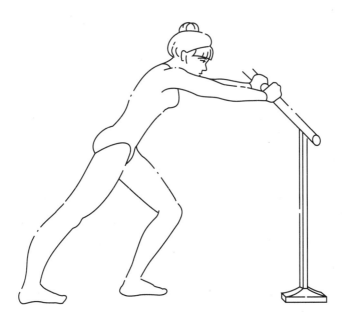

keeping it flat on the floor. Stretch the right leg out behind you, keeping the knee straight, and the ball of the foot on the floor, and push the right heel toward the floor until you feel a gentle stretching along the back of the leg. Hold for at least 5 seconds, then reverse and stretch the other calf. Repeat 2 or 3 times for each leg.

5. Put your feet together, both knees straight and heels on the floor. Bend your elbows, slowly lean toward the wall without lifting up your heels until you feel the stretch in both legs. Hold for 10 seconds.

6.   To stretch the thighs, use your right hand to support yourself. Holding your body erect, put your weight on your right foot and bend your left leg, bringing the foot up behind you and grasping your ankle or toes with your

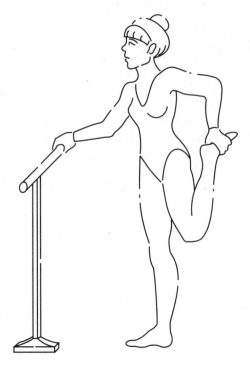

left hand. If you don't feel a gentle pull in the left thigh, press the left knee back a fraction until you do. Hold at least 5 seconds. Reverse and repeat the exercise with your right leg. Repeat on each side 2 or 3 times.

7.   Finally, still supporting yourself with one hand, lift one foot and rotate it at the ankle, gently circling around to the right 8 or 10 times, then circling to the left. Repeat with the other foot.

    To repeat, this last part of the warm-up is the most important, since your legs and ankles bear the brunt of the exercise. We advise 3 to 5 minutes of stretching before beginning each session of a walking program. For jogging, take a few extra minutes on the legs, because jogging puts greater stress on them; warm-up stretching for jogging should take from 5 to 8 minutes. We also advise that you follow your walking or jogging with some final, gentle stretching of the calves and thighs, using the exercises just described. This will help keep your muscles from tightening up.

    From week 13 on, continue to check your pulse periodically to make sure you are exercising within your target zone. As you get into shape, try exercising in the 70 to 75 percent range of your target zone. Well before

Level 1 Fitness: A Sample Walking Program
Each session should be repeated at least three times per week

WEEK	WARM-UP	TARGET ZONE	COOL-DOWN	TOTAL TIME
1	Walk slowly 5 min.	Walk briskly 5 min.	Walk slowly 5 min.	15 min.
2	Walk slowly 5 min.	Walk briskly 7 min.	Walk slowly 5 min.	17 min.
3	Walk slowly 5 min.	Walk briskly 9 min.	Walk slowly 5 min.	19 min.
4	Walk slowly 5 min.	Walk briskly 11 min.	Walk slowly 5 min.	21 min.
5	Walk slowly 5 min.	Walk briskly 13 min.	Walk slowly 5 min.	23 min.
6	Walk slowly 5 min.	Walk briskly 15 min.	Walk slowly 5 min.	25 min.
7	Walk slowly 5 min.	Walk briskly 18 min.	Walk slowly 5 min.	28 min.
8	Walk slowly 5 min.	Walk briskly 20 min.	Walk slowly 5 min.	30 min.
9	Walk slowly 5 min.	Walk briskly 23 min.	Walk slowly 5 min.	33 min.
10	Walk slowly 5 min.	Walk briskly 26 min.	Walk slowly 5 min.	36 min.
11	Walk slowly 5 min.	Walk briskly 28 min.	Walk slowly 5 min.	38 min.
12	Walk slowly 5 min.	Walk briskly 30 min.	Walk slowly 5 min.	40 min.

you reach your thirteenth week, you'll have a sense of how far you can walk in a given period. By the twelfth week, you're likely to be covering a mile and a half during the brisk walking portion of your workout. For the 35-plus woman who weighs less than 150 pounds, this will expend about 200 calories. For the woman between 150 and 200 pounds, it will use up about 250 calories. If you get inspired, you may want to raise your goal to 2 miles, bringing the brisk-walking portion up to about forty minutes and increasing the number of calories burned by one-third. But take the program more slowly if you need to; your goal is to enjoy yourself while you get in shape.

Level 1 Fitness: A Sample Jogging Program
Each session should be repeated at least three times per week

WEEK	WARM-UP	TARGET ZONE	COOL-DOWN	TOTAL TIME
1	Stretch and limber 5 min.	Walk 10 min.	Walk slowly 3 min., stretch 2 min.	20 min.
2	Stretch and limber 5 min.	Walk 5 min., jog 1 min., walk 5 min., jog 1 min.	Walk slowly 3 min., stretch 2 min.	22 min.
3	Stretch and limber 5 min.	Walk 5 min., jog 3 min., walk 5 min., jog 3 min.	Walk slowly 3 min., stretch 2 min.	26 min.
4	Stretch and limber 5 min.	Walk 4 min., jog 5 min., walk 4 min., jog 5 min.	Walk slowly 3 min., stretch 2 min.	28 min.
5	Stretch and limber 5 min.	Walk 4 min., jog 5 min., walk 4 min., jog 5 min.	Walk slowly 3 min., stretch 2 min.	28 min.
6	Stretch and limber 5 min.	Walk 4 min., jog 6 min., walk 4 min., jog 6 min.	Walk slowly 3 min., stretch 2 min.	30 min.
7	Stretch and limber 5 min.	Walk 4 min., jog 7 min., walk 4 min., jog 7 min.	Walk slowly 3 min., stretch 2 min.	32 min.
8	Stretch and limber 5 min.	Walk 4 min., jog 8 min., walk 4 min., jog 8 min.	Walk slowly 3 min., stretch 2 min.	34 min.
9	Stretch and limber 5 min.	Walk 4 min., jog 9 min., walk 4 min., jog 9 min.	Walk slowly 3 min., stretch 2 min.	36 min.
10	Stretch and limber 5 min.	Walk 4 min., jog 13 min.	Walk slowly 3 min., stretch 2 min.	27 min.
11	Stretch and limber 5 min.	Walk 4 min., jog 15 min.	Walk slowly 3 min., stretch 2 min.	29 min.
12	Stretch and limber 5 min.	Walk 4 min., jog 17 min.	Walk slowly 3 min., stretch 2 min.	31 min.
13	Stretch and limber 5 min.	Walk 2 min., jog slowly 2 min., jog 17 min.	Walk slowly 3 min., stretch 2 min.	31 min.
14	Stretch and limber 5 min.	Walk 1 min., jog slowly 3 min., jog 17 min.	Walk slowly 3 min., stretch 2 min.	31 min.
15	Stretch and limber 5 min.	Jog slowly 3 min., jog 17 min.	Walk slowly 3 min., stretch 2 min.	30 min.

From week 16 on, continue to check your pulse periodically to make sure you are exercising in your target zone. As you become more fit, start to exercise the upper range of your target zone.

Well before you reach the fifteenth week, you'll have a sense of how much ground you can cover in a given period. These distances will gradually increase; by the fifteenth week you'll probably be covering better than a mile and a half during the jogging portion of each session. For the 35-plus woman who weighs under 150 pounds, this will expend nearly 280 calories per session; for the woman between 150 and 200 pounds, it will expend about 340. As you become conditioned you may find it convenient and also more interesting to think of your goals in terms of distances, slowly increasing the distance you jog during each session.

The programs that follow are for moderately active women with no health risks. These will bring you up to a good maintenance level more quickly than the Level 1 programs: Level 2 walking takes five weeks to reach maintenance; Level 2 jogging takes seven weeks.

Level 2 Fitness: A Sample Walking Program

Each session should be repeated at least three times per week

	ACTIVITY	TIME (MINUTES)	TOTAL TIME
Week 1	Stretching	5	25 min.
	Slow walk (2 m.p.h.)	5	
	Accelerated walk (4 m.p.h.)	10	
	Slow walk	5	
Week 2	Stretching	5	30 min.
	Slow walk	5	
	Accelerated walk	15	
	Slow walk	5	
Week 3	Stretching	5	40 min.
	Slow walk	5	
	Accelerated walk	20	
	Slow walk	10	
Week 4	Stretching	5	40 min.
	Slow walk	5	
	Accelerated walk	25	
	Slow walk	5	
Week 5	Stretching	5	45 min.
	Slow walk	5	
	Accelerated walk	30	
	Slow walk	5	

By the fifth week, you will probably be covering a mile and a half during the accelerated portion of your walk. For the 35-plus woman who weighs under 150 pounds, this will expend nearly 200 calories per session. For a woman between 180 and 200 pounds, the calories burned reach approximately 250 per session.

Level 2 Fitness: A Sample Jogging Program

Each session should be repeated at least three times per week

	ACTIVITY	TIME (MINUTES)	TOTAL TIME
Week 1	Stretching	5	21 min.
	Walk	5	
	Jog	2	
	Walk	2	
	Jog	2	
	Walk	3	
	Stretching	2	
Week 2	Stretching	5	26 min.
	Walk	4	
	Jog	4	
	Walk	4	
	Jog	4	
	Walk	3	
	Stretching	2	
Week 3	Stretching	5	30 min.
	Walk	4	
	Jog	6	
	Walk	4	
	Jog	6	
	Walk	3	
	Stretching	2	
Week 4	Stretching	5	34 min.
	Walk	4	
	Jog	8	
	Walk	4	
	Jog	8	
	Walk	3	
	Stretching	2	
Week 5	Stretching	5	38 min.
	Walk	4	
	Jog	10	
	Walk	4	
	Jog	10	
	Walk	3	
	Stretching	2	
Week 6	Stretching	5	31 min.
	Walk	4	
	Jog	15	
	Walk	5	
	Stretching	2	

Level 2 Fitness: A Sample Jogging Program
(continued)
Each session should be repeated at least three times per week

	ACTIVITY	TIME (MINUTES)	TOTAL TIME
Week 7	Stretching	5	37 min.
	Walk	5	
	Jog	20	
	Walk	5	
	Stretching	2	

By the seventh week, you will probably be covering over a mile during the jogging portion of each session; by the twelfth week you're likely to be doing ten-minute miles. For a 35-plus woman under 150 pounds, this will expend approximately 280 calories per session. For a woman 150–180 pounds, calories spent are approximately 340 per session.

Safety Hints for Aerobics

1. Always spend at least five minutes warming up and at least five minutes cooling down after you have exercised in your target zone, so that your heart rate increases and decreases gradually.
2. In any fitness program, the warm-up should always include stretching. Stretching exercises are crucial to long-term health and for reducing the risk of muscle, tendon, and ligament injuries. Consistency—exercising at least three times a week—is essential not only to achieve good cardiovascular conditioning but also to minimize injury—the strains and sprains so common to "weekend athletes."
3. Wear a pair of well-fitted shoes that will cushion and support your feet. A good shoe store or sporting goods store will be able to help you select a shoe that's appropriate for your sport. The importance of excellent footwear cannot be overstressed, and it must be changed when signs of wear appear.
4. Build up your program gradually. It takes about six months to reach peak conditioning with any given aerobic activity. For the very vigorous sports listed on page 355, begin with no more than a few minutes of exercise in your target zone for the first few sessions, increasing warm-up and cool-down times to fill out twenty to thirty minutes of exercise. Increase no more than a couple of minutes each week after that, until you reach the maximum time of fifteen to twenty minutes in your target zone. Moderately vigorous sports may be increased by five minutes a week, building up to thirty minutes in your target zone.
5. Listen to your body. If you are overdoing it, stop. If you feel very

tired, stop. Cut back to a pace that is comfortable. You should always be able to speak and breathe comfortably at any point during your exercise session.

6. Stop if you feel any pain. While it is unlikely that you will push yourself too far using the very gradual introductions to exercise in our sample walking and jogging programs, be alert to signs that could spell heart problems. If you break out in a cold sweat, faint, or have chest pains or pains in the left neck, shoulder or arm, consult your doctor immediately.

7. If you miss a few exercise sessions, don't take it as a defeat. Pick up again at an earlier pace and get back into your routine. If you miss one day, review your schedule and try to fit it in the next day. Even —or maybe *especially*—at the beginner's level, consider each block of exercise time a big achievement. It is, and you deserve the credit.

8. Nothing is forever, certainly not your life sport. If you get bored with one form of exercise after two or three months, or no longer find it enjoyable, try another. When changing over to something new, remember that the muscles you'll be using are probably different from those you used before, and you'll need to start up again slowly, building up to fifteen to thirty minutes of target-zone exercise.

The Conditioning Effect

As your body gradually becomes conditioned in a jogging program (for example), you'll discover that you can jog for longer periods of time and it will take less and less exertion to move faster and farther than you did as a beginner. As this happens it will take more exercise to bring your heart up to the 60 to 75 percent target range. You can pick up the pace a bit to keep things interesting—especially if you're losing weight along the way—but the real benefit comes from exercising for at least twenty, and preferably thirty, minutes at a stretch. If you can cover more ground in the same time than you could at the outset, it's better to cover more ground than to cut down on the time.

Is Three Times a Week Enough?

Three times a week is the minimum requirement for aerobic conditioning, and if you're new to this, three times a week may be all you want to contemplate. That's fine; it's far better to stick to a modest program than to burn out on an ambitious one. Depending on the vigor of the sport, you may well need days off just to let your muscles recover from the exertion. But many fitness experts say that exercising four to five times a week is a much more efficient way to get into peak condition. If you can get an extra session in on the weekend, do it. If you can augment your program by riding a bicycle or walking to work a few times during the week, do it. Wear your walking or running shoes and tote your dress shoes. Having exercise serve another purpose—getting you someplace you want to go—is a good motivator.

PHASE TWO: PHYSICAL FITNESS

While our main focus is on aerobic sports that bring a host of benefits, the sport you choose may not condition and strengthen all your muscles. Ideally, you will want to balance out muscle strength in those muscle groups you don't use during your aerobic workout. Take a look at the sports listed below; you'll see what parts of the body are conditioned in each instance:

SPORT	MUSCLES USED
Bicycling	Lower body: legs and lower back
Cross-country skiing	Upper and lower body
Jogging/running	Lower body
Walking	Lower body
Jumping rope	Primarily lower body, secondarily arms
Swimming	Upper body, chest, legs
Tennis (singles)	Upper and lower body

Even if you choose a sport that can condition both the upper and lower body, your style may have an impact on how effective the conditioning is for specific muscle groups. For instance, if you're a novice tennis player and spend more time running around the court than hitting the ball, you may want to put in a little extra time on upper-body conditioning; if you do more work with your arms than your legs when you swim, you may want to spend some extra time on specific conditioning for the lower body.

Supplementary Exercise

Isometric exercise—working the muscles against some form of resistance—strengthens and tones the muscles. Isometrics are a good and relatively simple way to round out your exercise program, to balance out muscle strength and to further strengthen the muscles you use in your regular sport, so as to prevent injury. You can use ankle or wrist weights, but with some exercises—sit-ups, push-ups, and leg lifts, for example—gravity and your own body weight supply enough resistance to give you a workout.

There are many excellent books and videotapes featuring fitness programs with a variety of isometric (and other) exercises: *Jane Fonda's Workout Book* and her videotapes range from beginning to advanced levels of isometrics and stretching exercises, with some attention to aerobics; *The*

Athlete Within, by Harvey D. Simon, M.D., and Steven R. Levisohn, M.D., is an excellent all-around book on life sports for men and women that includes stretching and exercises with weights; *Peak Condition* by James G. Garrick, M.D., and Peter Radetsky goes into the specifics of preventing (and rehabilitating) sports injuries; and *Sports Fitness and Training* by Richard Mangi, M.D., Peter Jokl, M.D., and O. William Dayton, A.T.C., shows how to condition specific muscle groups. And there are dozens of books on running, tennis, aerobics, and calisthenics. Browse your local bookstore; there are many books to choose from that can help you further shape your fitness program. You might also enjoy a class or like working out at a fitness center (see information on Nautilus equipment, page 362).

It's possible, however, to attain a good level of overall fitness with just a few basic exercises that you can do in a few minutes a day to supplement your aerobic workout. Some of the old standards—sit-ups and push-ups— exercise the upper body and the all-important abdominal muscles. But there are better ways of doing them than the traditional way. Deep knee bends are another exercise not particularly useful or good for the knees, but there's a modified version that's easier on the knees and gives a good workout to the thighs and, to a lesser extent, the buttocks. On your "off days" do these along with a series of stretches: those we've described on pages 346–348, plus windmills, touching your toes, side stretches, and floor stretches. Don't forget stretches for the lower back. These exercises will take just a few minutes, and they'll not only condition unused muscles, they'll give you a good pickup. If you're in reasonably good shape, try doing them immediately after your aerobic workout, then follow with a series of slow, gentle stretches for your cool-down, including again stretches for your lower back. Then just lie back quietly for a minute or two with your eyes closed, and totally *relax*. You'll feel wonderful afterward.

A Brief Workout for Specific Muscle Groups

ABDOMINAL CURLS.   Though some aerobic sports like tennis can strengthen arms and shoulders, few aerobic sports do very much for the abdominal muscles, and they're important balancing muscles that help to protect your back. Specific isometric exercise is the best way to strengthen them and help flatten your stomach. But old-fashioned sit-ups, where someone holds your feet down and you come up to a full sitting position, bring back and hip muscles into play, and not always in good ways.

Abdominal curls, done correctly, make the abdominal muscles do almost all the work, making curls a more efficient way to exercise these muscles and putting far less strain on the back. Start by lying flat on your back, legs extended, arms crossed over your chest. Press the small of your

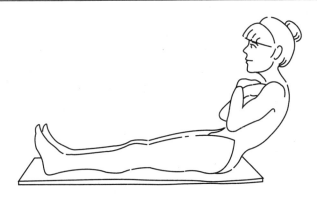

back toward the floor. Slowly raise your upper torso until it's at a 30 to 45 degree angle from the floor. How high you go doesn't really matter, so long as you feel the pull in the muscles beginning in the lower abdomen and running up to the middle of the ribcage. Don't arch your back. Try to keep the lower abdominals flat by pulling your stomach in and pressing your lower back toward the floor as you lift the upper torso. Lift up slowly to a count of three, hold the position for two counts, then lie back slowly to a count of three. Exhale as you lift, inhale as you lower. Repeat the curl five times each session of the first week. If you get sore, drop back to three. As an alternative the curl can be done with the knees bent, feet flat on the floor. If it's more comfortable for your back, do them this way. The advantage of doing them with legs extended is that you'll get a little bit of a workout in the thighs at the same time.

MODIFIED PUSH-UPS. Full extension push-ups are difficult for women, who have less upper body strength and a lower center of gravity than men do. But modified push-ups will help strengthen and tone your shoulders, arms (especially the triceps), and pectoral muscles. There are two ways to do them. The less strenuous is to do your push-ups against a heavy table, counter or desk (something that won't move). Stand about three feet back from the edge, leaning your weight on your arms. Keeping your hips, torso, and legs aligned, lower your body toward the table by bending your arms, then slowly push back up. At the lowest point your body should touch the table at chest height; adjust your stance accordingly. A slightly more strenuous version, but still easier than full push-ups, is to do push-ups from the floor but with your weight on your hands and knees. Start on all fours, then, bring your feet up behind you, crossing them comfortably at the ankles, and lower your hips until your torso and thighs are aligned, your back flat. Without bending at the waist or hips, slowly lower your upper body to the floor and slowly push back up. With either of these, repeat five times per session for the first week. Drop back to three times if it seems too much.

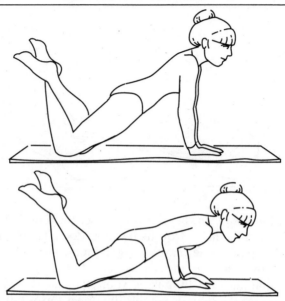

MODIFIED KNEE BENDS.   If you have had any acquaintance with ballet, you will recognize that these are basically pliés. Stand with your heels about two feet apart, toes turned slightly out—a wide second position.

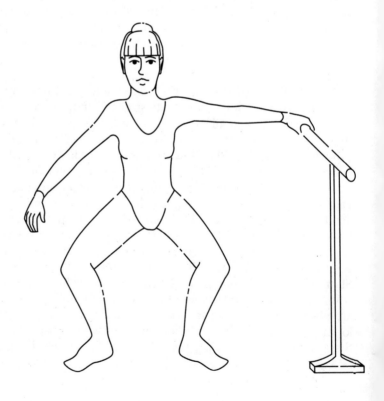

Hold your upper body erect, back straight and buttocks tucked in. Put one hand on the back of a chair for balance. Slowly bend the knees until you feel a gentle stretch in the back of the thighs, then slowly straighten. Keep the torso erect—don't lean forward. If you don't feel the stretch, try moving your feet slightly farther apart. If you tighten the buttocks and do these slowly, you'll work both the quadriceps, the iliopsoas (back thigh muscles) and the buttocks to some extent as well. Repeat these five times each session, the first week. Bend as deeply as you can *without* putting an uncomfortable strain on your knees.

SIDE LEG RAISES. Lie on your right side with your right arm under you to raise your trunk from the floor, your left hand a bit in front of your chest for balance. Your left leg is on top of your right. Raise the left leg slowly to a count of three, until it's at about a 45 degree angle from the floor. Hold it there for one count, then lower to a count of three. Keep your left knee straight, and check to be sure that your hips, torso, and legs are in a straight line. As you lift, keep the knee facing forward—don't rotate it so that it faces the ceiling. Repeat five or six times. This works the muscles along the outer part of the thigh. Now for the hard part: After the last lift, cross your left leg over your right with your knee up and foot flat on the floor. Now raise the lower (right) leg, keeping the knee straight and using the inner thigh muscles to lift it. Remember to keep your hips, torso, and legs in a straight line, and don't roll forward. If you can only do three at

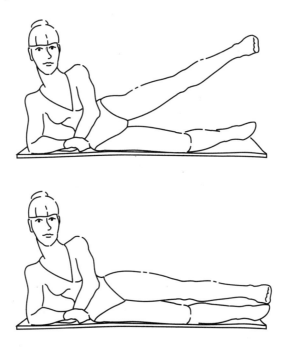

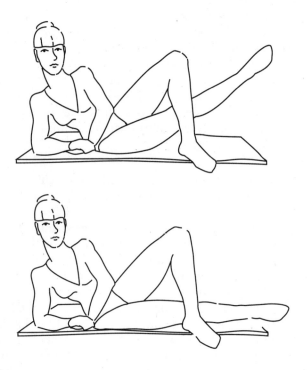

first, that's okay. When you're finished roll over to the other side and repeat the whole series.

PELVIC TILTS. These help stretch and limber the lower back muscles, and work the gluteus maximus (the buttocks) muscles as well. Lie on your back, knees up and about eight inches apart (or at hip width), feet flat on the floor, arms comfortably at your sides. Using your abdominal muscles, press your lower back to the floor, tucking the buttocks in and tilting

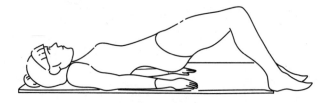

the pelvis up slightly. To a count of four, lift the buttocks slightly off the floor without arching or lifting your back. Keep the lower back pressed to the floor. Lower the buttocks without completely relaxing—that is, keep them tucked, keep the abdominals sucked in and keep the back pressed to the floor. Repeat, slowly, six or eight times.

FINAL BACK STRETCHES.   Finish these exercises by extending both legs out flat, then bringing one knee up to the chest, hugging it to your chest with your arms for a count of five. Gently lower that leg, bring the other knee up to the chest and hug it there for a count of five. Then lower

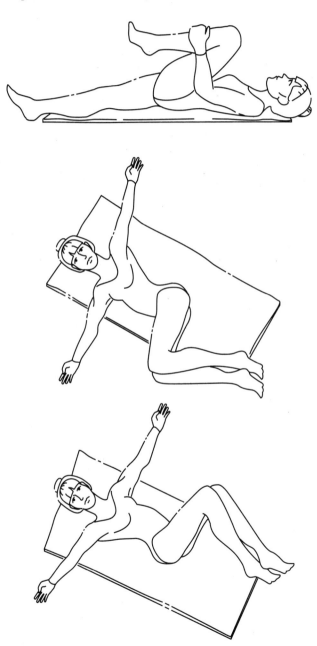

that leg and spread your arms out directly to the sides. Bring both knees up to your chest. Try to keep both shoulders flat on the floor as you let your lower body roll over to the left, so that your knees rest on the floor. Hold for a few seconds. Then bring the knees back up and let them gently drop to the other side. Again hold for a few seconds. You probably won't be able to keep your shoulders absolutely flat during this, and you must not strain to do so. But keep the opposite arm stretched out and keep the upper body as flat as you *comfortably* can. This stretch can really help work out the kinks.

Nautilus Equipment

The 35-plus woman who prefers a structured program and likes the discipline and sociability of a club setting may find the programs using Nautilus equipment very beneficial. The equipment is well designed, and if used properly can improve muscle tone and overall conditioning. The caveat here is to receive instruction on *each* piece of equipment and to work with the club's fitness personnel. Nautilus should not be a "do it yourself" program. All top-quality health clubs not only have fitness personnel to assist you, they require an introduction to all equipment used. The workouts should be regular, and you can use our muscle-group exercises as a home supplement on "days off." Whatever route is chosen—a home fitness program, a club program, or a mix—the issues of care and consistency remain the same.

Cross Training

Although our major thrust has been on choosing a life sport and sticking with it, the concept of cross training should be considered as well. Serious runners (competitors, who may run up to 50 miles a week) were among the first to start varying their programs, owing to chronic fatigue and decreased motivation, which lead to decreased performance. Once you have attained a good aerobic fitness level in your first sport, you may then wish to branch out—for runners, often to cycling and swimming—spending part of your exercise time on a secondary sport. Serious athletes have found that cross training improves their performance in their primary sport, even though they spend less time training in that specific area.

The advantages of cross training are many. Cross training conditions different muscle groups and decreases the risk of overusing one group; a greater variety in your program combats boredom, and cross training can lead to a more balanced level of overall fitness. It is especially beneficial if your exercise goes from three times a week to five or six times. Keep this concept in mind as your fitness program evolves. Fitness should never be a "static" part of your life; it can and should change as you change.

A NUTRITIONIST'S REFLECTIONS
ON STRENUOUS SPORTS

Good nutrition and plenty of fluids are an essential part of physical fitness, particularly for those who take their exercise seriously. For those women who move on to meet the challenge of marathons and other competitive events, certain aspects of your diet assume particular importance.

Fluids

On average, a woman needs 2½ quarts of fluid a day to maintain body temperature, blood circulation, and urine production. This should include six to eight glasses of plain water; the rest can come from other nonalcoholic beverages and food. These needs increase depending on how much and how long you exercise.

Because the body can only absorb eight to ten ounces of fluids every twenty minutes, the ideal way to replace fluid during and after exercising is in small amounts of plain water. Drink plenty of it, and hold off on other sources of fluid until after a competitive event. Plain water is absorbed faster than drinks that contain sugar, such as soda or juice, which tend to be retained in the stomach. Cold water is absorbed faster than warm water.

With strenuous exercise at marathon levels, loss of fluids can be deceptive. Without proper replacement, it can result in dehydration, or worse. The body does not trigger the thirst mechanism until fluid loss reaches 1 percent of the body weight. When fluid loss reaches 2 to 3 percent, performance begins to decline; at 7 to 10 percent heat stroke can occur. This can be fatal, as it was for two amateur runners competing in a race in New York City during the hot summer of 1988.

A marathoner can actually lose three quarts of fluid through perspiration per hour, equivalent to six pounds of body weight. If you are bitten by a marathon bug, you need:

- at least twenty-one ounces (nearly a pint and a half) of water two hours before such an event
- fourteen to seventeen ounces (about 1 pint) just before it starts
- three to seven ounces every ten to fifteen minutes during the race
- enough water afterward to replace lost weight

After the event, remember that the body can't absorb more than eight or ten ounces of water every twenty minutes. It doesn't absorb water as fast as it loses it. Here again, thirst is unreliable, as it is satisfied long before true fluid needs are met. Most persons voluntarily drink about two-thirds of the fluid they have lost, and then stop. The only sure way to know how much fluid to drink is to compare body weight before and after exercising. This is of particular importance if you're engaging in serious endurance competitions—marathons, triathlons, bike races, and the like—but everyone who exercises should be aware of it.

What about the athlete who comes in from a big event feeling she deserves a few beers? She's not doing herself any favors, nor is her male counterpart, by reaching into the ice chest for a six-pack. Alcohol can hinder performance and cause dehydration, so it should not be used for fluid replacement before, during, or immediately after participating in any sports event.

Beer contains carbohydrates, but it is not a good choice for carbohydrate loading, either, if that is a strategy you're interested in.

Carbohydrate Loading

Carbohydrate loading is a technique that was developed in Sweden in 1960 to increase muscle stamina. The primary way the body stores carbohydrates is in the form of glycogen, which is stored in the muscles (see page 273). When an athlete trains hard, he or she depletes these stores. After exercising the body replaces them—with more glycogen than was present before. This is why training is so important to performance. Greater amounts of glycogen in the muscles mean more strength and greater stamina in the sorts of endurance tests posed by marathons and other long-distance competitions. Carbohydrate loading is a way to capitalize on this effect, providing more available carbohydrate for conversion to glycogen. Studies have shown that with training and an adequate diet, you can actually double or triple the amount of glycogen normally found in the muscles.

In the absence of training, of course, extra carbohydrates will simply be converted to fat.

Carbohydrate loading is of no benefit to a sprinter or to anyone who exercises for less than ninety minutes at a time, which makes it useless for the 35-plus woman who exercises for half an hour three or four times a week. Consistent workouts, as we've pointed out, will increase your speed and stamina no matter what form of exercise you choose, but at this very moderate level the carbohydrates you get from a well-balanced diet are more than adequate for your needs. Any extra carbohydrates you take in will likely be converted to fat.

For those who do train for longer periods or are involved in competition, a moderate increase in complex carbohydrates the night before and the day of a race can help. For example, if you were going to be in a ten kilometer race, which is about six miles, a bit of extra pasta at dinner the night before, and a good breakfast including whole grain cereal and toast the next morning, would be enough to see you through. Note that these are complex carbohydrates, not simple sugars. You should also be careful to allow at least two hours between eating a full meal and strenuous exercising.

Caffeine "Loading"

Many serious athletes find that caffeine enhances athletic performance, and so it can, apparently by increasing the number of free fatty acids in the blood, which are then preferentially used for energy over glycogen. This prolongs endurance by decreasing the rate at which glycogen is used by the muscles. Caffeine is controversial in light of the health risks posed by excessive caffeine in the body, but for the competitive athlete two cups of coffee, tea, or cola a day are probably not detrimental, depending on the individual's tolerance to caffeine, and may be beneficial if included in the meal just prior to the event. Amounts beyond this may cancel out benefits, however, as coffee and tea have been shown to interfere with thiamine and iron absorption, two nutrients of particular importance to athletes. These beverages are also diuretics, and can precipitate dehydration. Taken immediately before an event, quantities of caffeine that exceed an individual's tolerance may also hinder performance by overstimulating the nervous system.

Fructose

As with protein powders, people are also buying fructose in health food stores assuming it is an ideal precompetition source of carbohydrate. Like most sugar, fructose is easily digested, but it does not trigger the release of insulin and therefore does not cause as rapid a rise in blood sugar as glucose. Because it sustains blood sugar at a more constant level for a longer period of time than sucrose does, some athletes take fructose before competition in the belief that it will spare muscle glycogen and permit longer endurance. While the logic is tempting, subsequent miracles have yet to occur, although real problems with diarrhea following large intakes of fructose *have* been reported, and for that reason I don't recommend it.

Protein Powders

Protein powders sell briskly in health food stores—mainly to young people who think these will help build muscles and in turn help them perform better when they exercise. This is not the case, and excessive protein can actually be harmful. The best "fuel" for the athlete is a well-balanced diet that includes complex carbohydrates. An excessive amount of protein upsets the body in three ways: It increases water requirements and puts a load on the kidneys to excrete urea; it decreases the absorption of calcium, an important nutrient for maintaining good bone density; and it actually decreases the body's efficiency in converting protein to muscle tissue.

For these reasons, serious athletes (indeed anyone) should avoid eating large quantities of meat—more than 12 to 16 ounces a day—or taking protein powders, which are actually a low quality protein source.

Vitamins and Minerals

Some athletes feel strongly that as they increase levels of exercise, they need to take large doses of vitamins and minerals. This isn't necessary. Usually the extra calories burned by serious athletes are balanced by certain increases in their diet, so that vitamins and minerals are kept up to good levels. If they eat a balanced diet, they need no more than the sort of daily vitamin-mineral supplement described on page 286. Iron needs are the exception here.

Iron

Loss of iron has been linked to sports anemia, a condition that can occur in women who run more than ten or fifteen miles a week. They lose blood cells through tiny hemorrhages caused by the impact of the feet pounding a hard surface, which is coupled with the normal losses of menstruation. Whether committed to strenuous exercise or not, most women need an iron supplement anyway to ensure they get their quota of 18 mg. a day.

Other Vitamins and Minerals

B COMPLEX.   Theoretically these are the vitamins most likely to help performance, since they aid in the conversion of calories to energy. But while studies have shown that a deficiency in the B vitamins can decrease athletic performance, it does not necessarily follow that by taking more B vitamins performance is going to be any better, and an excessive amount of any one vitamin or group of vitamins can interfere with the utilization of other nutrients.

THIAMINE AND RIBOFLAVIN.   Thiamine is particularly important for energy metabolism. It has been suggested but not confirmed that thiamine supplementation can increase endurance, especially if an athlete loads up on carbohydrates, as discussed. There is limited evidence that exercise may increase the body's requirement for riboflavin; a diet that provides enough calories and plenty of whole grains, milk and cheese should provide an adequate supply of both these nutrients.

VITAMIN C.   There have been dubious reports of increased endurance and decreased muscular fatigue with large (1,000 milligrams a day) doses of vitamin C, attributed to its effect on the heart rate and oxygen consumption. However, the studies that led to this claim were not controlled well enough to eliminate the placebo effect. While most excessive vitamin C is excreted, negative side effects of very large doses may include kidney stones, diarrhea, increased serum cholesterol, and iron overload.

VITAMIN E. One poorly controlled study has suggested that vitamin E increases blood flow to the tissues and aids their oxygen uptake, but a more recent, better designed study indicates it has no effect on athletic performance at all and suggests that the placebo effect is responsible for any marked improvement. However, there is a good possibility that vitamin E is beneficial in increasing oxygen intake at high altitudes, so that if you are a mountain climber you might find supplements helpful. The rest of us who exercise or run at 5,000 or 6,000 feet above sea level, maximum, are fine without vitamin E supplements.

VITAMINS A AND D. These have no benefits for athletic performance, and both are *toxic* at levels that are only 5 to 20 times the recommended dietary allowance.

POTASSIUM AND SODIUM. Losses of these minerals are not significant unless more than 6 pounds of body weight are lost, as they may be in a marathon. To replace these losses, you can add a little salt to your diet over the next two or three days following an event, and eat plenty of fresh fruit and vegetables, which are high in potassium. Salt tablets are not recommended, as they can be dangerous—upsetting the body's fluid-electrolyte balance, actually exacerbating dehydration and increasing potassium loss.

MAGNESIUM. Like sodium and potassium, magnesium is an electrolyte that is lost in sweat, but the amount lost is not enough to be significant and is easily replaced by eating a balanced diet. Researchers have demonstrated that severe prolonged muscle exertion—running a twenty-six-mile marathon, for example—leads to a depleted magnesium level, which can cause muscle cramping. However, it is not known whether the occasional muscle cramps that might occur after a less prolonged or strenuous exercise are a symptom of magnesium deficiency or the result of mild dehydration.

RISKS OF EXCESSIVE EXERCISE

Excessively strenuous exercise causes some women to stop menstruating. It has been commonly thought that so-called "athletic amenorrhea" was triggered by a lower than normal percent of body fat, but recent studies indicate that a specific decrease in estrogen levels is responsible for the condition. If that is the case, it puts these women almost in a post-menopausal state, and at risk of decreased bone mineralization which can lead to osteoporosis as well as to stress fractures. Any woman who exercises so strenuously that she stops menstruating should discuss the situation with her physician or gynecologist.

COMMON SPORTS INJURIES

Although there is a broad range of exercise-related injuries, the most common involve the foot, ankle, knee, and elbow.

General stress on the feet and lower body can be alleviated by doing your exercise on a good surface. Jogging or running on packed earth or even asphalt is easier on your body than running on concrete. Calisthenics and aerobics classes are better on a wooden floor than on concrete (even if it's covered with carpeting) for the same reason—these surfaces are more resilient and will absorb some of the impact your body would otherwise absorb. Here are some specific injuries and how to recognize them.

1. *Foot problems* usually result from overuse—strain, with or without inflammation. Pain under the heel may be due to a bruise, pain along the bottom of the foot to an inflammation of the connective tissue such as plantar fasciitis (an inflammation of the connective tissue in the arch of your foot). A rigid plastic heel cup, available in many shoestores that carry running gear, may relieve the pain of a bruise. A well-fitted arch support may relieve plantar fasciitis, but not if it supports your arch at the very place that hurts. Both bruises and fasciitis respond to rest and anti-inflammatory medications, either aspirin or prescription medications such as ibuprofen (Motrin) or indomethacin (Indocin). If the problem persists, a small fracture of the bone or bones must be ruled out, and it's a good idea to get an evaluation by an experienced podiatrist or an orthopedist with special interest in foot problems. As we've said before, excellent and well-fitting shoes are a must to help protect your feet from injury.

2. *Ankle problems* are usually due to sprains—stretching and sometimes tearing of the connective tissue that binds the ankle bones together (the ligaments) or anchors muscle to bone (tendons). Simple sprains should respond to rest—that is, keeping your weight off the ankle—but as with foot injuries, pain and swelling should be further evaluated by a qualified consultant if it continues for more than three days.

3. *Knee problems*—usually the result of overuse—can produce inflammation of the bursal sacs, tendons, ligaments, or joint lining, with attendant pain, stiffness, and swelling. Treatment for these minor injuries includes using cold packs, compression, and aspirin, and stopping or cutting back on exercise until the condition improves before gradually working back up to previous levels. Cartilage tears and injury to the ligaments are more serious, and may require surgery. Fortunately, these injuries are relatively rare except in downhill skiers and professional athletes. If your knee locks or buckles, a cartilage problem is a real possibility, and you should get prompt attention from an orthopedist, but any persistent pain, swelling, or

problem with function that doesn't respond to rest calls for medical attention. Arthritis may also be a cause; if severe you may need to be on specific
medication, and you may have to switch from high-impact exercise (including running) to swimming.

Often an examination in the office leads to a diagnosis, but more extensive examination with an arthrogram or arthroscope may be needed. In an
arthrogram, dye is injected into the knee joint and X-rays are taken; in
arthroscopy the insertion of a small-caliber fiberoptic scope allows your
doctor to look at the joint and cartilage directly.

4. *Elbow problems*—often the so-called tennis elbow—usually result from
overuse of the joint in racquet sports. Rest and anti-inflammation medications—sometimes including a cortisone injection—are the mainstays of
treatment. But it's better to take care of tennis elbow before it gets to that
point. Exercises that gently stretch and strengthen the muscles in the forearm will help prevent tennis elbow. In their book *Peak Condition*, James
Garrick and Peter Radetsky suggest two that are useful. For strengthening,
rest your arm on a table with the wrist just over the edge. Curl your wrist
back as far as you can. Try three sets of 10 each day for a few days. If you
can do this without pain, increase the resistance by holding a small weight,
gradually increasing the weight as your forearm muscles grow stronger; a 1-
to 2-pound weight may be all you want to use. Follow these with some
stretches. Hold the arm out in front of you, palm down. With your other
hand gently pull the hand on the bad side downward, bending the wrist in
as far as is comfortable. You should feel a stretch along the top of your
forearm. Hold for five seconds, then relax. Repeat two to three times.

For virtually all exercise-caused muscle or joint strains and sprains,
complete rest, followed by resumption of the activity at a slow and careful
pace, is the treatment of choice. Don't ignore persistent pain! If pain persists or recurs, a careful evaluation by your physician and an appropriate
consultant is in order. In the case of recurring tennis elbow, the *Peak
Condition* authors suggest that one of your consultations be with a tennis
pro! They point out that professional players almost never get tennis elbow
because their fundamentals are sound. Correcting your service and back-
hand may go a long way toward preventing elbow pain.

SUMMING UP

Time and motivation are the chief hurdles for most people in maintaining
an exercise program, but once you've gotten motivated, finding the time
for fitness becomes a simpler task than you may have thought. We've reit-
erated the many benefits of regular exercise at the beginning of this chapter,

and indeed these have been a recurrent theme throughout the book, but if anything bears repeating it's this: consistent exercise can become one of life's real pleasures, one that truly makes a difference in your overall sense of well-being. Go for it!

AFTERWORD

We may sometimes feel so bombarded with news of frightening diseases and new health risks that we hardly know what's safe to do or eat. But in truth the role of prevention, nutrition, and exercise in maintaining health has been mapped out well enough that each succeeding generation in this country has increased its life expectancy and is, on average, taller, stronger, and healthier than the generations before it. There are great scourges still facing us—cancer, AIDS, and, on a global scale, the pervasive problem of world hunger—but many other ills that devastated past generations, such as cholera, smallpox, and typhoid, to name a few, have all but disappeared from the developed countries and, with few exceptions, are rapidly receding everywhere. Other diseases, like bacterial pneumonia, tuberculosis, and syphilis, have been successfully brought under control, and the usual prognosis for those who do fall prey to them is bright: complete cure. For most of us, the state of our health really does hinge on personal choices: to eat a healthy diet, to exercise, to avoid deliberately introducing toxins to our bodies (with cigarettes, alcohol, drugs), and to protect ourselves from toxins that have been introduced to the environment. The challenges we face in curbing pollution and feeding the world are enormous; what we've addressed in this book is the more manageable challenge of improving individual health prospects and quality of life. We hope we've made the task a bit easier.

J.P.S.
D.P.C.

INDEX